Update on Diagnosis and Management of Preeclampsia and Fetal Growth Restriction

Update on Diagnosis and Management of Preeclampsia and Fetal Growth Restriction

Editor

Silvia Lobmaier

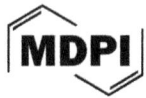

Basel • Beijing • Wuhan • Barcelona • Belgrade • Novi Sad • Cluj • Manchester

Editor
Silvia Lobmaier
Technical University of Munich
München, Germany

Editorial Office
MDPI
St. Alban-Anlage 66
4052 Basel, Switzerland

This is a reprint of articles from the Special Issue published online in the open access journal *Journal of Clinical Medicine* (ISSN 2077-0383) (available at: https://www.mdpi.com/journal/jcm/special_issues/update_preeclampsia_fetal_growth_restriction).

For citation purposes, cite each article independently as indicated on the article page online and as indicated below:

Lastname, A.A.; Lastname, B.B. Article Title. *Journal Name* **Year**, *Volume Number*, Page Range.

ISBN 978-3-0365-9923-6 (Hbk)
ISBN 978-3-0365-9924-3 (PDF)
doi.org/10.3390/books978-3-0365-9924-3

© 2024 by the authors. Articles in this book are Open Access and distributed under the Creative Commons Attribution (CC BY) license. The book as a whole is distributed by MDPI under the terms and conditions of the Creative Commons Attribution-NonCommercial-NoDerivs (CC BY-NC-ND) license.

Contents

Anne Karge, Linus Desing, Bernhard Haller, Javier U. Ortiz, Silvia M. Lobmaier, Bettina Kuschel and Oliver Graupner
Performance of sFlt-1/PlGF Ratio for the Prediction of Perinatal Outcome in Obese Pre-Eclamptic Women
Reprinted from: *J. Clin. Med.* **2022**, *11*, 3023, doi:10.3390/jcm11113023 1

Anne Karge, Silvia M. Lobmaier, Bernhard Haller, Bettina Kuschel and Javier U. Ortiz
Value of Cerebroplacental Ratio and Uterine Artery Doppler as Predictors of Adverse Perinatal Outcome in Very Small for Gestational Age at Term Fetuses
Reprinted from: *J. Clin. Med.* **2022**, *11*, 3852, doi:10.3390/jcm11133852 15

Jon G. Steller, Diane Gumina, Camille Driver, Emma Peek, Henry L. Galan, Shane Reeves and John C. Hobbins
Patterns of Brain Sparing in a Fetal Growth Restriction Cohort
Reprinted from: *J. Clin. Med.* **2022**, *11*, 4480, doi:10.3390/jcm11154480 25

Salman Hussain, Ambrish Singh, Benny Antony, Jitka Klugarová, M. Hassan Murad, Aarthi S. Jayraj, et al.
Proton Pump Inhibitors Use and Risk of Preeclampsia: A Meta-Analysis
Reprinted from: *J. Clin. Med.* **2022**, *11*, 4675, doi:10.3390/jcm11164675 37

Sylwia Sławek-Szmyt, Katarzyna Kawka-Paciorkowska, Aleksandra Ciepłucha, Maciej Lesiak and Mariola Ropacka-Lesiak
Preeclampsia and Fetal Growth Restriction as Risk Factors of Future Maternal Cardiovascular Disease—A Review
Reprinted from: *J. Clin. Med.* **2022**, *11*, 6048, doi:10.3390/jcm11206048 53

Katarzyna Pankiewicz, Ewa Szczerba, Anna Fijałkowska, Janusz Sierdziński, Tadeusz Issat and Tomasz Mikołaj Maciejewski
The Impact of Coexisting Gestational Diabetes Mellitus on the Course of Preeclampsia
Reprinted from: *J. Clin. Med.* **2022**, *11*, 6390, doi:10.3390/jcm11216390 69

Daniel Boroń, Jakub Kornacki, Paweł Gutaj, Urszula Mantaj, Przemysław Wirstlein and Ewa Wender-Ozegowska
Corin—The Early Marker of Preeclampsia in Pregestational Diabetes Mellitus
Reprinted from: *J. Clin. Med.* **2023**, *12*, 61, doi:10.3390/jcm12010061 81

Carmen Garrido-Giménez, Mónica Cruz-Lemini, Francisco V. Álvarez, Madalina Nicoleta Nan, Francisco Carretero, Antonio Fernández-Oliva, et al.
Predictive Model for Preeclampsia Combining sFlt-1, PlGF, NT-proBNP, and Uric Acid as Biomarkers
Reprinted from: *J. Clin. Med.* **2023**, *12*, 431, doi:10.3390/jcm12020431 91

Xianjing Xie, Dan Chen, Xingyu Yang, Yunyun Cao, Yuna Guo and Weiwei Cheng
Combination of Maternal Serum ESM-1 and PLGF with Uterine Artery Doppler PI for Predicting Preeclampsia
Reprinted from: *J. Clin. Med.* **2023**, *12*, 459, doi:10.3390/jcm12020459 105

Charlotte Lößner, Anna Multhaup, Thomas Lehmann, Ekkehard Schleußner and Tanja Groten
Sonographic Flow-Mediated Dilation Imaging versus Electronic EndoCheck Flow-Mediated Slowing by VICORDER in Pregnant Women—A Comparison of Two Methods to Evaluate Vascular Function in Pregnancy
Reprinted from: *J. Clin. Med.* **2023**, *12*, 1719, doi:10.3390/jcm12051719 115

Piotr Tousty, Magda Fraszczyk-Tousty, Anna Golara, Adrianna Zahorowska, Michał Sławiński, Sylwia Dzidek, Hanna Jasiak-Jóźwik, et al.
Screening for Preeclampsia and Fetal Growth Restriction in the First Trimester in Women without Chronic Hypertension
Reprinted from: *J. Clin. Med.* **2023**, *12*, 5582, doi:10.3390/jcm12175582 . . . . **123**

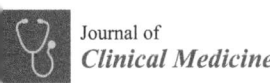

Article

Performance of sFlt-1/PlGF Ratio for the Prediction of Perinatal Outcome in Obese Pre-Eclamptic Women

Anne Karge [1,*], Linus Desing [1], Bernhard Haller [2], Javier U. Ortiz [1], Silvia M. Lobmaier [1], Bettina Kuschel [1,†] and Oliver Graupner [1,3,†]

1 Department of Obstetrics and Gynecology, University Hospital Rechts der Isar, Technical University of Munich, 80333 Munich, Germany; linus.desing@mri.tum.de (L.D.); javier.ortiz@mri.tum.de (J.U.O.); silvia.lobmaier@mri.tum.de (S.M.L.); bettina.kuschel@mri.tum.de (B.K.); ograupner@ukaachen.de (O.G.)
2 Institute of AI and Informatics in Medicine, University Hospital Rechts der Isar, Technical University of Munich, 80333 Munich, Germany; bernhard.haller@mri.tum.de
3 Department of Obstetrics and Gynecology, University Hospital Aachen, RWTH University, 52062 Aachen, Germany
* Correspondence: anne.karge@mri.tum.de; Tel.: +49-89-4140-2430; Fax: +49-89-4140-2447
† These authors contributed equally to this work.

Citation: Karge, A.; Desing, L.; Haller, B.; Ortiz, J.U.; Lobmaier, S.M.; Kuschel, B.; Graupner, O. Performance of sFlt-1/PlGF Ratio for the Prediction of Perinatal Outcome in Obese Pre-Eclamptic Women. *J. Clin. Med.* **2022**, *11*, 3023. https://doi.org/10.3390/jcm11113023

Academic Editor: Erich Cosmi

Received: 28 April 2022
Accepted: 24 May 2022
Published: 27 May 2022

Publisher's Note: MDPI stays neutral with regard to jurisdictional claims in published maps and institutional affiliations.

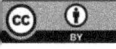

Copyright: © 2022 by the authors. Licensee MDPI, Basel, Switzerland. This article is an open access article distributed under the terms and conditions of the Creative Commons Attribution (CC BY) license (https://creativecommons.org/licenses/by/4.0/).

Abstract: Obese women are at high risk of developing pre-eclampsia (PE). As an altered angiogenic profile is characteristic for PE, measurement of soluble fms-like tyrosine kinase-1 (sFlt-1)/placental growth factor (PlGF) ratio in the maternal serum can be helpful for PE diagnosis, as well as for adverse perinatal outcome (APO) prediction. There is growing evidence that obesity might influence the level of sFlt-1/PlGF and, therefore, the aim of the study was the evaluation of sFlt-1/PlGF as an APO predictor in obese women with PE. Pre-eclamptic women who had an sFlt-1/PlGF measurement at the time of diagnosis were retrospectively included. Women were classified according to their pre-pregnancy body mass index (BMI) as normal weight (BMI < 25 kg/m^2), overweight (BMI > 25–29.9 kg/m^2) or obese (BMI ≥ 30 kg/m^2). APO was defined as the occurrence of one of the following outcomes: Small for gestational age, defined as a birthweight < 3rd centile, neonatal mortality, neonatal seizures, admission to neonatal unit required (NICU) or respiratory support. A total of 141 women were included. Of them, 28 (20%) patients were obese. ROC (receiver operating characteristic) analysis revealed a high predictive value for sFlt-1/PlGF and APO across the whole study cohort (AUC = 0.880, 95% CI: 0.826–0.936); $p < 0.001$). However, the subgroup of obese women showed a significantly lower level of sFlt-1 and, therefore, the performance of sFlt-1/PlGF as APO predictor was poorer compared to normal or overweight PE women (AUC = 0.754, 95% CI: 0.552–0.956, $p = 0.025$). In contrast to normal or overweight women, a ratio of sFlt-1/PlGF < 38 could not rule out APO in women with obesity.

Keywords: preeclampsia; (anti-)angiogenic factors; placental growth factor; soluble fms-like tyrosine kinase 1; obesity

1. Introduction

Pre-eclampsia (PE) is a disease affecting 2–8% of all pregnancies and a major cause for fetal and maternal morbidity [1–3]. An altered inflammatory and angiogenic profile is a main finding in the pathophysiology of PE and serum markers, such as soluble fms-like tyrosine kinase-1 (sFlt-1) and placental growth factor (PlGF), are now established for the diagnosis of PE [4,5].

Around a third of pregnant women in Western countries are affected by overweight and the percentage is steadily increasing [6,7]. In 2017, 15% of pregnant women in Germany were obese compared to 12% in 2003 [8]. Obesity is a risk factor for the development of

PE [9] and is, as well as PE, characterized by an endothelial dysfunction and a proinflammatory microenvironment [10]. Therefore, the evaluation of the established predictive marker of PE, sFlt-1/PlGF ratio, is of the utmost importance in this high-risk cohort. Recent guidelines recommend the use of sFlt-1/PlGF for diagnosis or exclusion of PE [11]. The PROGNOSIS study, which evaluated and established sFlt-1/PlGF as a diagnostic tool, did not differentiate between obese or normal-weight women and did not, therefore, examine if different cutoffs are necessary or not [12].

The ratio of sFlt-1/PlGF is not only used for diagnosing or excluding PE, but also for the prediction of adverse perinatal outcome (APO) and adverse maternal outcome (AMO) [13–16]. Specifically, highly elevated levels of sFlt-1/PlGF correlate with APO and might be helpful for estimating the mean time until delivery [12,17–20]. Likewise, published data do not discriminate between different BMI groups.

It is important to notice that not only the severity of PE itself, but also other factors influence the serum level of sFlt-1/PlGF, such as twin pregnancies or, as mentioned above, BMI [21,22]. Levels of sFlt-1 seem to be inversely correlated with BMI and, therefore, APO prediction by sFlt-1/PlGF might be distorted [23].

The aim of this study was the evaluation of sFlt-1/PlGF as an APO and AMO predictor in obese women with PE and/or HELLP syndrome.

2. Materials and Methods

This is a retrospective single-center study from January 2018 to December 2020 at the University Hospital rechts der Isar, Department of Obstetrics and Gynecology (Technical University of Munich). All patients with diagnosed PE and/or HELLP syndrome were included if sFlt-1/PlGF was determined at the time of diagnosis. Cases with missing data on perinatal outcome as well as multiple pregnancies were excluded. Additionally, we included the study cohort of women with late-onset PE which was described before [24].

Elevated blood pressure was defined as a new onset hypertension with a systolic blood pressure of 140 mmHg and/or a diastolic blood pressure of 90 mmHg, on two occasions at least 4 h apart [25]. Large cuffs were used for obese women.

PE was defined as elevated blood pressure and one of the following symptoms: proteinuria ($\geq$300 mg/24 h), thrombocytopenia (platelet count less than 100.000/microliter), poor liver function (elevated blood levels of liver transaminases to twice the normal concentration), new-onset renal insufficiency (elevated serum creatinine greater than 1.1 mg/dL or a doubling of serum creatinine in the absence of other renal disease), pulmonary edema or new-onset cerebral or visual disturbances [26]. HELLP syndrome was defined as the occurrence of hemolysis (haptoglobin < 10 mg/L), elevated liver enzymes (twice the normal concentration) and low platelets (<100.000/microliter) [27].

Diagnosis of PE < 34 weeks was classified as early onset (eo) PE and diagnosis of PE $\geq$ 34 weeks as late-onset (lo) PE [28].

APO was defined as the presence of at least one of the following outcomes according to the Delphi consensus defining the core outcome of PE [29]: Small for gestational age defined as a birthweight < 3rd centile according to local standards [30], neonatal mortality, neonatal seizures, admission to neonatal unit required (NICU) or respiratory support. There was no case of stillbirth.

Adverse maternal outcome (AMO) was defined as the occurrence of at least one of the following core outcomes of PE: eclampsia, pulmonary edema, acute kidney injury (defined as elevated serum creatinine greater than 1.1 mg/dL or a doubling of serum creatinine in the absence of other renal disease), placental abruption, HELLP syndrome, admission to intensive care unit or the need of intubation and mechanical ventilation. There was no case of maternal mortality, cortical blindness, retinal detachment, liver capsule hematoma or rupture or stroke.

The sFlt-1/PlGF ratio was determined at the time of diagnosis according to our local chemistry guidelines as previously described [18].

We used the cutoff values for sFlt-1/PlGF, which are recommended by the consensus statement [31]: <38 exclusion of PE (gestational-age independent) for at least 1 week, >85 diagnosis of early onset (eo) PE (<34 week of gestation) and >110 diagnosis of late-onset (lo) PE ($\geq$34 week of gestation).

Overweight and obesity were defined according to the WHO guidelines as a BMI from 25 to 29.9 kg/m^2 or >30 kg/m^2, respectively [32]. A BMI <25 kg/m^2 was considered as normal weight. The pre-pregnancy BMI was used for classification.

2.1. Statistical Analysis

We used IBM SPSS Statistics for Windows, version 28 (IBM Corp., Armonk, NY, USA) and R version 4.1.2 (R Foundation for Statistical Computing, Vienna, Austria) for our statistical analysis. Quantitative data are shown as means and standard deviations or median and interquartile range; categorical data are presented as absolute and relative frequencies. Differences in distributions of quantitative data between the three weight groups were tested using the Kruskal–Wallis test. If a significant difference was found pairwise group comparisons were performed with Mann–Whitney U tests. Categorical data were compared between groups using Fisher's exact test. The predictive value of sFlt-1/PlGF for APO or AMO was analyzed with receiver operating characteristic (ROC) curves. Areas under the ROC curves were compared between groups using the method proposed by Delong et al. [33]. All statistical tests were conducted two sided and a p-value < 0.05 was considered statistically significant.

2.2. Ethical Approval

The study was approved by our local Institutional Ethics Board (Ethikkommission der Fakultät für Medizin der Technischen Universität München, protocol number 232/17). The study was not registered in a public trial registry.

3. Results

3.1. Baseline Characteristics and Perinatal Outcome

In total, 141 pregnancies with PE and/or HELLP were enrolled. Of these cases, 45 (32%) were diagnosed with early onset and 96 (68%) with late-onset PE and/or HELLP syndrome. Further, 84 women in our cohort had a normal pre-conceptional BMI (60%), 29 were overweight (20%) and 28 were obese (20%). Of all newborns, APO occurred in 69 cases (49%). Many newborns were affected by more than one event. The most common APO was admission to NICU in 55 cases (40%), followed by respiratory support in 42 cases (30%). There were 13 cases of newborns with a birthweight <3rd centile (9%), three cases of seizures (2%) and one case of neonatal death (0.7%).

AMO was observed in 36 cases (26%). The most common event was acute kidney injury in 15 cases (11%), followed by early onset HELLP syndrome affecting 10 pregnancies and late-onset HELLP syndrome affecting nine pregnancies (7% and 6%, respectively). Other AMO events were rarely observed.

Baseline characteristics of the study cohort and data on perinatal outcome are described in Tables 1 and 2.

3.2. Levels of Angiogenic Factors in Preeclamptic Women Depending on BMI

Figures 1–3 demonstrate the median level of sFlt-1/PlGF, sFlt-1 and PlGF in the different BMI subgroups. Obese women show a significantly lower sFlt-1 compared to normal-weight or overweight women (p = 0.001), whereas sFlt-1/PlGF and PlGF are not statistically different in the different subgroups.

Table 1. Baseline characteristics.

Baseline Characteristics	BMI < 25 n = 84	BMI > 25–29.9 kg/m² n = 29	BMI ≥ 30 kg/m² n = 28	p-Value
Age at diagnosis	33.5 (±5.4)	34.1 (±5.7)	33.2 (±4.6)	0.608
BMI	21.2 (±1.8)	27.3 (±1.5)	34.1 (±3.9)	<0.001 ***
Weight gain during pregnancy (in kg)	13.5 (±6.1)	12.6 (±5.4)	10.9 (±7.0)	0.216
Gestational age at diagnosis	34.8 (±3.8)	34.8 (±3.9)	34.5 (±3.3)	0.680
sFlt-1/PlGF level at diagnosis	125.1 (IQR: 64.4–213.1)	116.0 (IQR: 45.3–233.0)	99.30 (IQR: 30.36–187.0)	0.275
PlGF level at diagnosis	93.9 (IQR: 54.6–93.9)	86.3 (IQR: 46.1–130.4)	89.35 (IQR: 51.0–130.9)	0.810
sFlt-1 level at diagnosis	12,024.8 (IQR: 7472.0–13,544.8)	8756.0 (IQR: 5708.5–13,040.0)	7014.0 (IQR: 3668.6–11,347.3)	0.003 **
Gestational age at delivery	35.5 (±3.3)	35.7 (±3.9)	35.9 (±3.0)	0.684
Nullipara	57 (68%)	17 (58%)	17 (61%)	0.396
ASS prophylaxis	10 (12%)	11 (38%)	9 (32%)	0.005 *
Chronic hypertension	8 (10%)	3 (10%)	3 (11%)	0.844
Early-onset PE/HELLP	24/84 (29%)	10/28 (36%)	10/29 (35%)	0.430
Late-onset PE/HELLP	60 (71%)	19 (66%)	17 (61%)	0.272
RDS Prophylaxis	27 (32%)	8 (28%)	11 (39%)	0.637
Status after PE/HELLP/FGR	16 (19%)	9 (31%)	8 (29%)	0.205
Magnesium sulfate prophylaxis	44 (52%)	16 (55%)	15 (54%)	0.868

BMI body mass index, sFlt-1 soluble fms-like tyrosine kinase-1, PlGF placental growth factor, ASS acetylsalicylic acid, PE pre-eclampsia, RDS respiratory distress syndrome, FGR fetal growth restriction. Data are presented as n (%) or mean ± SD or median and interquartile range. A p-value < 0.05 was considered as statistically significant (* $p < 0.05$; ** $p < 0.005$; *** $p < 0.001$).

Table 2. Perinatal outcome.

Perinatal Outcome	BMI < 25 kg/m² n = 84	BMI > 25–29.9 kg/m² n = 29	BMI ≥ 30 kg/m² n = 28	p-Value
APO	46/84 (55%)	12/29 (41%)	11/28 (39%)	0.110
Respiratory support	27/84 (33%)	8/29 (28%)	7/28 (25%)	0.421
Admission to NICU	34/84 (41%)	10/29 (35%)	11/28 (39%)	0.764
Birthweight (g)	2243.2 (±48.4)	2422.1 (±932.5)	2456.3 (±841.3)	0.404
Birthweight < 3. centile	9/84 (11%)	2/29 (7%)	2/28 (7%)	0.751
Neonatal mortality	0/84 (0%)	0/29 (0%)	1/28 (4%)	0.080
Fetal growth restriction	24/84 (29%)	7/29 (24%)	5/28 (18%)	0.257
Seizures	1/84 (1%)	2/29 (7%)	0/28 (0%)	0.167
AMO	29/84 (35%)	3/29 (10%)	4/28 (14%)	0.010 *
Early-onset HELLP	8/84 (10%)	0/29 (0%)	2/28 (7%)	0.406
Late-onset HELLP	7/84 (8%)	1/29 (3%)	1/28 (4%)	0.297
Postpartum haemorrhage	1/84 (1%)	0/29 (0%)	1/28 (4%)	0.005 *
Eclampsia	0/84 (0%)	1/29 (3%)	0/28 (0%)	0.619
Acute kidney injury	12/84 (14%)	2/29 (7%)	1/28 (4%)	0.085
Abruption	3/84 (4%)	0/29 (0%)	0/28 (0%)	0.187

BMI body mass index, APO adverse perinatal outcome, NICU neonatal intensive care unit, AMO adverse maternal outcome. Data are presented as n (%) or mean ± SD or median and interquartile range. A p-value < 0.05 was considered as statistically significant (* $p < 0.05$).

3.3. APO Prediction by sFlt-1/PlGF

For the whole study cohort, ROC analysis revealed a significant predictive value for sFlt-1/PlGF and APO (AUC = 0.880, 95% CI: 0.824–0.936; $p < 0.001$), as well as for PlGF or sFlt-1 alone (AUC = 0.866, 95% CI: 0.807–0.925, $p < 0.001$ and AUC = 0.721, 95% CI: 0.637–0.804, $p < 0.001$, respectively). The area under the ROC curve (AUC) was significantly larger for sFlt-1/PlGF and for PlGF than for sFlt-1 alone ($p < 0.001$ and $p = 0.005$).

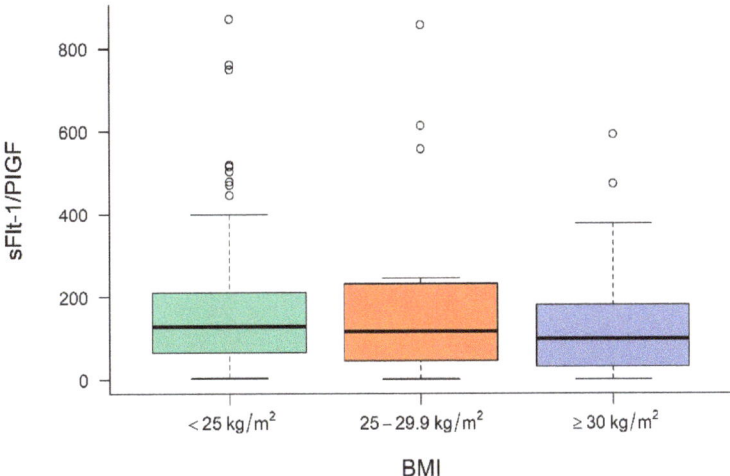

Figure 1. Level of sFlt-1/PlGF at diagnosis in normal-weight, overweight and obese women. BMI body mass index, sFlt-1 soluble fms-like tyrosine kinase-1, PlGF placental growth factor.

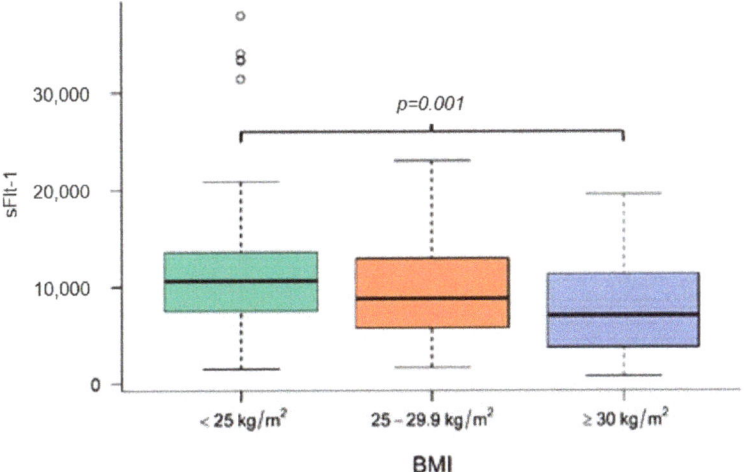

Figure 2. Level of sFlt-1 at diagnosis in normal-weight, overweight and obese women. BMI body mass index, sFlt-1 soluble fms-like tyrosine kinase-1.

In all the subgroups of normal weight, overweight and obese women, sFlt-1/PlGF was significantly associated with APO, although the prognostic value was reduced in obese women compared to the other two subgroups (AUC = 0.914, 95% CI: 0.857–0.972, $p < 0.001$; AUC = 0.931, 95% CI: 0.845–0.999, $p < 0.001$; AUC = 0.754, 95% CI: 0.552–0.956, $p = 0.025$). In contrast, sFlt-1 failed to be statistically significant as an outcome predictor in obese women (AUC = 0.642, 95% CI: 0.428–0.855, $p = 0.213$).

The results are presented in Figures 4–7.

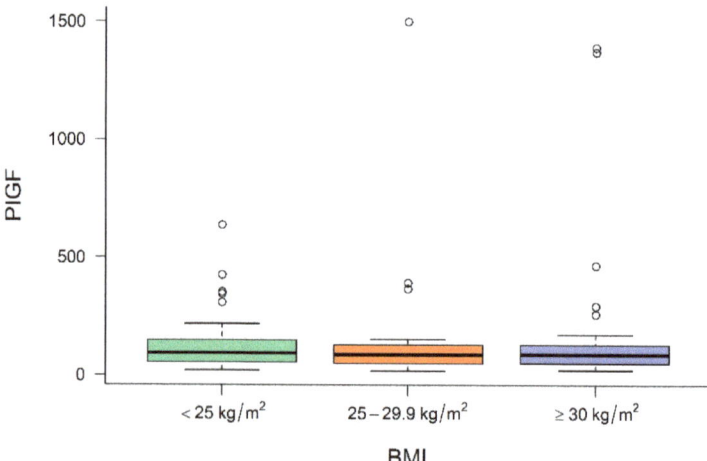

Figure 3. Level of PlGF at diagnosis in normal-weight, overweight and obese women. BMI body mass index, PlGF placental growth factor.

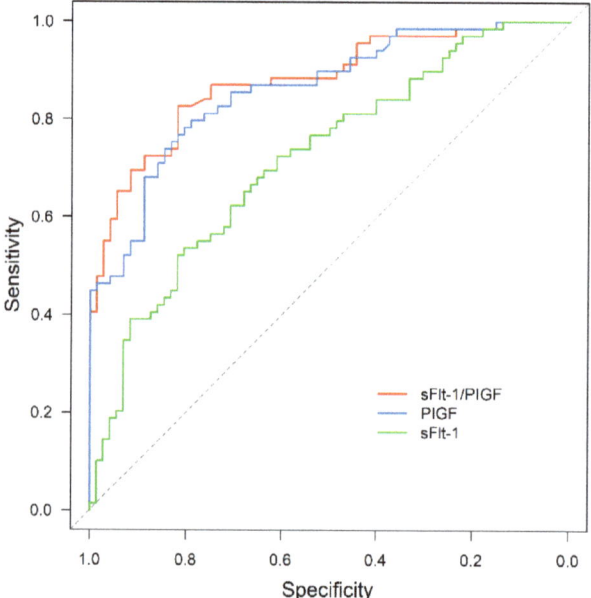

Figure 4. ROC curve for APO prediction by sFlt-1 (AUC = 0.721, 95% CI: 0.637–0.804, $p < 0.001$), PlGF (AUC = 0.866, 95% CI: 0.807–0.925, $p < 0.001$) and sFlt-1/PlGF (AUC = 0.880, 95% CI: 0.824–0.936, $p < 0.001$). ROC receiver operating characteristic, APO adverse perinatal outcome, sFlt-1 soluble fms-like tyrosine kinase-1, PlGF placental growth factor.

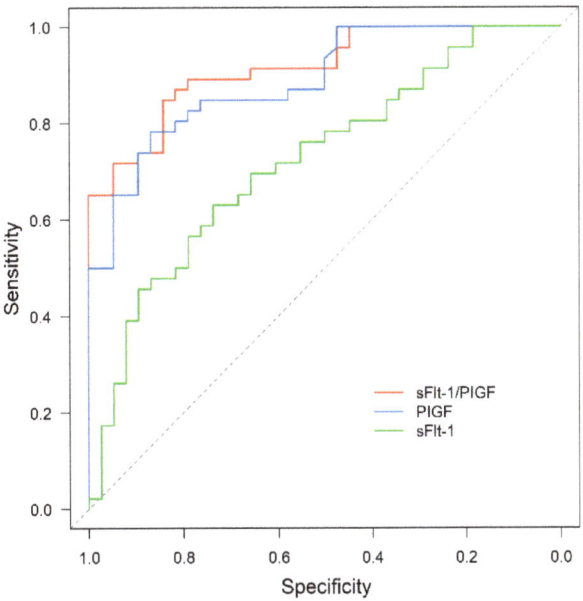

Figure 5. ROC curve for APO prediction in the subgroup of normal-weight women by sFlt-1 (AUC = 0.723, 95% CI: 0.615–0.832, $p < 0.001$), PlGF (AUC = 0.892, 95% CI: 0.826–0.958, $p < 0.001$) and sFlt-1/PlGF (AUC = 0.914, 95% CI: 0.857–0.972, $p < 0.001$). ROC receiver operating characteristic, APO adverse perinatal outcome, sFlt-1 soluble fms-like tyrosine kinase-1, PlGF placental growth factor.

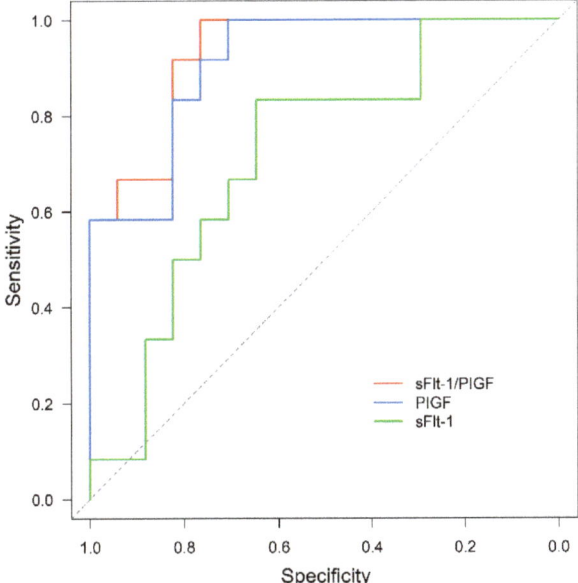

Figure 6. ROC curve for APO prediction in the subgroup of overweight women by sFlt-1 (AUC = 0.721, 95% CI: 0.531–0.910, $p = 0.046$), PlGF (AUC = 0.912, 95% CI: 0.811–1.000, $p < 0.001$) and sFlt-1/PlGF (AUC = 0.931, 95% CI: 0.845–0.999, $p < 0.001$). ROC receiver operating characteristic, APO adverse perinatal outcome, sFlt-1 soluble fms-like tyrosine kinase-1, PlGF placental growth factor.

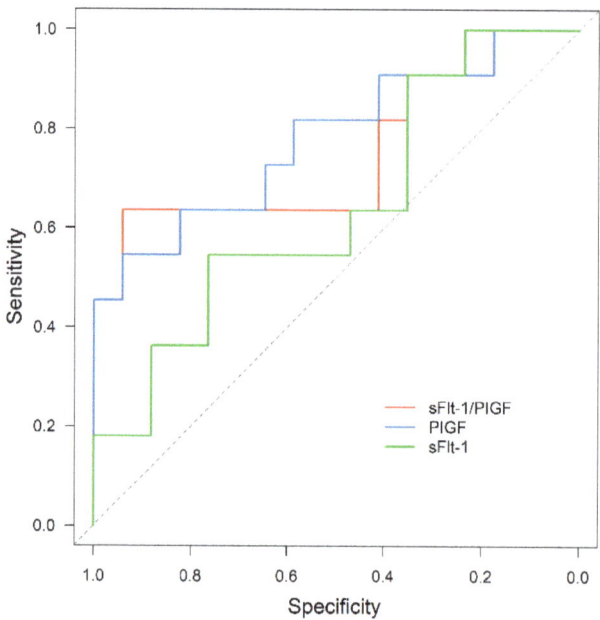

Figure 7. ROC curve for APO prediction in the subgroup of obese women by sFlt-1 (AUC = 0.642, 95% CI: 0.428–0.855, p = 0.213), PlGF (AUC = 0.781, 95% CI: 0.596–0.966, p = 0.014) and sFlt-1/PlGF (AUC = 0.754, 95% CI: 0.552–0.956, p = 0.025). ROC receiver operating characteristic, APO adverse perinatal outcome, sFlt-1 soluble fms-like tyrosine kinase-1, PlGF placental growth factor.

3.4. AMO Prediction by sFlt-1/PlGF

For the whole study cohort, ROC analysis revealed a predictive value for sFlt-1/PlGF and AMO (AUC = 0.667, 95% CI: 0.566–0.768; p = 0.003), as well as for sFlt-1 (AUC = 0.694, 95% CI: 0.598–0.790; p = 0.001), but not for PlGF (AUC = 0.605, 95% CI: 0.495–0.715, p = 0.061). Due to the small number of events, we did not perform a subgroup analysis. ROC analysis is shown in Figure 8.

3.5. Exclusion of APO by sFlt-1/PlGF

In the group of normal-weight women, 8 of 84 (10%) women showed an sFlt-1/PlGF level < 38 and in the overweight cohort, 5 of 29 (17%) women. None of these women were affected by APO. In contrast, 7 of 28 (25%) obese women showed an sFlt-1/PlGF level < 38, but two of them were affected by APO. Both women developed superimposed PE and high blood pressure despite their antihypertensive medications, which led to iatrogenic preterm delivery with admission of the newborn to NICU.

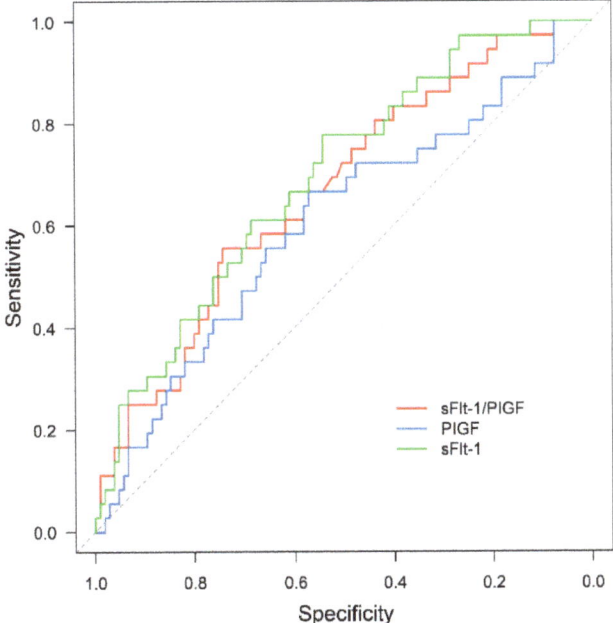

Figure 8. ROC curve for AMO prediction by sFlt-1 (AUC = 0.694, 95% CI: 0.598–0.790, p = 0.001), PIGF (AUC = 0.605, 95% CI: 0.495–0.715, p = 0.061) and sFlt-1/PIGF (AUC = 0.667, 95% CI: 0.566–0.768, p = 0.003). ROC receiver operating characteristic, APO adverse perinatal outcome, sFlt-1 soluble fms-like tyrosine kinase-1, PIGF placental growth factor.

4. Discussion

This study confirmed that obese women with PE show significantly lower levels of sFlt 1 compared to normal or overweight women. However, APO prediction by sFlt-1/PIGF is still possible, although with a poorer prognostic value compared to normal or overweight women.

As obesity is an epidemic disease affecting more and more pregnancies, outcome prediction in this subgroup is of urgent need. Outcome prediction in pre-eclamptic women using (anti-)angiogenic factors, especially sFlt-1/PIGF, was evaluated over the last decade [16,19,34]. In our study cohort, sFlt-1/PIGF had a high prognostic value for APO, a finding in line with previous publications of our working group [20,24]. Saleh et al. recently suggested a model using sFlt-1/PIGF, proteinuria and gestational age for outcome prediction in pregnancies diagnosed with PE [35]. Patients with normal sFlt-1/PIGF were affected by APO in less than 5%. However, in several studies APO prediction by sFlt-1/PIGF remains inconclusive or with a reduced prognostic value compared to our data [36,37]. One explanation for this observation might be the inconsistency in the reported outcome data; therefore, we decided to define APO according to the recently published Delphi consensus by Duffy et al. [29]. Another reason might be the focus on special cohorts, such as twin pregnancies [38]. Our results suggest that it might be necessary to investigate obese women as an independent subgroup to avoid a distorted result.

The main finding of our study is that APO can be predicted by sFlt-1/PIGF, not only in the group of normal and overweight women, but also in women with obesity, considering the decreasing prognostic value. This should be taken into account, especially if sFlt-1/PIGF levels are low. In contrast to normal and overweight women [39], obese women are at a higher risk of developing APO, even with sFlt-1/PIGF-levels < 38 and, therefore, these women might be in need of intensified clinical surveillance.

It is unclear why sFlt-1 levels are lower in obese women. In a Finnish case-control study, including 1450 women, sFlt-1 levels in pre-eclamptic obese women were significantly lower compared to women with normal BMI, whereas sFlt-1 levels in the first trimester did not differ [22]. In line with our own results, Suwaki et al. reported an inverse correlation of sFlt-1 and BMI in pre-eclamptic women [40], but no difference in the angiogenic profile of normotensive women. Lobmaier et al. could not find a significant influence of BMI on sFlt-1/PlGF levels, considering that the study group showed a relatively low BMI (22.5 (20.5–25.6) kg/m^2) [20]. The profile of sFlt-1/PlGF in obese women without PE remains controversial, as some studies report a higher level of sFlt-1 and PlGF, as well as the opposite [41,42]. A possible explanation might be the above-mentioned "low BMI" study cohorts. Nevertheless, obese women affected by AMO, APO or PE show elevated levels of sFlt-1/PlGF compared to obese women without further complications [43].

Increased plasma volume, as a confounder, might, at least, contribute to our finding of a lower sFlt-1 level, as animal studies rather implicate a higher sFlt-1 release in obese pregnancies [44,45]. On the other hand, TNF-α, a proinflammatory factor elevated in obese women, decreases the sFlt-1 expression in fat tissue [46]. Another reason might be the higher mass of extracellular matrix in fat tissue containing heparin sulfate proteoglycans, which leads to sequestration of sFlt-1 from blood circulation [47]. However, PlGF concentrations were not different in obese and normal-weight women, which is in line with other studies [40]. Therefore, further research needs to be conducted to analyze the role of adipose tissue in the processing of angiogenic factors in PE.

The ratio of sFlt-1 and PlGF was not only a predictor of APO, but also of AMO, although its prognostic value is limited due to the low incidence of AMO in our study cohort. HELLP syndrome, as well as acute kidney failure, were more common in normal-weight women and other events were rare. This finding was unexpected, as obesity itself is a risk factor for HELLP syndrome or other pregnancy complications [48]. One explanation for this finding might be that women with the risk factor of obesity are carefully observed during pregnancy and, therefore, AMO might be prevented in some cases. Rana et al. demonstrated that pre-eclamptic women with a normal angiogenic profile were more likely to be obese and AMO was rare, except for iatrogenic preterm delivery [49]. Therefore, there might be a subgroup of obese women diagnosed with only mild symptoms of PE in the late-onset group, as obesity especially increases the risk of late-onset PE [50].

The limitations of our study were the retrospective design and a relatively small sample size. Furthermore, data on weight gain during pregnancy were not available for all women. We used the levels of sFlt-1/PlGF at the time of diagnosis of PE, but another measurement prior to delivery might give further and more detailed information about the angiogenic profile in PE women. Further, clinicians were aware of the test results. Therefore, sFlt-1/PlGF might have influenced the decision making, especially regarding the timing of delivery. On the one hand, this might have prolonged pregnancies if a low sFlt-1/PlGF was measured and helped to prevent APO. On the other hand, it might have led to an iatrogenic delivery if high serum levels were detected, especially if the mother was severely affected by PE and, therefore, might have prevented AMO. An impact of sFlt-1/PlGF in the decision-making process regarding further therapy of women with PE was described before [51]. Pre-pregnancy BMI was used for the statistical analysis; however, weight gain during pregnancy might influence our results. Interestingly, mean weight gain during pregnancy was lower in obese women. These results might be biased, as severe PE is often accompanied by excessive oedema. Another effect might be the diatetic counselling all obese women received during pregnancy.

5. Conclusions

In conclusion, we could demonstrate that sFlt-1/PlGF is a helpful tool for APO prediction in normal and overweight, but also in obese women. However, for decisions on the timing of delivery and perinatal management, it should be taken into account that the performance is not as precise in obese women as it is in normal-weight women. Clinicians should be aware that normal sFlt-1/PlGF might not rule out APO and, therefore, obese women with PE are a subgroup of patients who should be managed carefully.

Author Contributions: Conceptualization, A.K., B.K. and O.G.; methodology, A.K., B.K. and O.G.; software, A.K. and B.H.; validation, A.K., L.D., J.U.O., S.M.L., B.K. and O.G.; formal analysis, A.K., L.D. and B.H.; investigation, A.K. and L.D.; resources, B.K.; data curation, A.K. and L.D.; writing—original draft preparation, A.K. and O.G.; writing—review and editing, A.K., L.D., J.U.O., S.M.L., B.K. and O.G.; visualization, A.K.; supervision, B.K. and O.G.; project administration A.K., B.K. and O.G. All authors have read and agreed to the published version of the manuscript.

Funding: This research received no external funding.

Institutional Review Board Statement: The study was approved by our local Institutional Ethics Board (Ethikkommission der Fakultät für Medizin der Technischen Universität München, protocol number 232/17). The study was not registered in a public trial registry.

Informed Consent Statement: In accordance with article §27, Section 4 of the Bavarian hospital law ("Bayrisches Krankenhausgesetz—BayKrG"), patient data, collected in the context of the hospital medical treatment relationship, may be used for training, further education, research purposes in the hospital, and statistics for the hospital. However, the patient data must remain in the custody of the hospital. For this reason, a separate declaration of informed consent of the patients in this retrospective hospital data collection was waived. There were no minors included in the study.

Data Availability Statement: Not applicable.

Conflicts of Interest: The authors declare no conflict of interest.

References

1. Khan, K.S.; Wojdyla, D.; Say, L.; Gülmezoglu, A.M.; Van Look, P.F. WHO analysis of causes of maternal death: A systematic review. *Lancet* **2006**, *367*, 1066–1074. [CrossRef]
2. van Esch, J.J.A.; van Heijst, A.F.; de Haan, A.F.J.; van der Heijden, O.W.H. Early-onset preeclampsia is associated with perinatal mortality and severe neonatal morbidity. *J. Matern. Fetal Neonatal Med.* **2017**, *30*, 2789–2794. [CrossRef] [PubMed]
3. WHO Guidelines Approved by the Guidelines Review Committee. In *WHO Recommendations: Policy of Interventionist versus Expectant Management of Severe Pre-Eclampsia before Term*; World Health Organization: Geneva, Switzerland, 2018.
4. Tomimatsu, T.; Mimura, K.; Endo, M.; Kumasawa, K.; Kimura, T. Pathophysiology of preeclampsia: An angiogenic imbalance and long-lasting systemic vascular dysfunction. *Hypertens. Res.* **2017**, *40*, 305–310. [CrossRef] [PubMed]
5. Verlohren, S.; Herraiz, I.; Lapaire, O.; Schlembach, D.; Moertl, M.; Zeisler, H.; Calda, P.; Holzgreve, W.; Galindo, A.; Engels, T.; et al. The sFlt-1/PlGF ratio in different types of hypertensive pregnancy disorders and its prognostic potential in preeclamptic patients. *Am. J. Obstet. Gynecol.* **2012**, *206*, 58.e1–58.e8. [CrossRef] [PubMed]
6. Gaillard, R. Maternal obesity during pregnancy and cardiovascular development and disease in the offspring. *Eur. J. Epidemiol.* **2015**, *30*, 1141–1152. [CrossRef]
7. Schaefer-Graf, U.; Ensenauer, R.; Gembruch, U.; Groten, T.; Flothkötter, M.; Hennicke, J.; Köhrle, J.; Möhler, J.; Kühnert, M.; Schmittendorf, A.; et al. Obesity and Pregnancy. Guideline of the German Society of Gynecology and Obstetrics (S3-Level, AWMF Registry No. 015-081, June 2019). *Geburtshilfe Frauenheilkd* **2021**, *81*, 279–303. [CrossRef]
8. Strauss, A.; Rochow, N.; Kunze, M.; Hesse, V.; Dudenhausen, J.W.; Voigt, M. Obesity in pregnant women: A 20-year analysis of the German experience. *Eur. J. Clin. Nutr.* **2021**, *75*, 1757–1763. [CrossRef]
9. Schummers, L.; Hutcheon, J.A.; Bodnar, L.M.; Lieberman, E.; Himes, K.P. Risk of Adverse Pregnancy Outcomes by Prepregnancy Body Mass Index. *Obstet. Gynecol.* **2015**, *125*, 133–143. [CrossRef]
10. Kwaifa, I.K.; Bahari, H.; Yong, Y.K.; Noor, S.M. Endothelial Dysfunction in Obesity-Induced Inflammation: Molecular Mechanisms and Clinical Implications. *Biomolecules* **2020**, *10*, 291. [CrossRef]
11. Hypertensive Pregnancy Disorders: Diagnosis and Therapy. Guideline of the German Society of Gynecology and Obstetrics (S2k-Level, AMWF Registry No. 015/018, March 2019). Available online: http://www.awmf.org/leitlinien/detail/II/015-018.html (accessed on 27 April 2022).
12. Verlohren, S.; Herraiz, I.; Lapaire, O.; Schlembach, D.; Zeisler, H.; Calda, P.; Sabria, J.; Markfeld-Erol, F.; Galindo, A.; Schoofs, K.; et al. New Gestational Phase–Specific Cutoff Values for the Use of the Soluble fms-Like Tyrosine Kinase-1/Placental Growth Factor Ratio as a Diagnostic Test for Preeclampsia. *Hypertension* **2014**, *63*, 346–352. [CrossRef]
13. Rana, S.; Salahuddin, S.; Mueller, A.; Berg, A.H.; Thadhani, R.I.; Karumanchi, S.A. Angiogenic biomarkers in triage and risk for preeclampsia with severe features. *Pregnancy Hypertens. Int. J. Women's Cardiovasc. Health* **2018**, *13*, 100–106. [CrossRef] [PubMed]
14. Chang, Y.-S.; Chen, C.-N.; Jeng, S.-F.; Su, Y.-N.; Chen, C.-Y.; Chou, H.-C.; Tsao, P.-N.; Hsieh, W.-S. The sFlt-1/PlGF ratio as a predictor for poor pregnancy and neonatal outcomes. *Pediatr. Neonatol.* **2017**, *58*, 529–533. [CrossRef] [PubMed]

15. Herraiz, I.; Llurba, E.; Verlohren, S.; Galindo, A.; on behalf of the Spanish Group for the Study of Angiogenic Markers in Preeclampsia. Update on the Diagnosis and Prognosis of Preeclampsia with the Aid of the sFlt-1/PlGF Ratio in Singleton Pregnancies. *Fetal Diagn. Ther.* **2018**, *43*, 81–89. [CrossRef] [PubMed]
16. Karge, A.; Beckert, L.; Moog, P.; Haller, B.; Ortiz, J.U.; Lobmaier, S.M.; Abel, K.; Flechsenhar, S.; Kuschel, B.; Graupner, O. Role of sFlt-1/PlGF ratio and uterine Doppler in pregnancies with chronic kidney disease suspected with Pre-eclampsia or HELLP syndrome. *Pregnancy Hypertens. Int. J. Women's Cardiovasc. Health* **2020**, *22*, 160–166. [CrossRef]
17. Gómez-Arriaga, P.I.; Herraiz, I.; López-Jiménez, E.A.; Escribano, D.; Denk, B.; Galindo, A. Uterine artery Doppler and sFlt-1/PlGF ratio: Prognostic value in early-onset pre-eclampsia. *Ultrasound Obstet. Gynecol.* **2014**, *43*, 525–532. [CrossRef]
18. Graupner, O.; Lobmaier, S.M.; Ortiz, J.U.; Karge, A.; Kuschel, B. sFlt-1/PlGF ratio for the prediction of the time of delivery. *Arch. Gynecol. Obstet.* **2018**, *298*, 567–577. [CrossRef]
19. Karge, A.; Seiler, A.; Flechsenhar, S.; Haller, B.; Ortiz, J.U.; Lobmaier, S.M.; Axt-Fliedner, R.; Enzensberger, C.; Abel, K.; Kuschel, B.; et al. Prediction of adverse perinatal outcome and the mean time until delivery in twin pregnancies with suspected pre-eclampsia using sFlt-1/PlGF ratio. *Pregnancy Hypertens. Int. J. Women's Cardiovasc. Health* **2021**, *24*, 37–43. [CrossRef]
20. Lobmaier, S.M.; Figueras, F.; Mercade, I.; Perello, M.; Peguero, A.; Crovetto, F.; Ortiz, J.U.; Crispi, F.; Gratacos, E. Angiogenic factorsvsDoppler surveillance in the prediction of adverse outcome among late-pregnancy small-for- gestational-age fetuses. *Ultrasound Obstet. Gynecol.* **2014**, *43*, 533–540. [CrossRef]
21. Dröge, L.; Herraiz, I.; Zeisler, H.; Schlembach, D.; Stepan, H.; Küssel, L.; Henrich, W.; Galindo, A.; Verlohren, S. Maternal serum sFlt-1/PlGF ratio in twin pregnancies with and without pre-eclampsia in comparison with singleton pregnancies. *Ultrasound Obstet. Gynecol.* **2015**, *45*, 286–293. [CrossRef]
22. Jääskeläinen, T.; Finnpec, F.T.; Heinonen, S.; Hämäläinen, E.; Pulkki, K.; Romppanen, J.; Laivuori, H. Impact of obesity on angiogenic and inflammatory markers in the Finnish Genetics of Pre-eclampsia Consortium (FINNPEC) cohort. *Int. J. Obes.* **2019**, *43*, 1070–1081. [CrossRef]
23. Zera, C.A.; Seely, E.W.; Wilkins-Haug, L.E.; Lim, K.-H.; Parry, S.I.; McElrath, T.F. The association of body mass index with serum angiogenic markers in normal and abnormal pregnancies. *Am. J. Obstet. Gynecol.* **2014**, *211*, 247.e1–247.e7. [CrossRef] [PubMed]
24. Graupner, O.; Karge, A.; Flechsenhar, S.; Seiler, A.; Haller, B.; Ortiz, J.U.; Lobmaier, S.M.; Axt-Fliedner, R.; Enzensberger, C.; Abel, K.; et al. Role of sFlt-1/PlGF ratio and feto-maternal Doppler for the prediction of adverse perinatal outcome in late-onset pre-eclampsia. *Arch. Gynecol. Obstet.* **2020**, *301*, 375–385. [CrossRef] [PubMed]
25. ACOG. Practice Bulletin No. 202: Gestational Hypertension and Preeclampsia. *Obstet. Gynecol.* **2019**, *133*, e1–e25. [CrossRef]
26. American College of Obstetricians and Gynecologists; Task Force on Hypertension in Pregnancy. Hypertension in pregnancy. Report of the American College of Obstetricians and Gynecologists' Task Force on Hypertension in Pregnancy. *Obstet. Gynecol.* **2013**, *122*, 1122–1131. [CrossRef]
27. Weinstein, L. Syndrome of hemolysis, elevated liver enzymes, and low platelet count: A severe consequence of hypertension in pregnancy. *Am. J. Obstet. Gynecol.* **1982**, *142*, 159–167. [CrossRef]
28. Von Dadelszen, P.; Magee, L.A.; Roberts, J.M. Subclassification of Preeclampsia. *Hypertens. Pregnancy* **2003**, *22*, 143–148. [CrossRef]
29. Duffy, J.M.; Cairns, A.E.; Richards-Doran, D.; Hooft, J.V.; Gale, C.; Brown, M.; Chappell, L.; Grobman, W.A.; Fitzpatrick, R.; Karumanchi, S.A.; et al. A core outcome set for pre-eclampsia research: An international consensus development study. *BJOG* **2020**, *127*, 1516–1526. [CrossRef]
30. Voigt, M.; Rochow, N.; Schneider, K.T.M.; Hagenah, H.-P.; Scholz, R.; Hesse, V.; Wittwer-Backofen, U.; Straube, S.; Olbertz, D. New percentile values for the anthropometric dimensions of singleton neonates: Analysis of perinatal survey data of 2007–2011 from all 16 states of Germany. *Z. Geburtshilfe Neonatol.* **2014**, *218*, 210–217. [CrossRef]
31. Stepan, H.; Herraiz, I.; Schlembach, D.; Verlohren, S.; Brennecke, S.; Chantraine, F.; Klein, E.; Lapaire, O.; Llurba, E.; Ramoni, A.; et al. Implementation of the sFlt-1/PlGF ratio for prediction and diagnosis of pre-eclampsia in singleton pregnancy: Implications for clinical practice. *Ultrasound Obstet. Gynecol.* **2015**, *45*, 241–246. [CrossRef]
32. WHO. *Obesity: Preventing and Managing the Global Epidemic*; Report of a WHO Consultation; WHO Technical Report Series; WHO: Geneva, Switzerland, 2000; Volume 894, pp. 1–253.
33. DeLong, E.R.; DeLong, D.M.; Clarke-Pearson, D.L. Comparing the areas under two or more correlated receiver operating charac-teristic curves: A nonparametric approach. *Biometrics* **1988**, *44*, 837–845. [CrossRef]
34. Graupner, O.; Enzensberger, C. Prediction of Adverse Pregnancy Outcome Related to Placental Dysfunction Using the sFlt-1/PlGF Ratio: A Narrative Review. *Geburtshilfe Frauenheilkd.* **2021**, *81*, 948–954. [CrossRef] [PubMed]
35. Saleh, L.; Alblas, M.M.; Nieboer, D.; Neuman, R.I.; Vergouwe, Y.; Brussé, I.A.; Duvekot, J.J.; Steyerberg, E.W.; Versendaal, H.J.; Danser, A.H.J.; et al. Prediction of pre-eclampsia-related complications in women with suspected or confirmed pre-eclampsia: Development and internal validation of clinical prediction model. *Ultrasound Obstet. Gynecol.* **2021**, *58*, 698–704. [CrossRef] [PubMed]
36. Stolz, M.; Zeisler, H.; Heinzl, F.; Binder, J.; Farr, A. An sFlt-1:PlGF ratio of 655 is not a reliable cut-off value for predicting perinatal outcomes in women with preeclampsia. *Pregnancy Hypertens. Int. J. Women's Cardiovasc. Health* **2018**, *11*, 54–60. [CrossRef] [PubMed]
37. Simón, E.; Permuy, C.; Sacristán, L.; Zamoro-Lorenci, M.J.; Villalaín, C.; Galindo, A.; Herraiz, I. sFlt-1/PlGF ratio for the prediction of delivery within 48 hours and adverse outcomes in expectantly managed early-onset preeclampsia. *Pregnancy Hypertens. Int. J. Women's Cardiovasc. Health* **2020**, *22*, 17–23. [CrossRef]

38. Saleh, L.; Tahitu, S.I.; Danser, A.J.; Meiracker, A.H.V.D.; Visser, W. The predictive value of the sFlt-1/PlGF ratio on short-term absence of preeclampsia and maternal and fetal or neonatal complications in twin pregnancies. *Pregnancy Hypertens. Int. J. Women's Cardiovasc. Health* **2018**, *14*, 222–227. [CrossRef]
39. Zeisler, H.; Llurba, E.; Chantraine, F.; Vatish, M.; Staff, A.C.; Sennström, M.; Olovsson, M.; Brennecke, S.P.; Stepan, H.; Allegranza, D.; et al. Predictive Value of the sFlt-1:PlGF Ratio in Women with Suspected Preeclampsia. *N. Engl. J. Med.* **2016**, *374*, 13–22. [CrossRef]
40. Suwaki, N.; Masuyama, H.; Nakatsukasa, H.; Masumoto, A.; Sumida, Y.; Takamoto, N.; Hiramatrsu, Y. Hypoadiponectinemia and circulating angiogenic factors in overweight patients complicated with pre-eclampsia. *Am. J. Obstet. Gynecol.* **2006**, *195*, 1687–1692. [CrossRef]
41. Mijal, R.S.; Holzman, C.B.; Rana, S.; Karumanchi, S.A.; Wang, J.; Sikorskii, A. Midpregnancy levels of angiogenic markers in relation to maternal characteristics. *Am. J. Obstet. Gynecol.* **2011**, *204*, 244.e1–244.e12. [CrossRef]
42. Faupel-Badger, J.M.; Staff, A.C.; Thadhani, R.; Powe, C.E.; Potischman, N.; Hoover, R.N.; Troisi, R. Maternal angiogenic profile in pregnancies that remain normotensive. *Eur. J. Obstet. Gynecol. Reprod. Biol.* **2011**, *158*, 189–193. [CrossRef]
43. Heimberger, S.; Mueller, A.; Ratnaparkhi, R.; Perdigao, J.L.; Rana, S. Angiogenic factor abnormalities and risk of peripartum complications and prematurity among urban predominantly obese parturients with chronic hypertension. *Pregnancy Hypertens. Int. J. Women Cardiovasc. Health* **2020**, *20*, 124–130. [CrossRef]
44. Spradley, F.T.; Palei, A.C.; Granger, J.P. Obese melanocortin-4 receptor-deficient rats exhibit augmented angiogenic balance and vasorelaxation during pregnancy. *Physiol. Rep.* **2013**, *1*, e00081. [CrossRef] [PubMed]
45. Spradley, F.T.; Palei, A.C.; Granger, J.P. Increased risk for the development of preeclampsia in obese pregnancies: Weighing in on the mechanisms. *Am. J. Physiol. Regul. Integr. Comp. Physiol.* **2015**, *309*, R1326–R1343. [CrossRef] [PubMed]
46. Herse, F.; Fain, J.N.; Janke, J.; Engeli, S.; Kuhn, C.; Frey, N.; Weich, H.A.; Bergmann, A.; Kappert, K.; Karumanchi, S.A.; et al. Adipose Tissue-Derived Soluble Fms-Like Tyrosine Kinase 1 Is an Obesity-Relevant Endogenous Paracrine Adipokine. *Hypertension* **2011**, *58*, 37–42. [CrossRef] [PubMed]
47. Mariman, E.C.M.; Wang, P. Adipocyte extracellular matrix composition, dynamics and role in obesity. *Cell. Mol. Life Sci.* **2010**, *67*, 1277–1292. [CrossRef]
48. Lisonkova, S.; Razaz, N.; Sabr, Y.; Muraca, G.M.; Boutin, A.; Mayer, C.; Joseph, K.; Kramer, M.S. Maternal risk factors and adverse birth outcomes associated with HELLP syndrome: A population-based study. *BJOG* **2020**, *127*, 1189–1198. [CrossRef]
49. Rana, S.; Schnettler, W.T.; Powe, C.; Wenger, J.; Salahuddin, S.; Cerdeira, A.S.; Verlohren, S.; Perschel, F.H.; Arany, Z.; Lim, K.-H.; et al. Clinical characterization and outcomes of preeclampsia with normal angiogenic profile. *Hypertens. Pregnancy* **2013**, *32*, 189–201. [CrossRef]
50. Mbah, A.K.; Kornosky, J.L.; Kristensen, S.; August, E.M.; Alio, A.P.; Marty, P.J.; Belogolovkin, V.; Bruder, K.; Salihu, H.M. Super-obesity and risk for early and late pre-eclampsia. *BJOG* **2010**, *117*, 997–1004. [CrossRef]
51. Klein, E.; Schlembach, D.; Ramoni, A.; Langer, E.; Bahlmann, F.; Grill, S.; Schaffenrath, H.; van der Does, R.; Messinger, D.; Verhagen-Kamerbeek, W.D.; et al. Influence of the sFlt-1/PlGF Ratio on Clinical Decision-Making in Women with Sus-pected Preeclampsia. *PLoS ONE* **2016**, *11*, e0156013. [CrossRef]

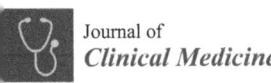

Article

Value of Cerebroplacental Ratio and Uterine Artery Doppler as Predictors of Adverse Perinatal Outcome in Very Small for Gestational Age at Term Fetuses

Anne Karge [1], Silvia M. Lobmaier [1], Bernhard Haller [2], Bettina Kuschel [1] and Javier U. Ortiz [1,*]

1 Division of Obstetrics and Perinatal Medicine, Department of Obstetrics and Gynecology, University Hospital Rechts der Isar, Technical University of Munich, 81675 Munich, Germany; anne.karge@mri.tum.de (A.K.); silvia.lobmaier@mri.tum.de (S.M.L.); bettina.kuschel@mri.tum.de (B.K.)
2 Institute of AI Medical Informatics in Medicine, University Hospital Rechts der Isar, Technical University of Munich, 81675 Munich, Germany; bernhard.haller@mri.tum.de
* Correspondence: javier.ortiz@mri.tum.de; Tel.: +49-89-4140-2430; Fax: +49-89-4140-2447

Abstract: The aim of this study was to evaluate the association between cerebroplacental ratio (CPR), mean uterine artery (mUtA) Doppler and adverse perinatal outcome (APO) and their predictive performance in fetuses with birth weight (BW) <3rd centile (very small for gestational age, VSGA) in comparison with fetuses with BW 3rd–10th centile (small for gestational age, SGA). This was a retrospective cohort study including singleton pregnancies delivered at term (37 + 0–41 + 6) in a single tertiary referral center over a six-year period. APO was defined as a composite of cesarean section for intrapartum fetal compromise (IFC), umbilical artery pH < 7.20, and admission to the neonatal intensive care unit for >24 h. The characteristics of the study population according to BW (VSGA and SGA) as well as the presence of composite APO were assessed. The prognostic performance of CPR and mUtA-PI was evaluated using receiver operating characteristic (ROC) analysis. In total, 203 pregnancies were included. Of these, 55 (27%) had CPR <10th centile, 25 (12%) mUtA-PI >95th centile, 65 (32%) VSGA fetuses, and 93 (46%) composite APO. VSGA showed a non-significantly higher rate of composite APO in comparison to SGA (52% vs. 43%; $p = 0.202$). The composite APO rate was significantly higher in SGA with CPR <10th centile (36% vs. 13%; $p = 0.001$), while in VSGA with CPR <10th centile was not (38% vs. 35%; $p = 0.818$). The composite APO rate was non-significantly higher both in VSGA (26% vs. 10%; $p = 0.081$) and SGA (14% vs. 6%; $p = 0.742$) with mUtA-PI >95th centile. The ROC analysis showed a significantly predictive value of CPR for composite APO in SGA only (AUC 0.612; $p = 0.025$). A low CPR was associated with composite APO in SGA fetuses. VSGA fetuses were more frequently affected by composite APO regardless of Doppler values. The predictive performance of CPR and uterine artery Doppler was poor.

Keywords: cerebroplacental ratio; uterine artery Doppler; small for gestational age; adverse perinatal outcome

Citation: Karge, A.; Lobmaier, S.M.; Haller, B.; Kuschel, B.; Ortiz, J.U. Value of Cerebroplacental Ratio and Uterine Artery Doppler as Predictors of Adverse Perinatal Outcome in Very Small for Gestational Age at Term Fetuses. *J. Clin. Med.* 2022, 11, 3852. https://doi.org/10.3390/jcm11133852

Academic Editor: Sylvie Girard

Received: 25 May 2022
Accepted: 29 June 2022
Published: 3 July 2022

Publisher's Note: MDPI stays neutral with regard to jurisdictional claims in published maps and institutional affiliations.

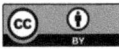

Copyright: © 2022 by the authors. Licensee MDPI, Basel, Switzerland. This article is an open access article distributed under the terms and conditions of the Creative Commons Attribution (CC BY) license (https://creativecommons.org/licenses/by/4.0/).

1. Introduction

Fetuses with a birthweight (BW) <10th centile are classified as small for gestational age (SGA) [1]. Among them, there is a subset of fetuses with different clinical behaviors. Compared to merely constitutional SGA, growth-restricted fetuses are more often affected by adverse perinatal outcomes (APOs) including operative delivery, low Apgar scores, low umbilical artery (UA) pH, neonatal intensive care unit (NICU) admissions, hypotension, poor thermoregulation, hypoglycemia, intrauterine fetal death, and neonatal death [2–4]. Maternal underperfusion of the placenta is a common finding in fetal growth restriction (FGR) and could explain the differences in the pathophysiology of constitutional SGA and FGR [5]. Since a low cerebroplacental ratio (CPR) reflects a redistribution of cardiac output towards the brain due to placental dysfunction, it may identify fetuses at higher risk of APO [6,7]. In addition, an elevated mean uterine artery pulsatility index (mUtA-PI) is associated with a higher risk of cesarean section for fetal distress as well as APO [8,9]. However, its main impact is still considered as a predictor for pre-eclampsia [10–12].

Very small for gestational age (VSGA) fetuses with BW <3rd centile represent a particular subgroup showing a higher risk of APO [13,14]. Doppler performance in these fetuses has rarely been evaluated. Although there is a large variety of literature focusing on CPR and mUtA-PI, their meaning for APO prediction in VSGA at term remains unclear. Our aim was therefore to evaluate the association between CPR, mUtA-PI, and APO and their predictive performance in VSGA compared to SGA.

2. Materials and Methods

2.1. Participants and Protocol

This was retrospective cohort study performed at the University Hospital rechts der Isar in January 2012 and December 2017. The inclusion criteria were singleton pregnancies, cephalic presentation, mUtA-PI measurements from 32 + 0 weeks of gestation onwards, CPR measurements within one week of delivery, and delivery of an alive newborn between 37 + 0 and 41 + 6 weeks of gestation with a birth weight <10th centile. VSGA and SGA were defined as a BW <3rd centile and a BW in the 3rd–9th centile, respectively [15]. Fetuses with anatomical or chromosomal abnormalities, pregnancies with elective CS and women with abnormal labor progression (protraction or arrest at the first or second stage of labor) were excluded.

Gestational age (GA) was calculated based on measurements of the crown–rump length in the first trimester. Either a Voluson E8 (GE Medical Systems, Solingen, NRW, Germany) or a Voluson E10 (GE Medical Systems, Solingen, NRW, Germany) with 4- to 6-MHz curvilinear abdominal transducer was used. Fetal biometry was performed by measuring the biparietal diameter, head circumference, abdominal circumference, and femur length. The EFW and its centiles were calculated [15,16]. Doppler assessment of UtA, UA, and MCA was routinely performed according to our protocol for pregnancies at $\geq 32 + 0$ weeks of gestation by doctors with at least two years' experience in obstetric ultrasound, adhering to standardized recommendations [17]. mUtA-PI was obtained by averaging the PI values from the right and left uterine arteries. An mUtA-PI >95th centile was considered abnormal. The CPR was calculated by using MCA-PI divided by UA-PI. A cutoff <10th centile was considered abnormal according to its better performance regarding APO as compared to CPR <5th centile or CPR < 1 [18].

Composite APO was defined as the occurrence of at least one of the following parameters: CS for intrapartum fetal compromise (IFC), umbilical artery pH < 7.20, or admission to the neonatal intensive care unit (NICU) for >24 h. IFC was defined as a persistent pathological CTG pattern or the combination of a pathological CTG pattern and a fetal scalp pH < 7.20. The CTG pattern was evaluated according to the International Federation of Gynecology and Obstetrics (FIGO) criteria [19]. A pathological CTG pattern was initially managed conservatively (left lateral decubitus position, intravenous tocolysis). Fetal scalp blood sampling was indicated at the discretion of the attending obstetrician. If fetal scalp blood sampling was not possible due to cervical conditions and if the CTG pattern persisted in being pathological for 10 min after starting conservative management, CS was indicated.

2.2. Data Collected

The following parameters were obtained and analyzed: maternal age, body mass index (BMI), parity, ethnicity, nicotine use, pre-existing conditions, GA at ultrasound, amniotic fluid index, mUtA-PI, UA-PI, MCA-PI, CPR, CPR centiles [20,21], induction of labor, CTG assessment, fetal scalp pH, mode of delivery, GA at delivery, sex, BW, BW centile, UA pH, and Apgar score at 5 min.

2.3. Statistical Analysis

We used IBM SPSS Statistics for Windows, version 26 (IBM Corp., Armonk, NY, USA) for analysis. Quantitative data were shown as median and interquartile range. Categorical data were presented as absolute and relative frequencies. Differences in the distributions of quantitative variables between groups were tested using the Mann–Whitney U test. Categorical data were compared between groups using Pearson's chi-square test or Fisher's exact test. All statistical tests were conducted two-sided and a p-value < 0.05 was considered statistically significant.

Characteristics of the study population according to BW (VSGA/SGA) as well as the presence of composite APO were analyzed. Moreover, univariate logistic regression analyses stratified by BW (VSGA/SGA) were carried out using maternal characteristics (age, BMI, parity, ethnicity, nicotine use, pre-existing conditions) and ultrasound parameters (EFW, EFW centile, CPR, CPR centile, CPR <10th centile, mUtA-PI, mUtA-PI centile, mUtA-PI >95th centile, sex) as independent variables with composite APO as a binary outcome. Statistically significant variables in the univariate analysis were considered in a multivariable logistic regression model. Finally, values of CPR and mUtA-PI, both alone and combined (multivariable logistic regression), for predicting composite APO were evaluated using receiver operating characteristics (ROC) analysis stratified by BW (VSGA/SGA).

3. Results

3.1. Baseline Characteristics and Perinatal Outcome

A total of 203 pregnancies were enrolled. Fourteen women had pre-existing conditions (four cases of systemic lupus erythematosus, four cases of essential hypertension, three cases of preeclampsia, two cases of thrombophilia, one case of type 1 diabetes). In the whole study group, 55 (27%) fetuses showed a CPR <10th centile, 25 (12%) women had a mUtA-PI >95th centile, and 10 (5%) pregnancies showed a CPR <10th centile and a mUtA-PI >95th centile. Induction of labor was performed in 131 (65%) pregnancies (93 dinoprostone vaginal insert, 38 intravaginal minprostin gel) and the most frequent indications were premature rupture of membranes $\geq$12 h, SGA with normal CPR from 40 + 0 weeks onwards or with low CPR from 37 + 0 weeks onward, or VSGA from 37 + 0 weeks onwards. APO included 33 (16%) cases of CS for IFC, 48 (24%) newborns with umbilical artery pH < 7.20, and 29 (14%) newborns admitted to NICU >24 h (reasons were hypoglycemia (11/29), respiratory distress (9/29), hypothermia (4/29), infection (3/29) or hyperbilirubinemia (2/29)). Composite APO occurred in 93 (46%) cases.

Overall, 65 (32%) newborns were VSGA and 138 (68%) SGA (Table 1). There were no significant differences in maternal age, BMI, nulliparity, ethnicity, nicotine use, pre-existing conditions, GA at measurement of mUtA-PI, and CPR measurement to delivery intervals between the groups. As expected, BW and BW centiles were lower in the VSGA group. In addition, VSGA showed a lower rate of UA pH < 7.20 and a higher rate of CS for IFC, admission to NICU >24 h, and composite APO in comparison to SGA.

Regarding perinatal outcome within the groups (Table 2), VSGA pregnancies with composite APO showed a significantly higher proportion of nulliparity and induction of labor as well as a significantly lower GA at delivery and BW. SGA pregnancies with composite APO showed a significantly lower BMI, a lower proportion of Caucasian women, and a higher proportion of male fetuses.

Table 1. Characteristics and outcomes of the study population according to birth weight.

	VSGA (n = 65)	SGA (n = 138)	p
Maternal age (years)	30.6 (7.1)	32 (6.4)	0.270
BMI (kg/m^2)	21.6 (3.4)	21.7 (4.3)	0.947
Nulliparity	49 (75)	91 (66)	0.175
Caucasian	61 (96)	133 (96)	0.471
Smoking	6 (9)	6 (4)	0.205
Pre-existing conditions	4 (6)	10 (7)	1.000
EFW (gram)	2699 (1530)	2890 (484)	0.011 *
EFW centile	5 (10)	9 (41)	0.014 *
CPR	1.53 (0.62)	1.61 (0.57)	0.079
CPR centile	24 (42)	33 (42)	0.040 *
CPR < 10th centile	24 (37)	31 (23)	0.031 *
mUtA-PI	0.69 (0.33)	0.68 (0.23)	0.998
mUtA-PI centile	50 (71)	46 (59)	0.709
mUtA-PI > 95th centile	12 (19)	13 (9)	0.067
Measurement of mUtA-PI (weeks)	37.3 (3.8)	36.5 (5.4)	0.210
Amniotic fluid index (cm)	9.9 (6.2)	11.5 (5.4)	0.114
Induction of labor	43 (66)	88 (64)	0.740
GA at delivery (weeks)	39.4 (2.2)	40.1 (1.8)	0.019 *
CPR to delivery interval (days)	2 (5)	2 (4)	0.362
Delivery at ≥40 weeks	23 (35)	75 (54)	0.012 *
Cesarean section for IFC	15 (23)	18 (13)	0.071
UA pH	7.26 (0.09)	7.27 (0.13)	0.558
UA pH < 7.20	14 (22)	34 (25)	0.628
Apgar 5 min	10 (1)	10 (1)	0.568
Apgar 5 min < 7	1 (2)	2 (1)	1.000
Male	35 (54)	83 (60)	0.396
Birthweight (g)	2725 (280)	2870 (210)	<0.001 *

Data are expressed as median (interquartile range) or n (%). VSGA very small for gestational age; SGA small for gestational age; BMI body mass index; EFW estimated fetal weight; CPR cerebroplacental ratio; mUtA-PI mean uterine artery pulsatility index; IFC intrapartum fetal compromise; UA umbilical artery; GA gestational age; NICU neonatal intensive care unit; APO adverse perinatal outcome. A p-value < 0.05 was considered as statistically significant (*).

Table 2. Characteristics of the entire study population according to the composite adverse perinatal outcome (APO).

	VSGA (n = 65)			SGA (n = 138)		
	Composite APO		p	Composite APO		p
	no (n = 31)	yes (n = 34)		no (n = 79)	yes (n = 59)	
Maternal age (years)	30.7 (9.1)	29.8 (6.1)	0.533	31.9 (7.2)	32.1 (5.8)	0.952
BMI (kg/m^2)	21.5 (3.7)	21.6 (4.6)	0.536	22.3 (4.5)	20.9 (4.5)	0.019 *
Nulliparity	17 (55)	32 (94)	<0.001 *	49 (62)	42 (71)	0.261
Caucasian	30 (97)	31 (91)	0.615	79 (100)	54 (92)	0.013 *
Smoking	3 (10)	3 (9)	1.000	4 (5)	2 (3)	1.000
Pre-existing conditions	0 (0)	4 (12)	0.115	5 (6)	5 (8)	0.744
EFW (gram)	2809 (460)	2568 (748)	0.176	2885 (513)	2890 (523)	0.679
EFW centile	5 (10)	5 (8)	0.642	9 (9)	10 (14)	0.833
CPR	1.49 (0.63)	1.61 (0.58)	0.834	1.62 (0.53)	1.59 (0.71)	0.025 *
CPR centile	25 (45)	18 (41)	0.773	35 (33)	32 (59)	0.039 *
CPR < 10th centile	11 (35)	13 (38)	0.818	10 (13)	21 (36)	0.001 *

Table 2. Cont.

	VSGA (n = 65)			SGA (n = 138)		
	Composite APO		p	Composite APO		p
mUtA-PI	0.64 (0.29)	0.73 (0.41)	0.053	0.68 (0.22)	0.67 (0.26)	0.735
mUtA-PI centile	41 (64)	66 (73)	0.054	49 (59)	46 (59)	0.919
mUtA-PI >95th centile	3 (10)	9 (26)	0.081	5 (6)	8 (14)	0.742
CPR <10th centile and mUtA-PI >95th centile	2 (6)	5 (15)	0.430	1 (1)	2 (3)	1.000
GA at measurement of UtA-PI	37.5 (4.0)	37.1 (1.9)	0.703	36.3 (5.9)	35.7 (5.1)	0.632
Amniotic fluid index (cm)	9.5 (6.3)	10.1 (7.0)	0.702	11.5 (5.9)	11.5 (5.8)	0.820
Induction of labor	16 (52)	27 (79)	0.018 *	45 (57)	43 (73)	0.054
GA at delivery (weeks)	39.8 (1.2)	39.0 (2.4)	0.035 *	40.0 (1.9)	40.1 (2.1)	0.514
CPR to delivery interval (days)	1.5 (7.0)	3.0 (5.0)	0.384	2.0 (5.0)	1.5 (3.0)	0.423
Delivery at ≥40 weeks	13 (42)	10 (29)	0.292	42 (53)	33 (56)	0.747
Male	14 (45)	16 (47)	0.878	25 (32)	30 (51)	0.023 *
Birthweight (g)	2760 (185)	2640 (370)	0.048 *	2855 (200)	2917 (220)	0.101
Birthweight centile	2 (0)	2 (0)	0.340	7 (2)	8 (2)	0.120

Data are expressed as median (interquartile range) or n (%). VSGA very small for gestational age; SGA small for gestational age; BMI body mass index; EFW estimated fetal weight; CPR cerebroplacental ratio; mUtA-PI mean uterine artery pulsatility index; GA gestational age. A p-value < 0.05 was considered as statistically significant (*).

3.2. Association between Doppler and Composite APO

VSGA fetuses with a CPR <10th centile or mUtA-PI >95th centile or CPR <10th centile and mUtA-PI >95th centile showed a non-significantly higher rate of composite APO (Table 2).

SGA fetuses with a CPR <10th centile had a significantly higher rate of composite APO (Table 2). In addition, SGA fetuses with composite APO showed a significantly lower CPR and CPR centile. On the contrary, mUtA-PI >95th centile or CPR <10th centile and mUtA-PI > 95th centile had a non-significantly higher rate of composite APO.

3.3. Logistic Regression Model

In the VSGA group, univariate logistic regression identified a significant association between one variable (nulliparity) and composite APO (Table 3). Nulliparity increased the odds of composite APO by about 13 times.

Table 3. Univariate and multivariable logistic regression of predictors of composite adverse perinatal outcome. Variables significantly associated with adverse perinatal outcome in univariate regression (p < 0.05) were included in the multivariable model.

	Univariate OR	95% CI	p	Multivariable OR	95% CI	p
VSGA						
Maternal age (years)	0.959	0.873–1.053	0.378			
BMI (kg/m^2)	0.997	0.883–1.125	0.958			
Nulliparity	13.17	2.676–64.87	0.002 *			
Caucasian	0.344	0.034–3.499	0.368			
Nicotin use	0.903	0.168–4.846	0.905			
Pre-existing conditions	3.759	0.717–19.074	0.117			
EFW	0.999	0.998–1.001	0.250			
EFW centile	1.001	0.951–1.053	0.968			
CPR	1.115	0.358–3.468	0.851			
CPR centile	0.998	0.981–1.016	0.855			
CPR <10th centile	1.126	0.410–3.090	0.818			
mUtA-PI	6.153	0.599–63.22	0.126			
mUtA-PI centile	1.013	0.999–1.027	0.078			
mUtA-PI >95th centile	3.360	0.817–13.812	0.093			
Male	1.079	0.406–2.866	0.878			

Table 3. Cont.

	Univariate OR	95% CI	p	Multivariable OR	95% CI	p
SGA						
Maternal age (years)	1.010	0.948–1.076	0.762			
BMI (kg/m^2)	0.897	0.814–0.988	0.027 *	0.918	0.834–1.010	0.078
Nulliparity	1.513	0.733–3.119	0.262			
Caucasian	0.171	0.019–1.571	0.119			
Nicotin use	0.658	0.116–3.718	0.636			
Pre-existing conditions	1.408	0.545–3.641	0.480			
EFW	1.000	0.999–1.001	0.688			
EFW percentile	1.004	0.968–1.042	0.819			
CPR	0.445	0.190–1.039	0.061			
CPR percentile	0.992	0.980–1.004	0.182			
CPR < 10th percentile	3.813	1.629–8.928	0.002 *	2.804	1.133–6.944	0.026 *
mUtA-PI	1.012	0.156–6.556	0.990			
mUtA-PI percentile	0.999	0.988–1.010	0.877			
mUtA-PI >95th percentile	0.822	0.255–2.653	0.743			
Male	2.234	1.113–4.485	0.024 *	2.227	1.035–4.792	0.040 *

OR odds ratio; CI confidence interval; VSGA very small for gestational age; SGA small for gestational age; BMI body mass index; EFW estimated fetal weight; CPR cerebroplacental ratio; mUtA-PI mean uterine artery pulsatility index. A p-value < 0.05 was considered as statistically significant (*).

In the SGA group, univariate logistic regression identified a significant association between three variables (BMI, CPR <10th centile, male) and composite APO. However, multivariable logistic regression showed that only CPR <10th centile and male fetuses were independent predictors of composite APO (Table 3); they increased the odds of composite APO by about threefold and twofold, respectively.

3.4. Prognostic Value for Composite APO

In the VSGA group, a ROC analysis revealed no relevant prognostic value of CPR or mUtA-PI for composite APO, but a significant prognostic value for nulliparity (Table 4). The combined model of CPR and mUtA-PI did not improve prediction compared to mUtA-PI alone, while the combined model including nulliparity did.

Table 4. Receiver operating characteristics analysis of Doppler parameters alone and combined to predict composite adverse perinatal outcome stratified by birthweight.

	AUC	95% CI	p
VSGA			
CPR	0.515	0.372–0.658	0.834
mUtA-PI	0.639	0.504–0.775	0.054
Nulliparity	0.696	0.565–0.828	0.007 *
CPR + mUtA-PI	0.641	0.506–0.777	0.051
CPR + nulliparity	0.706	0.576–0.836	0.004 *
mUtA-PI + nulliparity	0.814	0.710–0.917	<0.001 *
CPR + mUtA-PI + nulliparity	0.809	0.705–0.914	<0.001 *
SGA			
CPR	0.612	0.512–0.712	0.025 *
mUtA-PI	0.517	0.419–0.615	0.735
Male	0.596	0.500–0.692	0.054
CPR + mUtA-PI	0.611	0.511–0.711	0.026 *
CPR + male	0.647	0.550–0.743	0.003 *
mUtA-PI + male	0.590	0.492–0.688	0.071
CPR + mUtA-PI + male	0.649	0.552–0.745	0.003 *

AUC area under the curve; CI confidence interval; VSGA very small for gestational age; SGA small for gestational age; CPR cerebroplacental ratio; mUtA-PI mean uterine artery pulsatility index. A p-value < 0.05 was considered as statistically significant (*).

In the SGA group, the ROC analysis showed a significant prognostic value of CPR for composite APO, while for mUtA-PI or male fetal sex it did not (Table 4). Both the combined model of CPR and mUtA-PI and the combined models including fetal sex (male) did not improve the prediction substantially compared to CPR alone.

4. Discussion

This study showed a significant association between CPR and the occurrence of composite APO in SGA fetuses. VSGA fetuses were more frequently affected by composite APO regardless of CPR value. Furthermore, uterine artery Doppler was not significantly associated with composite APO in either SGA and in VSGA fetuses. The prognostic value for composite APO of CPR and/or mUtA-PI was poor.

In the last decade, the difference between fetal growth and fetal size has been highlighted. It is important to distinguish between constitutionally small fetuses and fetuses with signs of placental insufficiency, as the latter are often affected by APO such as IFC or stillbirth, whereas the former are not [13,22–24]. Measurements of CPR are a part of the surveillance for SGA fetuses. Recent data suggest that pregnancies with SGA fetuses and normal Doppler findings can be prolonged safely [13]. Conversely, CPR abnormalities are associated with APO. Likewise, our data showed a significant association between low CPR and composite APO in the cohort of SGA fetuses. Previous studies have reported a poor performance of CPR as an APO predictor except for perinatal death [25–27]. Furthermore, Di Mascio et al. recently reported a poor performance of CPR as well as of UCA (umbilicocerebral ratio) in late-onset FGR as outcome predictors [28]. Accordingly, our analysis confirmed a low predictive performance of CPR in the SGA group. Serum parameters reflecting placental insufficiency, such as sFlt-1/PlGF, might help detect cases of SGA with a higher risk of APO, but their meaning for APO prediction in high-risk cohorts is still controversial [29–33].

We found that CPR values were not associated with composite APO in VSGA fetuses. This is in-line with recent data suggesting that at term EFW <3rd centile is a better APO predictor than low CPR or pathological uterine Doppler in growth restricted fetuses [13]. Furthermore, in fetuses with normal Doppler parameters, those with EFW <3rd centile showed a higher rate of CS for fetal distress and longer neonatal hospitalization compared to those with EFW >3rd centile and BW >10th centile [14]. In addition, a prospective study including a large cohort pointed out that SGA fetuses with low abdominal circumference have a particularly higher risk of being affected by APO, indicating the importance of fetal size itself in detecting FGR situations [33]. Therefore, a BW <3rd centile reflects placental insufficiency in many cases and an EFW <3rd centile should be handled as an FGR independently of the fetal Doppler status as suggested by the Delphi consensus [12]. Nevertheless, it is important to be aware of the inaccuracy of EFW as measured by ultrasound and the matching of BW. Cohort studies on EFW reported a high intra- and interobserver variability and a detection rate of less than 50% of SGA newborns [34,35].

In our cohort, mUtA-PI was not significantly associated with composite APO, although there was a trend in the VSGA group. However, we acknowledge that the subgroup of pregnancies with pathological uterine Doppler was small. This result is controversial, as a recently published meta-analysis implicates a similar performance of uterine artery Doppler compared to CPR for the prediction of APO in late-onset SGA fetuses [5]. In particular, the association of perinatal death or stillbirth is noteworthy not only in SGA, but also in AGA fetuses [5,36]. Still, the current suggested definition of late FGR does not include mUtA-PI [12]. In contrast to CPR, uterine Doppler reflects the maternal site of the placenta, and its elevation might be caused by an insufficient invasion of the trophoblast in the first trimester [37,38]. De novo elevations in the third trimester are more likely explained by a maternal cardiovascular maladaptation [39]. The meaning of uterine artery Doppler in VSGA pregnancies remains unclear.

Our findings showed that nulliparity was a significant predictor of APO in the VSGA cohort. An explanation for this finding might be the longer duration of the second stage of labor in nulliparous women, which is associated with APO [40]. As VSGA are already affected by a reduced placental capacity, they are more likely to experience APO—especially when the placental oxygenation is further decreased by contractions [41].

Our study was limited by its retrospective design. Furthermore, our institution is a tertiary referral center which can lead to selection bias. Moreover, since ultrasound and Doppler examinations were performed by different operators, the internal validity may be limited. Finally, as we routinely recommend induction of labor ≥ 37 weeks gestation for FGR fetuses (VSGA irrespective of Doppler values, SGA with abnormal Doppler), but prolongation for SGA fetuses with normal Doppler parameters, this might distort the results of this study. However, this is a common problem affecting all studies investigating APO prediction in SGA cohorts.

5. Conclusions

In conclusion, low CPR was associated with composite APO in SGA fetuses, but not in VSGA fetuses. VSGA is a condition that requires particularly careful monitoring regardless of the Doppler parameters. Further clinical research is warranted to clarify the role of cerebral blood flow redistribution and uterine artery Doppler in the prediction of APO as well as in the pathophysiology of the underlying placental insufficiency in VSGA fetuses.

Author Contributions: Conceptualization, J.U.O. and A.K.; methodology, J.U.O.; software, A.K. and B.H.; validation, A.K., S.M.L., B.H., B.K. and J.U.O.; formal analysis, A.K., B.H. and J.U.O.; investigation, J.U.O. and A.K.; resources, B.K. and J.U.O.; data curation, J.U.O.; writing—original draft preparation, J.U.O. and A.K.; writing—review and editing, A.K., S.M.L., B.H., B.K. and J.U.O.; visualization, J.U.O., B.H. and A.K.; supervision, B.K. and J.U.O.; project administration, J.U.O. All authors have read and agreed to the published version of the manuscript.

Funding: This research received no external funding.

Institutional Review Board Statement: All procedures performed in studies involving human participants were in accordance with the ethical standards of the institutional and national research committee and with the 1964 Helsinki declaration and its later amendments or comparable ethical standards.

Informed Consent Statement: In accordance with article 27 Section 4 of the Bavarian hospital law ("Bayerisches Krankenhausgesetz—BayKrG"), patient data collected in the context of medical treatment at a hospital may be used for training, further education, research purposes, and statistics for the hospital. Patient data must remain in the custody of the hospital. For this reason, in this retrospective hospital data collection, a separate declaration of informed consent of the patients was waived. There were no minors included in this study.

Data Availability Statement: Not applicable.

Conflicts of Interest: The authors declare no conflict of interest.

Abbreviations

APO	Adverse perinatal outcome
BMI	Body mass index
BW	Birth weight
CI	Confidence interval
CPR	Cerebroplacental ratio
EFW	Estimated fetal weight
FGR	Fetal growth restriction
FIGO	Federation of Gynecology and Obstetrics
GA	Gestational age
IFC	Intrapartum fetal compromise
mUtA	Mean uterine artery
NICU	Neonatal intensive care unit

PI	Pulsatility index	
ROC	Receiver operating characteristic	
SGA	Small for gestational age	
UA	Umbilical artery	
VSGA	Very small for gestational age	

References

1. Beune, I.M.; Bloomfield, F.H.; Ganzevoort, W.; Embleton, N.D.; Rozance, P.J.; van Wassenaer-Leemhuis, A.G.; Wynia, K.; Gordijn, S.J. Consensus Based Definition of Growth Restriction in the Newborn. *J. Pediatr.* **2018**, *196*, 71–76. [CrossRef] [PubMed]
2. Zhang-Rutledge, K.; Mack, L.M.; Mastrobattista, J.M.; Gandhi, M. Significance and Outcomes of Fetal Growth Restriction Below the 5th Percentile Compared to the 5th to 10th Percentiles on Midgestation Growth Ultrasonography. *J. Ultrasound Med.* **2018**, *37*, 2243–2249. [CrossRef] [PubMed]
3. Zeve, D.; Regelmann, M.O.; Holzman, I.R.; Rapaport, R. Small at Birth, but How Small? The Definition of SGA Revisited. *Horm. Res. Paediatr.* **2016**, *86*, 357–360. [CrossRef] [PubMed]
4. Malin, G.L.; Morris, R.K.; Riley, R.; Teune, M.J.; Khan, K.S. When is birthweight at term abnormally low? A systematic review and meta-analysis of the association and predictive ability of current birthweight standards for neonatal outcomes. *BJOG* **2014**, *121*, 515–526. [CrossRef]
5. Martinez-Portilla, R.J.; Caradeux, J.; Meler, E.; Lip-Sosa, D.L.; Sotiriadis, A.; Figueras, F. Third-trimester uterine artery Doppler for prediction of adverse outcome in late small-for-gestational-age fetuses: Systematic review and meta-analysis. *Ultrasound Obstet. Gynecol.* **2020**, *55*, 575–585. [CrossRef]
6. Parra-Saavedra, M.; Crovetto, F.; Triunfo, S.; Savchev, S.; Peguero, A.; Nadal, A.; Gratacós, E.; Figueras, F. Association of Doppler parameters with placental signs of underperfusion in late-onset small-for-gestational-age pregnancies. *Ultrasound Obstet. Gynecol.* **2014**, *44*, 330–337. [CrossRef]
7. DeVore, G.R. The importance of the cerebroplacental ratio in the evaluation of fetal well-being in SGA and AGA fetuses. *Am. J. Obstet. Gynecol.* **2015**, *213*, 5–15. [CrossRef]
8. Morales-Roselló, J.; Khalil, A. Fetal cerebral redistribution: A marker of compromise regardless of fetal size. *Ultrasound Obstet. Gynecol.* **2015**, *46*, 385–388. [CrossRef]
9. Cruz-Martinez, R.; Savchev, S.; Cruz-Lemini, M.; Mendez, A.; Gratacos, E.; Figueras, F. Clinical utility of third-trimester uterine artery Doppler in the prediction of brain hemodynamic deterioration and adverse perinatal outcome in small-for-gestational-age fetuses. *Ultrasound Obstet. Gynecol.* **2015**, *45*, 273–278. [CrossRef]
10. Rizzo, G.; Mappa, I.; Bitsadze, V.; Słodki, M.; Khizroeva, J.; Makatsariya, A.; D'Antonio, F. Role of Doppler ultrasound at time of diagnosis of late-onset fetal growth restriction in predicting adverse perinatal outcome: Prospective cohort study. *Ultrasound Obstet. Gynecol.* **2020**, *55*, 793–798. [CrossRef]
11. Rolnik, D.L.; Wright, D.; Poon, L.C.Y.; Syngelaki, A.; O'Gorman, N.; de Paco Matallana, C.; Akolekar, R.; Cicero, S.; Janga, D.; Singh, M.; et al. ASPRE trial: Performance of screening for preterm pre-eclampsia. *Ultrasound Obstet. Gynecol.* **2017**, *50*, 492–495. [CrossRef] [PubMed]
12. Gordijn, S.J.; Beune, I.M.; Thilaganathan, B.; Papageorghiou, A.; Baschat, A.A.; Baker, P.N.; Silver, R.M.; Wynia, K.; Ganzevoort, W. Consensus definition of fetal growth restriction: A Delphi procedure. *Ultrasound Obstet. Gynecol.* **2016**, *48*, 333–339. [CrossRef] [PubMed]
13. Meler, E.; Mazarico, E.; Eixarch, E.; Gonzalez, A.; Peguero, A.; Martinez, J.; Boada, D.; Vellvé, K.; Gomez-Roig, M.D.; Gratacós, E.; et al. Ten-year experience of protocol-based management of small-for-gestational-age fetuses: Perinatal outcome in late-pregnancy cases diagnosed after 32 weeks. *Ultrasound Obstet. Gynecol.* **2021**, *57*, 62–69. [CrossRef] [PubMed]
14. Savchev, S.; Figueras, F.; Cruz-Martinez, R.; Illa, M.; Botet, F.; Gratacos, E. Estimated weight centile as a predictor of perinatal outcome in small-for-gestational-age pregnancies with normal fetal and maternal Doppler indices. *Ultrasound Obstet. Gynecol.* **2012**, *39*, 299–303. [CrossRef] [PubMed]
15. Hadlock, F.P.; Harrist, R.B.; Sharman, R.S.; Deter, R.L.; Park, S.K. Estimation of fetal weight with the use of head, body, and femur measurements–a prospective study. *Am. J. Obstet. Gynecol.* **1985**, *151*, 333–337. [CrossRef]
16. Marsál, K.; Persson, P.H.; Larsen, T.; Lilja, H.; Selbing, A.; Sultan, B. Intrauterine growth curves based on ultrasonically estimated foetal weights. *Acta Paediatr.* **1996**, *85*, 843–848. [CrossRef]
17. Bhide, A.; Acharya, G.; Bilardo, C.M.; Brezinka, C.; Cafici, D.; Hernandez-Andrade, E.; Kalache, K.; Kingdom, J.; Kiserud, T.; Lee, W.; et al. ISUOG practice guidelines: Use of Doppler ultrasonography in obstetrics. *Ultrasound Obstet. Gynecol.* **2013**, *41*, 233–239.
18. Bligh, L.N.; Alsolai, A.A.; Greer, R.M.; Kumar, S. Cerebroplacental ratio thresholds measured within 2 weeks before birth and risk of Cesarean section for intrapartum fetal compromise and adverse neonatal outcome. *Ultrasound Obstet. Gynecol.* **2018**, *52*, 340–346. [CrossRef]
19. Ayres-de-Campos, D.; Spong, C.Y.; Chandraharan, E. FIGO consensus guidelines on intrapartum fetal monitoring: Cardiotocography. *Int. J. Gynaecol. Obstet.* **2015**, *131*, 13–24. [CrossRef]
20. Baschat, A.A.; Gembruch, U. The cerebroplacental Doppler ratio revisited. *Ultrasound Obstet. Gynecol.* **2003**, *21*, 124–127. [CrossRef]

21. Palacio, M.; Figueras, F.; Zamora, L.; Jiménez, J.M.; Puerto, B.; Coll, O.; Cararach, V.; Vanrell, J.A. Reference ranges for umbilical and middle cerebral artery pulsatility index and cerebroplacental ratio in prolonged pregnancies. *Ultrasound Obstet. Gynecol.* **2004**, *24*, 647–653. [CrossRef] [PubMed]
22. Figueras, F.; Savchev, S.; Triunfo, S.; Crovetto, F.; Gratacos, E. An integrated model with classification criteria to predict small-for-gestational-age fetuses at risk of adverse perinatal outcome. *Ultrasound Obstet. Gynecol.* **2015**, *45*, 279–285. [CrossRef] [PubMed]
23. Gardosi, J.; Madurasinghe, V.; Williams, M.; Malik, A.; Francis, A. Maternal and fetal risk factors for stillbirth: Population based study. *BMJ* **2013**, *346*, f108. [CrossRef] [PubMed]
24. Kalafat, E.; Morales-Roselló, J.; Scarinci, E.; Thilaganathan, B.; Khalil, A. Risk of operative delivery for intrapartum fetal compromise in small-for-gestational-age fetuses at term: External validation of the IRIS algorithm. *J. Matern. Fetal Neonatal Med.* **2020**, *33*, 2775–2784. [CrossRef]
25. Conde-Agudelo, A.; Villar, J.; Kennedy, S.H.; Papageorghiou, A.T. Predictive accuracy of cerebroplacental ratio for adverse perinatal and neurodevelopmental outcomes in suspected fetal growth restriction: Systematic review and meta-analysis. *Ultrasound Obstet. Gynecol.* **2018**, *52*, 430–441. [CrossRef]
26. Lobmaier, S.M.; Graupner, O.; Ortiz, J.U.; Haller, B.; Ried, C.; Wildner, N.; Abel, K.; Kuschel, B.; Rieger-Fackeldey, E.; Oberhoffer, R.; et al. Perinatal Outcome and its Prediction Using Longitudinal Feto-Maternal Doppler Follow-Up in Late Onset Small for Gestational Age Fetuses—A Prospective Cohort Study. *Ultraschall Med.* **2021**. [CrossRef]
27. Ortiz, J.U.; Graupner, O.; Karge, A.; Flechsenhar, S.; Haller, B.; Ostermayer, E.; Abel, K.; Kuschel, B.; Lobmaier, S.M. Does gestational age at term play a role in the association between cerebroplacental ratio and operative delivery for intrapartum fetal compromise? *Acta Obstet. Gynecol Scand.* **2021**, *100*, 1910–1916. [CrossRef]
28. Di Mascio, D.; Herraiz, I.; Villalain, C.; Buca, D.; Morales-Roselló, J.; Loscalzo, G.; Sileo, F.G.; Finarelli, A.; Bertucci, E.; Facchinetti, F.; et al. Comparison between Cerebroplacental Ratio and Umbilicocerebral Ratio in Predicting Adverse Perinatal Outcome in Pregnancies Complicated by Late Fetal Growth Restriction: A Multicenter, Retrospective Study. *Fetal Diagn. Ther.* **2021**, *48*, 448–456. [CrossRef]
29. Lobmaier, S.M.; Figueras, F.; Mercade, I.; Perello, M.; Peguero, A.; Crovetto, F.; Ortiz, J.U.; Crispi, F.; Gratacós, E. Angiogenic factors vs Doppler surveillance in the prediction of adverse outcome among late-pregnancy small-for- gestational-age fetuses. *Ultrasound Obstet. Gynecol.* **2014**, *43*, 533–540. [CrossRef]
30. Graupner, O.; Karge, A.; Flechsenhar, S.; Seiler, A.; Haller, B.; Ortiz, J.U.; Ortiz, J.U.; Crispi, F.; Gratacós, E. Role of sFlt-1/PlGF ratio and feto-maternal Doppler for the prediction of adverse perinatal outcome in late-onset pre-eclampsia. *Arch Gynecol. Obstet.* **2020**, *301*, 375–385. [CrossRef]
31. Karge, A.; Beckert, L.; Moog, P.; Haller, B.; Ortiz, J.U.; Lobmaier, S.M.; Abel, K.; Flechsenhar, S.; Kuschel, B.; Graupner, O. Role of sFlt-1/PlGF ratio and uterine Doppler in pregnancies with chronic kidney disease suspected with Pre-eclampsia or HELLP syndrome. *Pregnancy Hypertens* **2020**, *22*, 160–166. [CrossRef] [PubMed]
32. Ciobanou, A.; Jabak, S.; De Castro, H.; Frei, L.; Akolekar, R.; Nicolaides, K.H. Biomarkers of impaired placentation at 35-37 weeks' gestation in the prediction of adverse perinatal outcome. *Ultrasound Obstet. Gynecol.* **2019**, *54*, 79–86. [CrossRef] [PubMed]
33. Karge, A.; Seiler, A.; Flechsenhar, S.; Haller, B.; Ortiz, J.U.; Lobmaier, S.M.; Axt-Fliedner, R.; Enzensberger, C.; Abel, K.; Kuschel, B.; et al. Prediction of adverse perinatal outcome and the mean time until delivery in twin pregnancies with suspected pre-eclampsia using sFlt-1/PlGF ratio. *Pregnancy Hypertens* **2021**, *24*, 37–43. [CrossRef] [PubMed]
34. Choi, S.K.Y.; Gordon, A.; Hilder, L.; Henry, A.; Hyett, J.A.; Brew, B.K.; Joseph, F.; Jorm, L.; Chambers, G.M. Performance of six birthweight and estimated fetal weight standards for predicting adverse perinatal outcomes: A 10-year nationwide population-based study. *Ultrasound Obstet. Gynecol.* **2020**, *58*, 264–277. [CrossRef] [PubMed]
35. Ego, A.; Monier, I.; Skaare, K.; Zeitlin, J. Antenatal detection of fetal growth restriction and risk of stillbirth: Population-based case-control study. *Ultrasound Obstet. Gynecol.* **2020**, *55*, 613–620. [CrossRef]
36. Khalil, A.; Morales-Roselló, J.; Townsend, R.; Morlando, M.; Papageorghiou, A.; Bhide, A.; Thilaganathan, B. Value of third-trimester cerebroplacental ratio and uterine artery Doppler indices as predictors of stillbirth and perinatal loss. *Ultrasound Obstet. Gynecol.* **2016**, *47*, 74–80. [CrossRef]
37. Fisher, S.J. Why is placentation abnormal in preeclampsia? *Am. J. Obstet. Gynecol.* **2015**, *213*, S115–S122. [CrossRef]
38. Llurba, E.; Turan, O.; Kasdaglis, T.; Harman, C.R.; Baschat, A.A. Emergence of late-onset placental dysfunction: Relationship to the change in uterine artery blood flow resistance between the first and third trimesters. *Am. J. Perinatol.* **2013**, *30*, 505–512. [CrossRef]
39. Thilaganathan, B. Pre-eclampsia and the cardiovascular-placental axis. *Ultrasound Obstet. Gynecol.* **2018**, *51*, 714–717. [CrossRef]
40. Grobman, W.A.; Bailit, J.; Lai, Y.; Reddy, U.M.; Wapner, R.J.; Varner, M.W.; Caritis, S.N.; Prasad, M.; Tita, A.T.N.; Saade, G.; et al. Association of the Duration of Active Pushing With Obstetric Outcomes. *Obstet. Gynecol.* **2016**, *127*, 667–673. [CrossRef]
41. Turner, J.M.; Mitchell, M.D.; Kumar, S.S. The physiology of intrapartum fetal compromise at term. *Am. J. Obstet. Gynecol.* **2020**, *222*, 17–26. [CrossRef] [PubMed]

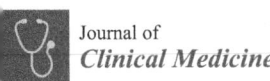

Article

Patterns of Brain Sparing in a Fetal Growth Restriction Cohort

Jon G. Steller *,†, Diane Gumina, Camille Driver, Emma Peek, Henry L. Galan, Shane Reeves and John C. Hobbins

Division of Maternal Fetal Medicine, Department of Obstetrics and Gynecology, University of Colorado School of Medicine, Aurora, CO 80045, USA; diane.gumina@cuanschutz.edu (D.G.); camille.elizabeth.driver@gmail.com (C.D.); emma.peek@cuanschutz.edu (E.P.); henry.galan@cuanschutz.edu (H.L.G.); shane.reeves@cuanschutz.edu (S.R.); jchobbins@gmail.com (J.C.H.)
* Correspondence: jsteller@hs.uci.edu; Tel.: +1-714-456-6810 or +1-559-360-8845
† Current address: Division of Maternal Fetal Medicine, Department of Obstetrics and Gynecology, University of California Irvine, 333 City Blvd W Ste 1400, Orange, CA 92868, USA.

Abstract: Objective: Our objective was to compare differences in Doppler blood flow in four fetal intracranial blood vessels in fetuses with late-onset fetal growth restriction (FGR) vs. those with small for gestational age (SGA). Methods: Fetuses with estimated fetal weight (EFW) <10th percentile were divided into SGA ($n = 30$) and FGR ($n = 51$) via Delphi criteria and had Doppler waveforms obtained from the middle cerebral artery (MCA), anterior cerebral artery (ACA), posterior cerebral artery (PCA), and vertebral artery (VA). A pulsatility index (PI) <5th centile was considered "abnormal". Outcomes included birth metrics and neonatal intensive care unit (NICU) admission. Results: There were more abnormal cerebral vessel PIs in the FGR group versus the SGA group (36 vs. 4; $p = 0.055$). In FGR, ACA + MCA vessel abnormalities outnumbered PCA + VA abnormalities. All 8 fetuses with abnormal VA PIs had at least one other abnormal vessel. Fetuses with abnormal VA PIs had lower BW (1712 vs. 2500 g; $p < 0.0001$), delivered earlier (35.22 vs. 37.89 wks; $p = 0.0052$), and had more admissions to the NICU (71.43% vs. 24.44%; $p = 0.023$). Conclusions: There were more anterior vessels showing vasodilation than posterior vessels, but when the VA was abnormal, the fetuses were more severely affected clinically than those showing normal VA PIs.

Keywords: fetal growth restriction; intrauterine growth restriction; middle cerebral artery; small for gestational age; uteroplacental insufficiency; vertebral artery

1. Introduction

Fetal growth restriction (FGR) is associated with significant fetal morbidity and mortality. Early-onset FGR (diagnosed prior to 32 weeks) is characterized by severe oxygen and nutritional deprivation leading to elevated risks of neonatal morbidity and intrauterine fetal demise (IUFD). Late-onset FGR fetuses (diagnosed after 32 weeks of gestation) are still vulnerable to long-term neurological [1,2], cardiovascular [3,4], and metabolic morbidity [5]. In late-onset FGR, management considerations regarding the timing of Doppler studies, antepartum fetal heart rate testing, and delivery, vary appreciably. To differentiate fetuses with low estimated fetal weights (EFWs) who are at greatest risk for complications from those who are not overtly deprived, a group of international experts convened and drafted criteria via Delphi consensus [6] that have been endorsed by the International Society of Ultrasound in Obstetrics and Gynecology (ISUOG) [7]. ISUOG defines small for gestational age (SGA) as a fetus between the 3rd and 10th percentile with normal Dopplers and defines FGR as a fetus with an EFW or abdominal circumference (AC) < 3rd centile or an SGA fetus with abnormal Dopplers (as outlined in Table 1). Although the clinical value of the Delphi/ISUOG criteria for identifying fetuses at greatest risk of adverse outcomes has been well formulated [6], the concept has not been endorsed by some official bodies [8,9].

Table 1. Delphi consensus-based definitions for late growth restriction [6,7].

Early FGR: GA < 32 Weeks with No Congenital Abnormalities	Late FGR: GA ≥ 32 Weeks with No Congenital Abnormalities
AC or EFW less than 3rd centile or UA-AEDF	AC or EFW less than 3rd centile
Or AC or EFW < 10th centile combined with	Or at least two of the three:
1. Uterine artery PI > 95th centile and/or 2. UAPI > 95th centile	3. AC or EFW less than 10th centile 4. AC or EFW crossing centiles greater than 2 quartiles on growth centiles 5. CPR less than 5th centile *or* UAPI greater than 95th centile *

Abbreviations: GA = gestational age; AC = fetal abdominal circumference; EFW = estimated fetal weight; AEDF = absent end diastolic flow; PI = pulsatility index; UA = umbilical artery; CPR = cerebroplacental ratio. * Growth centiles are non-customized centiles.

An important component of ISUOG criteria is the evaluation of the cerebroplacental ratio (CPR). This requires Doppler waveform assessments of the umbilical artery (UA), a reflector of placental resistance, and the middle cerebral artery (MCA), which reflects "brain sparing" as an adaptive reaction to counter fetal hypoxia [10]. Since the MCA perfuses the cerebral cortex, and its direction of flow within the brain lends itself to easy ultrasound sampling, it has been the principal source of information about the protective process of circulatory redistribution. However, other vessels emanate from the circle of Willis. The anterior cerebral artery (ACA), the posterior cerebral artery (PCA), and the vertebral artery (VA), which arrives in the brain via the subclavian artery on the right side and the aorta directly on the left, have been only sparsely investigated in the setting of FGR. There is evidence that these other vessels are involved in brain sparing and, in keeping with the concept of "gradual hypoxia" in FGR, may undergo vasodilatation at different times during the pathogenesis of mild-to-severe oxygen deprivation [11]. However, most investigations have been focused on the individual vessels [12–14] rather than how these vessels adapt collectively to "spare" the brain, especially in late-onset FGR, the more common form of clinical growth restriction.

Therefore, our objectives were:

1. To determine how often each study vessel (MCA, ACA, PCA, and VA) had pulsatility index (PI) values below the 5th percentile in fetuses whose estimated fetal weights were below the 10th percentile and who were defined as having FGR or SGA using Delphi (ISUOG) criteria.
2. To compare average cerebral vessel PI values in FGR and SGA fetuses with postnatal outcomes.
3. To determine if any of the fetal cerebral vessels yielded additional useful information regarding perinatal outcome above that provided by the MCA as used in the CPR.

2. Methods

A prospective observational cohort study was undertaken in an off-campus university outpatient high risk center in Denver, CO, USA. Patients between 31 and 39 weeks gestational age were enrolled onsite from the center's private referral base or from our on-campus perinatal practice. Inclusion criteria included fetuses with EFWs < 10th centile for gestational age with no obvious anatomical abnormalities and no absent/reversed end diastolic flow on umbilical artery Doppler assessment. Dating was established per ACOG (American College of Obstetricians & Gynecologists) criteria [15]. All initial dating was performed by the University of Colorado team unless the patients were referred from outside private clinics, for whom their dating was validated by our investigators at enrollment. The study was approved by the Colorado Multiple Institutional Review Board and informed consent was obtained from all study participants (IRB number 14-1360, date of approval 29 May 2015).

Estimated fetal weights were calculated from measurements of the head circumference (HC), biparietal diameter (BPD), abdominal circumference (AC), and femur length (FL) using Hadlock nomograms [16]. Percentiles for EFW were assigned according to the population-based fetal growth curve by Hadlock [17], used consistently in our perinatal practice for its applicability to our study population. Following ISUOG guidelines, fetuses measuring less than the 10th percentile by EFW or AC were classified as either FGR or SGA (Table 1). Further, cerebral placental ratios (CPRs) were computed by dividing pulsatility indices (PI) of MCA and UA (MCA PI/UA PI), which were converted to percentiles using Ebbing's nomogram [18–20]. Any fetus with an EFW or AC < 10th %ile with an abnormal umbilical artery Doppler (>95th %ile) or CPR (<5th %ile) or AC or EFW < 3rd percentile was defined as having FGR per ISUOG criteria. Those with EFWs between the 3rd and 10th percentiles with normal UA and MCA Dopplers were considered small for gestational age (SGA).

All examinations were performed during fetal quiescence. Both umbilical arteries were sampled from a free loop of umbilical cord, and the average PI was used for analysis. The cerebral vessels were imaged with directional color Doppler and waveforms obtained with pulsed Doppler. While an ideal angle of insonation for the UA and MCA of <20 degrees was obtained (Figure 1), a more liberal angle of <30 degrees was tolerated for the ACA, PCA, and vertebral arteries. All vessels emanating from the circle of Willis were sampled within the proximal third of the vessel, and although initially the near side vessel was preferentially chosen, the far side vessel occasionally provided a better waveform for analysis. The VA was approached posteriorly by obtaining a mid-sagittal view of the cervical spine and occiput (Figure 2). The vertebral artery most clearly visualized was sampled. Although only a small portion of the vessel can be imaged as it courses towards the posterior fossa just above the level of the first cervical vertebrae, the operator was aided by its distinctive directional Doppler signature (Figure 2). While every study parameter was attempted to be collected at each study visit, the results from the last, most complete exam before delivery were used for this analysis. Results from all 4 vessels were compared against control data from the literature, and the MCA, ACA, PCA, and VA were considered abnormal if the PI was <5th percentile using these control data [13,14,18–21]. All four vessels could not be perfectly visualized in all patients and some measures were excluded in images that were not of appropriate quality. Only the MCA was used in clinical decision-making such as the frequency of antepartum follow up and fetal heart rate testing, frequency of Doppler evaluation, or timing of delivery.

A retrospective analysis was performed in this cohort of growth restricted pregnancies that had all clinical and Doppler information collected in a prospective fashion. Cerebral vessels from the Circle of Willis as well as birth outcomes were compared between FGR and SGA fetuses. Since the MCA, as used in the CPR, is the only cerebral vessel currently being used in FGR management, fetuses were further stratified according to whether the VA PI and CPR fell below the 5th centile.

When evaluating outcomes, a cesarean delivery rate was calculated for all patients who attempted labor (i.e., not a scheduled repeat or elective cesarean section). We also reported rates of admission to the neonatal intensive care unit (NICU).

Graphpad Prism Version 9 (San Diego, CA, USA) was used for statistical analyses. Fisher's exact tests were used for categorical variables. Independent samples t-tests or Mann-Whitney U tests were used following a normality test to compare patient characteristics or Doppler measurements between groups.

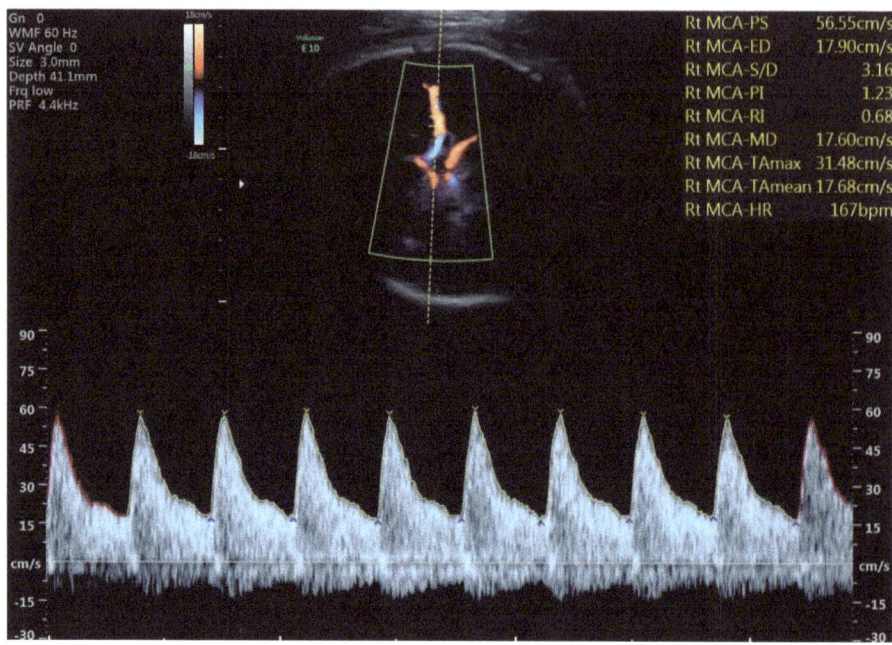

Figure 1. Mid cerebral artery Doppler with brain sparing.

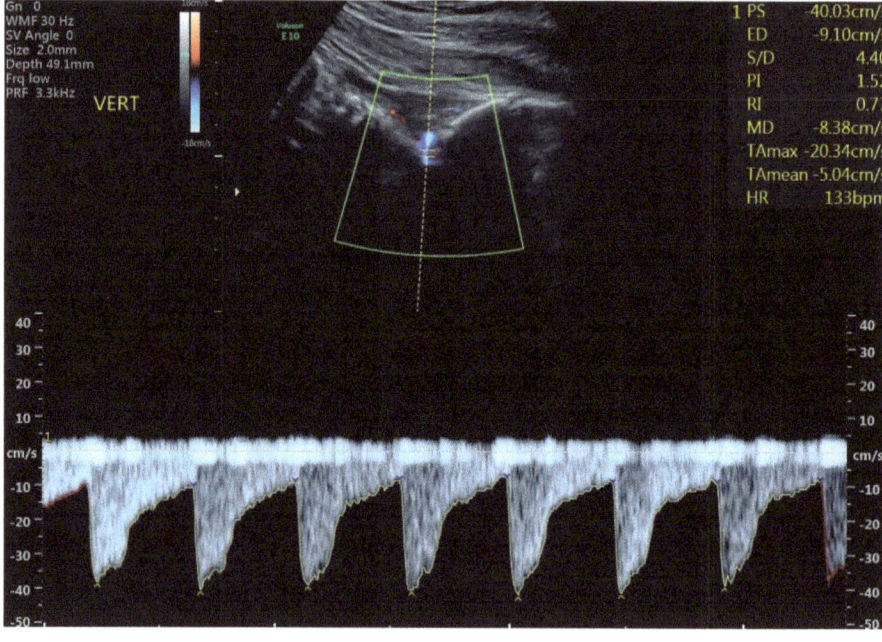

Figure 2. Vertebral artery Doppler. Example of vertebral artery Doppler measurement in a fetus affected by fetal growth restriction.

3. Results

During the study period, 81 patients were identified who met inclusion criteria. Thirty fetuses were classified as SGA and 51 patients as FGR. FGR pregnancies did not deliver significantly earlier than SGAs (37.3 weeks vs. 37.8 weeks, $p = 0.186$), but had significantly lower birthweights (2247 g vs. 2636 g, $p < 0.0001$) (Table 2). The average PIs of the ACA, MCA, and PCAs were all lower in FGR fetuses compared to SGA, but not enough to attain statistical significance (Table 2). The vessels most commonly having PIs below the 5th centiles in FGR were: the ACA (11/46), MCA (10/51), PCA (7/46), and VA (8/43) (Table 3). While the mean PI values were similar between the FGR and SGA groups, the number of abnormal PIs (<5th percentile) for the MCA and VA were significantly different between SGA and FGR groups (Table 3). In addition, whenever the VA PI was abnormal, it was never the only vessel showing brain sparing. Most of these fetuses (6/8) had abnormalities in 2 or more other cerebral vessels, and 3/8 had abnormalities in all 4 cerebral vessels.

Table 2. Comparison of patient characteristics in FGR and SGA cohorts.

Cerebral Dopplers between ISUOG Grouping	SGA Mean ± SEM (n = 30)	FGR Mean ± SEM (n = 51)	p Value
Mean MCA PI centile †	41.36% ± 4.86%	41.05% ± 4.46%	0.787
Mean ACA PI centile †	37.80% ± 5.75%	32.38% ± 4.26%	0.377
Mean PCA PI centile †	44.00% ± 4.51%	34.93% ± 4.25%	0.104
Mean UA PI centile †	63.47% ± 3.70%	77.41% ± 3.18%	0.0008 ***
Clinical Variables			
GA at Analysis (wks) †	35.82 ± 0.27	35.94 ± 0.22	0.710
GA at Delivery (wks) †	37.84 ± 0.22	37.29 ± 0.23	0.186
Birthweight (g) ‡	2636 ± 59.86	2247 ± 65.06	<0.0001 ***
Cesarean Section Rate §	4/26 (15.38%)	10/37 (27.03%)	0.362
Fenton Birthweight (%) ‡	20.61% ± 2.88%	6.91% ± 0.78%	<0.0001 ***
NICU Admission §	4/22 (18.18%)	13/36 (36.11%)	0.234

Mann-Whitney U † or independent samples t-tests ‡ were used following a normality test. Fisher's exact tests § were used for categorical variables. Because standard deviation equations were not published with the VA PI nomogram, we are unable to calculate PI centile for VA Dopplers. Abbreviations: SEM: standard error of the mean; MCA: middle cerebral artery; PI: pulsatility index; ACA: anterior cerebral artery; PCA: posterior cerebral artery; UA: umbilical artery; GA: gestational age; wks: weeks; NICU: neonatal intensive care unit. "* indicates statistical significance (* $p < 0.05$; ** $p < 0.01$; *** $p < 0.001$)."

Table 3. Comparison of cerebral Dopplers in FGR and SGA cohorts.

Number of Abnormal Dopplers in ISUOG Groups	SGA (n = 30)	FGR (n = 51)	p-Value
Total # of abnormal Dopplers † (1 pt each for MCA, ACA, PCA, VA; max: 4 pts/fetus)	4	36	0.055
# of fetuses with ≥1 abnormal cerebral Doppler ‡	4/30	15/51	0.113
# of fetuses with MCA PI < 5th centile ‡	1/30	10/51	0.047 *
# of fetuses with ACA PI < 5th centile ‡	2/27	11/46	0.113
# of fetuses with PCA PI < 5th centile ‡	1/29	7/46	0.141
# of fetuses with VA PI < 5th centile ‡	0/26	8/43	0.021 *

Comparisons of cerebral dopplers were performed with Mann-Whitney U † and Fisher's exact ‡ tests. Full Doppler information was not available on all 81 patients; thus, the N varies by Doppler study performed as evident above. Abbreviations: MCA: middle cerebral artery; PI: pulsatility index; ACA: anterior cerebral artery; PCA: posterior cerebral artery; VA: vertebral artery. "* indicates statistical significance (* $p < 0.05$)."

In patients with an abnormal VA, the differences between the mean PI percentiles for all the other cerebral vessels were strikingly lower compared with those with normal VAs (Table 4). Further, newborns with an abnormal VA in utero delivered on average significantly earlier (35.2 versus 37.9 weeks, $p = 0.0052$), had lower birthweights (1712 g versus 2500 g, $p < 0.0001$), had a higher rate of cesarean section (CSR) (71.4% vs. 16.3% $p = 0.005$), and were more frequently admitted to the NICU (71.4% vs. 24.4% $p = 0.023$) (Table 4). Of fetuses admitted to the NICU within this study cohort, two were only for a brief transitionary period lasting less than 24 h; one of these fetuses with FGR with a normal CPR and normal VA PI, and the other fetus was SGA with a normal CPR and no VA PI measurement. All other admissions were greater than 24 h.

Table 4. Comparison of patient characteristics in fetuses with and without abnormal VA Doppler (<5th centile).

Cerebral Dopplers in Fetuses with Normal and Abnormal VA	Pts w/Abnormal VA Dopplers Mean ± SEM ($n = 8$)	Pts w/Normal VA Dopplers Mean ± SEM ($n = 61$)	p-Value
Mean MCA PI %ile [†]	9.96% ± 5.56%	44.02% ± 3.81%	0.0002 ***
Mean ACA PI %ile [†]	3.41% ± 0.56%	37.44% ± 3.62%	<0.0001 ***
Mean PCA PI %ile [†]	7.72% ± 3.22%	41.09% ± 3.35%	<0.0001 ***
Clinical Variables			
GA at Analysis (wks) [†]	34.64 ± 0.71	36.13 ± 0.17	0.023 *
GA at Delivery (wks) [‡]	35.22 ± 0.63	37.89 ± 0.14	0.0052 **
Birthweight (g) [‡]	1712 ± 151.71	2500 ± 48.85	<0.0001 ***
Cesarean Section Rate [§]	5/7 (71.43%)	8/49 (16.32%)	0.005 **
Fenton Birthweight (%) [†]	4.64% ± 1.37%	13.37% ± 1.80%	0.036 *
Admission to NICU [§]	5/7 (71.43%)	11/45 (24.44%)	0.023 *

Mann-Whitney U [†] or independent samples t-tests [‡] were used following a normality test. Fisher's exact tests [§] were used for categorical variables. Because standard deviation equations were not published with the VA PI nomogram, we are unable to calculate PI centile for VA Dopplers. For this study, VA PI is assessed as a categorical variable that is either normal (>5th centile) or abnormal (<5th centile). Abbreviations: SEM: standard error of the mean; VA: vertebral artery; MCA: middle cerebral artery; PI: pulsatility index; ACA: anterior cerebral artery; PCA: posterior cerebral artery; GA: gestational age; wks: weeks; NICU: neonatal intensive care unit. "* indicates statistical significance (* $p < 0.05$; ** $p < 0.01$; *** $p < 0.001$)."

The mean PIs of the cerebral vessels were significantly lower in fetuses with an abnormal CPR compared to those with a normal CPR (Table 5). However, fetuses with an abnormal VA PI still had lower PIs in the other cerebral vessels than those fetuses with an abnormal CPR (Tables 4 and 5). These findings strongly indicate that while the MCA is not alone in brain sparing activity, that the VA seemed to be associated with a greater degree of overall vasodilatation. For example, when the VA was abnormal, the PIs were lower for ACAs (3.4% versus 12.8%) and PCAs (7.7% versus 21.2%) compared with those fetuses having abnormal CPRs (Tables 4 and 5). Furthermore, those with abnormal VAs delivered earlier on average (35.2 vs. 36.7 weeks) and had lower BWs (1712 g vs. 2009 g) than the fetuses with abnormal CPRs. However, when corrected for gestational age, the BW percentiles were similar (4.64% vs. 3.93%) (Tables 4 and 5). Finally, those with abnormal VAs had a higher CSR and a higher percentage of admissions to the NICU (Tables 4 and 5). As anterior cerebral vessel abnormalities were more frequently seen than in the posterior vessels (11 ACAs and 10 MCAs vs. 7 PCAs and 8 VAs) and fetuses with abnormal VA were the most severely affected with concomitant abnormalities in other vessels, the combination of these findings indirectly endorse the concept of front-to-back brain sparing in FGR (Table 3).

Table 5. Comparison of patient characteristics in fetuses with and without abnormal CPR (<5th centile).

Cerebral Dopplers in Fetuses with Normal and Abnormal CPR	Pts w/Abnormal CPR Dopplers Mean ± SEM (n = 14)	Pts w/Normal CPR Dopplers Mean ± SEM (n = 67)	p-Value
Mean MCA PI %ile [†]	7.83% ± 2.14%	48.14% ± 3.42%	<0.0001 ***
Mean ACA PI %ile [†]	12.78% ± 3.29%	39.06% ± 3.84%	0.0011 **
Mean PCA PI %ile [†]	21.19% ± 6.16%	42.05% ± 3.44%	0.006 **
# of VA PI < 5th centile [§]	5/12	3/57	0.003 **
Clinical Variables			
GA at Analysis (wks) [†]	35.68 ± 0.48	35.94 ± 0.18	0.350
GA at Delivery (wks) [†]	36.73 ± 0.52	37.69 ± 0.16	0.037 *
Birthweight (g) [‡]	2009 ± 135.31	2492 ± 47.67	0.0001 ***
Cesarean Section Rate [§]	4/11 (36.36%)	10/52 (19.23%)	0.243
Fenton Birthweight (%) [†]	3.93% ± 1.05%	14.30% ± 1.71%	<0.0001 ***
Admission to NICU [§]	5/12 (41.67%)	12/46 (26.09%)	0.307

Mann-Whitney U [†] or independent samples t-tests [‡] were used following a normality test. Fisher's exact tests [§] were used for categorical variables. Because standard deviation equations were not published with the VA PI nomogram, we are unable to calculate PI centile for VA Dopplers. For this study, VA PI is assessed as a categorical variable that is either normal (>5th centile) or abnormal (<5th centile). Abbreviations: SEM: standard error of the mean; CPR: cerebroplacental ratio; MCA: middle cerebral artery; PI: pulsatility index; ACA: anterior cerebral artery; PCA: posterior cerebral artery; VA: vertebral artery; GA: gestational age; wks: weeks; NICU: neonatal intensive care unit. "* indicates statistical significance (* $p < 0.05$; ** $p < 0.01$; *** $p < 0.001$)."

4. Discussion

Principle Findings

- While fetuses defined by ISUOG as FGR were not associated with earlier deliveries than those defined as SGA (37.3 weeks vs. 37.8 weeks $p = 0.186$), they did have significantly lower average birthweights (2247 g vs. 2636 g, $p < 0.0001$) and lower birthweight percentiles (6.91% vs. 20.61% $p < 0.0001$). Although FGR fetuses were more frequently admitted to the NICU than SGA fetuses, this did not attain statistical significance.
- The total numbers of abnormal PIs from the cerebral vessels studied were strikingly different between SGA and FGR (4 vs. 36, $p = 0.055$). However, the number of cerebral vessel PIs below the 5th centile was only significant between FGR and SGA groups for the MCA and VA (Table 3). All 8 fetuses in the study with abnormal VA PIs were FGR.
- Fetuses with an abnormal VA PI stood out as being different in birth metrics and in their distinct tendency to be linked with lower PIs in each vessel emanating from the circle of Willis, compared with those with normal VA PIs (Table 4).
- When comparing in utero cerebral Dopplers and neonatal outcome data between fetuses with abnormal VAs and the commonly used CPR, the VA was associated with lower average PIs from the companion vessels, earlier delivery, lower birthweight, higher rates of cesarean section, and more frequent admission to the NICU, suggesting a more specific measure for adverse perinatal outcome than MCA. However, birthweight centiles were not different between groups when corrected for gestational age (Tables 4 and 5).

In the early 2000s, investigators began to explore patterns of circulatory redistribution in the cerebral vessels in FGR [11,22–24] with one that utilized a sophisticated method to assess fractional moving blood volume [24]. These studies pointed to a front-to-back pathway of vasodilation with the frontal lobe receiving preferential initial attention, as evidenced by earlier or more frequent signs of ACA vasodilation than the MCA [11,23]. Our findings, using standard pulsed Doppler methods, support previous observations of a front-to-back pattern of brain sparing in FGR with those vessels feeding the anterior and middle portions of the brain frequently showing lower average PIs than those perfusing the posterior portion. When the VA PI was below the 5th centile, brain sparing had occurred in at least one other vessel for every fetus and in 3/8 patients all four cerebral vessels were abnormal. Assuming a front-to-back pattern of circulatory redistribution, by the time the

VA had been compromised, all fetuses had lower average birthweights and birthweight centiles, earlier deliveries, and higher rates of admission to the NICU compared to other fetuses in the study (Table 4). Morales Roselló et al. [25] showed the vertebral artery to be more predictive of lower birthweight in FGR than the middle cerebral artery, a standard measurement in FGR management. The VA supplies the cerebellar hemispheres, vermis, and brain stem, and our findings suggest that fetuses with an abnormal VA may be at risk for more severe compromise and worse perinatal outcome. Furthermore, in these eight cases the average PIs (suggesting the degree of vasodilation and, therefore, hypoxia) were the lowest for all the three accompanying cerebral vessels studied, thus inferring a higher degree of hypoxia or deprivation. (Table 4).

FGR is a placentally-mediated condition. The effects on the fetus are dependent upon the degree of placental pathology and the ability of the fetus to adapt in the setting of placental insufficiency. Clinicians have historically depended upon the UA to indirectly assess the extent of placental pathology based on the concept that a substantial proportion of the small villus circulation of the placenta is compromised before the UA PI becomes abnormal [26]. In early-onset FGR, the placenta is so severely affected that an elevated UA PI is often one of the first clues to nutritional and hypoxic deprivation [27–29]. Yet, in the more common late-onset FGR, diagnosed after 32 weeks, the UA PI is frequently unaffected, even when cardiac deformation and abnormal myocardial contractility has been noted [30,31]. Thus, to help to distinguish between pathologic and 'constitutional' growth restriction, many clinicians have turned diagnostically to the MCA and, with it, the CPR (MCA PI/UA PI) to determine if undergrown fetuses have turned to brain sparing as a protective mechanism in dealing with fetal hypoxia. This approach has been effective in predicting the need for cesarean section for fetal distress [32], combined adverse neonatal outcome [33], and identifying those fetuses who are at greater risk for childhood and adulthood cardiovascular [3,4] and neurobehavioral morbidities [1,2]. Yet, the role of the MCA has not been uniformly accepted in the management of FGR [9], which has been primarily focused on avoiding intrauterine demise or severe perinatal morbidity via timely delivery predicated on information from the UA PI, fetal heart rate monitoring, and, in severe FGR, ductus venosus waveforms [34].

We addressed the question of whether any vessel or combination of vessels provided added value beyond that provided by the MCA or the commonly used CPR, in which the MCA contributes 50% to the result. Fetuses with abnormal VAs had lower average birthweights (1712 g vs. 2009 g), delivered at an earlier average gestational age (35.2 weeks versus 36.7 weeks), but had a slightly higher average birthweight centile (4.6% vs. 3.93%) compared to the average abnormal CPR BW percentile (Table 5). Despite the latter finding, there were 3 infants in the study who had abnormal VA PIs but whose CPRs were low but in normal range. Two of these infants appeared to be seriously compromised, having spent 5 and 26 days in the NICU and delivering at 36.14 and 33 weeks, respectively.

Although some information is available linking brain sparing, as indicated by MCA PIs linking to abnormal neurobehavioral outcomes, few studies have addressed the ability of other cerebral vessels to predict long-term outcomes [12,35]. One study did compare the vessel most often showing vasodilation in FGR (the ACA in their study) with the MCA in predicting neurobehavioral outcome in children using the Neonatal Neurobehavioral Adjustment Scale (NBAS). The authors found that more abnormalities were detected via abnormal MCA PI than ACA PI [12]. Our findings suggest that tracking long-term neurobehavioral abnormalities in fetuses with abnormal VA PIs might represent a more clinically important vessel for further investigation.

Another clinical finding revealed in Table 2 is that the SGA group had an average birthweight in the 20th centile as defined by the Fenton birthweight population curve used in our nursery and by many centers around the country. Since our entry criterion was simply to have EFWs below the 10th percentile, this result might question the accuracy of the in-utero ultrasound method to separate out undergrown fetuses. However, this type of neonatal curve cannot be cleanly used for comparisons to EFW because data from this neonatal population did not exclude fetuses affected by growth restriction, thereby pulling the 10th centile of neonatal weight downward [36]. Nicolaides et al. [36] corrected for this by constructing a compatible Fetal Medicine Foundation BW curve which only included BWs of infants who, as fetuses, had rigidly dated pregnancies in the first trimester and no evidence of any maternal or fetal complications along the way. Since all patients chosen to construct the curve delivered at between 39–40.86 weeks, this excluded EFW data points from fetuses who were not necessarily "normal". In fact, we found the average BW (2636 g) of those in the SGA group fell between the 5th and 10th percentiles in the Nicolaides curve, rather than the 20th percentile in the Fenton neonatal curve as reported in Table 2.

Another reason for the birthweights to sometimes exceed the 10th percentile neonatally is that we adhered to a type of "intention to treat" concept in fetuses who entered the study with EFWs below the 10th percentile by keeping those in the study who later exceeded this threshold. This allowed our team to follow those who at some time during pregnancy had growth trajectories that rose above the arbitrary 10th percentile threshold and into a subcategory of the lower quartile (10th to 25th percentile). In a large study, Morales-Roselló et al. [37] found that 6.7% of fetuses with BWs between the 10th and 25th percentile had abnormal CPRs (their study definition of "FGR"). This strongly suggests that many fetuses designated as AGA in this category did not live up to their growth potential.

Each strength of the study was balanced with potential liabilities. For example, one strength was that data could be accumulated on 68 patients who had adequate images and Doppler waveforms of all 4 cerebral vessels and 74 patients in whom 3 of the 4 vessels could be evaluated on the last scan before their deliveries. Unfortunately, this left us with different denominators in each vessel category. Additionally, since there was a small number of fetuses with abnormal VA waveforms, the relationships to outcomes in our study will need to be addressed in future studies with, hopefully, larger numbers. Further, although we were able to retrieve outcome data on all infants delivering at the University Hospital, extracting information from records on a few infants delivering at outside hospitals was unsuccessful. This left us with dissimilar denominators in some outcome categories. We adapted our analysis to account for both issues.

Another possible strength was an ability, based on the nature on our referral patient population, to study a cohort heavily weighted towards late-onset FGR, a category less frequently studied. This also was a limitation since a higher risk population which contained more seriously affected FGR fetuses might have yielded even more dramatic results.

A weakness of the study is that one of our goals could only be reached indirectly. The results only inferred a front-to-back process of cerebral dilatation, which appeared to coincide with worsening fetal condition, but this type of progressive response to gradual fetal hypoxia can better be proven via longitudinal studies.

FGR and brain sparing have been linked to hypoxia-related morbidities. Our goal was to search for information provided by lesser-studied cerebral vessels to determine the extent of hypoxia pan-cerebrally. Our results allow us to hypothesize that Doppler of the VA (which may be more specific for a later occurring, more severe phenotype), used in conjunction with the MCA Doppler (a more sensitive, earlier screening modality for brain sparing), may be useful in providing information about the duration and extent of the hypoxia and should provide an incentive for future studies to apply this concept to a larger study group containing both late-onset and early-onset FGR, with emphasis on the identification or prevention of immediate as well as long term morbidities.

5. Conclusions

FGR fetuses defined by ISUOG guidelines deliver earlier, have lower birthweights, and have a much higher rate of abnormal cerebral vessel PIs than SGA fetuses. This study suggests that there are varying degrees of brain redistribution, with abnormal posterior brain blood flow being associated with more severe outcomes. We postulate that the VA, used in conjunction with the MCA, may be a useful adjunctive method to identify the duration and severity of FGR.

Author Contributions: Conceptualization, J.G.S., S.R., H.L.G. and J.C.H.; methodology, J.G.S., D.G., H.L.G., S.R. and J.C.H.; validation, J.G.S., H.L.G., S.R., D.G., C.D., E.P. and J.C.H.; formal analysis, J.G.S., H.L.G., D.G., S.R., C.D., E.P. and J.C.H.; investigation, J.G.S., H.L.G., S.R. and J.C.H.; data curation, D.G., C.D. and E.P.; writing—original draft preparation, J.G.S., H.L.G., D.G., S.R., C.D., E.P. and J.C.H.; writing—review and editing, J.G.S., H.L.G., D.G., S.R., C.D., E.P. and J.C.H.; visualization, J.G.S., J.C.H. and E.P.; supervision, S.R., H.L.G., J.G.S. and J.C.H.; project administration, J.C.H.; funding acquisition, J.C.H. All authors have read and agreed to the published version of the manuscript.

Funding: The Perelman Family Foundation provided financial support for this project but did not have any role in the study.

Institutional Review Board Statement: The study was conducted according to the guidelines of the Declaration of Helsinki and approved by the Colorado Multiple Institutional Review Board IRB number 14-1360, date of approval 29 May 2015.

Informed Consent Statement: Informed consent was obtained from all subjects involved in the study.

Data Availability Statement: The data that support the findings of this study are available from the corresponding author upon reasonable request.

Acknowledgments: We appreciate the support and peer review by Odessa Hamidi. Name: Odessa Hamidi. Place of Employment: Division of Maternal Fetal Medicine, Department of Obstetrics and Gynecology, University of Colorado School of Medicine, Aurora, CO.

Conflicts of Interest: The authors declare no conflict of interest.

References

1. Savchev, S.; Sanz-Cortes, M.; Cruz-Martinez, R.; Arranz, A.; Botet, F.; Gratacos, E.; Figueras, F. Neurodevelopmental outcome of full-term small-for-gestational-age infants with normal placental function. *Ultrasound Obstet. Gynecol.* **2013**, *42*, 201–206. [CrossRef] [PubMed]
2. Baschat, A.A. Neurodevelopment following fetal growth restriction and its relationship with antepartum parameters of placental dysfunction. *Ultrasound Obstet. Gynecol.* **2011**, *37*, 501–514. [CrossRef] [PubMed]
3. Rueda-Clausen, C.F.; Morton, J.S.; Davidge, S.T. Effects of hypoxia-induced intrauterine growth restriction on cardiopulmonary structure and function during adulthood. *Cardiovasc. Res.* **2009**, *81*, 713–722. [CrossRef] [PubMed]
4. Crispi, F.; Miranda, J.; Gratacos, E. Long-term cardiovascular consequences of fetal growth restriction: Biology, clinical implications, and opportunities for prevention of adult disease. *Am. J. Obstet. Gynecol.* **2018**, *218*, S869–S879. [CrossRef] [PubMed]
5. Hales, C.N.; Barker, D.J. The thrifty phenotype hypothesis. *Br. Med. Bull.* **2001**, *60*, 5–20. [CrossRef] [PubMed]
6. Gordijn, S.J.; Beune, I.M.; Thilaganathan, B.; Papageorghiou, A.; Baschat, A.A.; Baker, P.N.; Silver, R.M.; Wynia, K.; Ganzevoort, W. Consensus definition of fetal growth restriction: A Delphi procedure. *Ultrasound Obstet. Gynecol.* **2016**, *48*, 333–339. [CrossRef] [PubMed]
7. Lees, C.C.; Stampalija, T.; Baschat, A.; da Silva Costa, F.; Ferrazzi, E.; Figueras, F.; Hecher, K.; Poon, L.C.; Salomon, L.J.; Unterscheider, J. ISUOG Practice Guidelines: Diagnosis and management of small-for-gestational-age fetus and fetal growth restriction. *Ultrasound Obstet. Gynecol.* **2020**, *56*, 298–312. [CrossRef]
8. American College of Obstetricians and Gynecologists. ACOG Practice Bulletin No. 204: Fetal growth restriction. *Obstet. Gynecol.* **2019**, *133*, e97–e109. [CrossRef]
9. Martins, J.G.; Biggio, J.R.; Abuhamad, A. Society for Maternal-Fetal Medicine (SMFM. Society for Maternal-Fetal Medicine Consult Series# 52: Diagnosis and management of fetal growth restriction: (replaces clinical guideline number 3, April 2012). *Am. J. Obstet. Gynecol.* **2020**, *223*, B2–B17. [PubMed]
10. Giussani, D.A. The fetal brain sparing response to hypoxia: Physiological mechanisms. *J. Physiol.* **2016**, *594*, 1215–1230. [CrossRef]
11. Figueroa-Diesel, H.; Hernandez-Andrade, E.; Acosta-Rojas, R.; Cabero, L.; Gratacos, E. Doppler changes in the main fetal brain arteries at different stages of hemodynamic adaptation in severe intrauterine growth restriction. *Ultrasound Obstet. Gynecol.* **2007**, *30*, 297–302. [CrossRef] [PubMed]
12. Oros, D.; Figueras, F.; Cruz-Martinez, R.; Padilla, N.; Meler, E.; Hernandez-Andrade, E.; Gratacos, E. Middle cerebral versus anterior cerebral Doppler for prediction of prenatal outcome and behavior in term small for gestational age fetuses with normal umbilical artery Dopplers. *Ultrasound Obstet. Gynecol.* **2010**, *35*, 456–461. [CrossRef] [PubMed]

13. Benavides-Serralde, J.A.; Hernandez-Andrade, E.; Cruz-Martinez, R.; Cruz-Lemini, M.; Scheier, M.; Figueras, F.; Mancilla, J.; Gratacos, E. Doppler evaluation of the posterior cerebral artery in normally grown and growth restricted fetuses. *Prenat. Diagn.* **2014**, *34*, 115–120. [CrossRef]
14. Morales-Roselló, J.; Hervas Marin, D.; Perales Marin, A. The vertebral artery Doppler might be an alternative to the middle cerebral artery Doppler in the follow-up of the early onset growth-restricted fetus. *Prenat. Diagn.* **2014**, *34*, 109–114. [CrossRef] [PubMed]
15. American College of Obstetricians and Gynecologists. Committee Opinion No 700: Methods for Estimating the Due Date. *Obstet. Gynecol.* **2017**, *129*, e150–e154. [CrossRef] [PubMed]
16. Hadlock, F.P.; Harrist, R.B.; Martinez-Poyer, J. In utero analysis of fetal growth: A sonographic weight standard. *Radiology* **1991**, *181*, 129–133. [CrossRef]
17. Hadlock, F.P.; Harrist, R.B.; Sharman, R.S.; Deter, R.L.; Park, S.K. Estimation of fetal weight with the use of head, body, and femur measurements—A prospective study. *Am. J. Obstet. Gynecol.* **1985**, *151*, 333–337. [CrossRef]
18. Ebbing, C.; Rasmussen, S.; Kiserud, T. Middle cerebral artery blood flow velocities and pulsatility index and the cerebroplacental pulsatility ratio: Longitudinal reference ranges and terms for serial measurements. *Ultrasound Obstet. Gynecol.* **2007**, *30*, 287–296. [CrossRef]
19. DeVore, G.R. The importance of the cerebroplacental ratio in the evaluation of fetal well-being in SGA and AGA fetuses. *Am. J. Obstet. Gynecol.* **2015**, *213*, 5–15. [CrossRef]
20. DeVore, G.R. Computing the Z score and centiles for cross-sectional analysis: A practical approach. *J. Ultrasound Med.* **2017**, *36*, 459–473. [CrossRef]
21. Benavides-Serralde, J.A.; Hernandez-Andrade, E.; Figueroa-Diesel, H.; Oros, D.; Feria, L.A.; Scheier, M.; Figueras, F.; Gratacos, E. Reference values for Doppler parameters of the fetal anterior cerebral artery throughout gestation. *Gynecol. Obstet. Investig.* **2010**, *69*, 33–39. [CrossRef] [PubMed]
22. Hernandez-Andrade, E.; Figueroa-Diesel, H.; Jansson, T.; Rangel-Nava, H.; Gratacos, E. Changes in regional fetal cerebral blood flow perfusion in relation to hemodynamic deterioration in severely growth-restricted fetuses. *Ultrasound Obstet. Gynecol.* **2008**, *32*, 71–76. [CrossRef] [PubMed]
23. Dubiel, M.; Gunnarsson, G.O.; Gudmundsson, S. Blood redistribution in the fetal brain during chronic hypoxia. *Ultrasound Obstet. Gynecol.* **2002**, *20*, 117–121. [CrossRef] [PubMed]
24. Cruz-Martinez, R.; Figueras, F.; Hernandez-Andrade, E.; Puerto, B.; Gratacós, E. Longitudinal brain perfusion changes in near-term small-for-gestational-age fetuses as measured by spectral Doppler indices or by fractional moving blood volume. *Am. J. Obstet. Gynecol.* **2010**, *203*, 42-e1. [CrossRef] [PubMed]
25. Morales Roselló, J.; Hervás Marín, D.; Fillol Crespo, M.; Perales Marín, A. Doppler changes in the vertebral, middle cerebral, and umbilical arteries in fetuses delivered after 34 weeks: Relationship to severity of growth restriction. *Prenat. Diagn.* **2012**, *32*, 960–967. [CrossRef]
26. Trudinger, B.J.; Stevens, D.; Connelly, A.; Hales, J.R.; Alexander, G.; Bradley, L.; Fawcett, A.; Thompson, R.S. Umbilical artery flow velocity waveforms and placental resistance: The effects of embolization of the umbilical circulation. *Am. J. Obstet. Gynecol.* **1987**, *157*, 1443–1448. [CrossRef]
27. Ferrazzi, E.; Bozzo, M.; Rigano, S.; Bellotti, M.; Morabito, A.; Pardi, G.; Battaglia, F.C.; Galan, H.L. Temporal sequence of abnormal Doppler changes in the peripheral and central circulatory systems of the severely growth-restricted fetus. *Ultrasound Obstet. Gynecol.* **2002**, *19*, 140–146. [CrossRef]
28. Hecher, K.; Bilardo, C.M.; Stigter, R.H.; Ville, Y.; Hackelöer, B.J.; Kok, H.J.; Senat, M.V.; Visser, G.H. Monitoring of fetuses with intrauterine growth restriction: A longitudinal study. *Ultrasound Obstet. Gynecol.* **2001**, *18*, 564–570. [CrossRef]
29. Turan, O.M.; Turan, S.; Gungor, S.; Berg, C.; Moyano, D.; Gembruch, U.; Nicolaides, K.H.; Harman, C.R.; Baschat, A.A. Progression of Doppler abnormalities in intrauterine growth restriction. *Ultrasound Obstet. Gynecol.* **2008**, *32*, 160–167. [CrossRef]
30. Hobbins, J.C.; Gumina, D.L.; Zaretsky, M.V.; Driver, C.; Wilcox, A.; DeVore, G.R. Size and shape of the four-chamber view of the fetal heart in fetuses with an estimated fetal weight less than the tenth centile. *Am. J. Obstet. Gynecol.* **2019**, *221*, 495.e1–495.e9. [CrossRef]
31. DeVore, G.R.; Gumina, D.L.; Hobbins, J.C. Assessment of ventricular contractility in fetuses with an estimated fetal weight less than the tenth centile. *Am. J. Obstet. Gynecol.* **2019**, *221*, 498.e1–498.e22. [CrossRef] [PubMed]
32. Cruz-Martínez, R.; Figueras, F.; Hernandez-Andrade, E.; Oros, D.; Gratacos, E. Fetal brain Doppler to predict cesarean delivery for nonreassuring fetal status in term small-for-gestational-age fetuses. *Obstet. Gynecol.* **2011**, *117*, 618–626. [CrossRef] [PubMed]
33. Makhseed, M.; Jirous, J.; Ahmed, M.A.; Viswanathan, D.L. Middle cerebral artery to umbilical artery resistance index ratio in the prediction of neonatal outcome. *Int. J. Gynaecol. Obstet.* **2000**, *71*, 119–125. [CrossRef]
34. Alfirevic, Z.; Stampalija, T.; Dowswell, T. Fetal umbilical Doppler ultrasound in high-risk pregnancies. *Cochrane Database Syst. Rev.* **2017**. [CrossRef] [PubMed]
35. Eixarch, E.; Meler, E.; Iraola, A.; Illa, M.; Crispi, F.; Hernandez-Andrade, E.; Gratacos, E.; Figueras, F. Neurodevelopmental outcome in 2-year-old infants who were small-for-gestational age term fetuses with cerebral blood flow redistribution. *Ultrasound Obstet. Gynecol.* **2008**, *32*, 894–899. [CrossRef] [PubMed]

36. Nicolaides, K.H.; Wright, D.; Syngelaki, A.; Wright, A.; Akolekar, R. Fetal Medicine Foundation population weight charts. *Ultrasound Obstet. Gynecol.* **2018**, *52*, 44–51. [CrossRef] [PubMed]
37. Morales-Roselló, J.; Khalil, A.; Morlando, M.; Papageorghiou, A.; Bhide, A.; Thilaganathan, B. Changes in fetal Doppler indices as a marker of failure to reach growth potential at term. *Ultrasound Obstet. Gynecol.* **2014**, *43*, 303–310. [CrossRef]

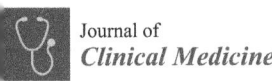

Article

Proton Pump Inhibitors Use and Risk of Preeclampsia: A Meta-Analysis

Salman Hussain [1,*], Ambrish Singh [2], Benny Antony [2], Jitka Klugarová [1], M. Hassan Murad [3], Aarthi S. Jayraj [4], Alena Langaufová [1] and Miloslav Klugar [1,*]

1. Czech National Centre for Evidence-Based Healthcare and Knowledge Translation (Cochrane Czech Republic, Czech EBHC: JBI Centre of Excellence, Masaryk University GRADE Centre), Institute of Biostatistics and Analyses, Faculty of Medicine, Masaryk University, Brno, Czech Republic, Kamenice 5, 62500 Brno, Czech Republic
2. Menzies Institute for Medical Research, University of Tasmania, 17 Liverpool St, Hobart, TAS 7000, Australia
3. Division of Public Health, Infectious Diseases and Occupational Medicine, Mayo Clinic, 200 1st St SW, Rochester, MN 55905, USA
4. Department of Obstetrics & Gynaecology, All India Institute of Medical Sciences, New Delhi 110029, India
* Correspondence: mohammad.hussain@med.muni.cz (S.H.); klugar@med.muni.cz (M.K.)

Abstract: Evidence from preclinical studies suggests a preventive effect of proton pump inhibitors (PPIs) in preeclampsia. Recently, several epidemiological studies have described a conflicting association between the use of PPIs during pregnancy and preeclampsia risk. This study aimed to evaluate the association between PPI use and the risk of preeclampsia. We searched databases, including MEDLINE, Embase, Scopus, Web of Science Core Collection, Emcare, CINAHL, and the relevant grey literature from inception until 13 September 2021. Studies reporting the preeclampsia risk with the use of PPIs were eligible for inclusion. Literature screening, data extraction, and the risk of bias assessment were performed independently by two investigators. Random-effect meta-analysis was performed to generate relative risks (RR) and 95% confidence intervals (CI). The risk of preeclampsia and preterm preeclampsia among women receiving PPIs during pregnancy were the primary outcomes of interest. This meta-analysis comprised three studies involving 4,877,565 pregnant women, of whom 119,017 were PPI users. The included studies were judged to have a low risk of bias. The risk of preeclampsia among pregnant women who received PPIs anytime during pregnancy was significantly increased (RR 1.27 (95% CI: 1.23–1.31)), although the increase was trivial in absolute terms (2 per 1000). The subgroup analysis revealed that the risk was increased in each of the three trimesters. The risk of preterm preeclampsia among pregnant women receiving PPIs anytime during pregnancy was not significantly increased (RR 1.04 (95% CI: 0.70–1.55)). The certainty evaluated by GRADE in these estimates was low. PPI use may be associated with a trivial increase in the risk of preeclampsia in pregnant women. There is no evidence supporting that PPI use decreases the risk of preeclampsia or preterm preeclampsia.

Keywords: hypertension; preeclampsia; proton pump inhibitors; PPIs; pregnancy; meta-analysis

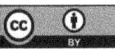

1. Introduction

Preeclampsia is one of the most severe complications of pregnancy characterized by high blood pressure. It is one of the leading causes of maternal morbidity and mortality worldwide. The global burden of preeclampsia is continuously rising; epidemiological trends showed a 10.9% increase in the incidence of preeclampsia from 1990 to 2019 [1]. Preeclampsia leads to adverse maternal and perinatal outcomes, including preterm birth, prolonged hospital stays, low birthweight babies, and a higher risk of neonatal intensive care unit admission [2]. Preterm birth imposes a significant mortality risk on the mother and the baby [3]. Several database studies have reported a positive association between preterm birth and mortality and morbidity in both the mother and the baby [4,5]. There are no definitive treatment options available for preeclampsia management, except for the timely delivery of the fetus and placenta.

Evidence from preclinical studies suggests a plausible preventive effect of proton pump inhibitors (PPIs) in preeclampsia [6–8]. The potential mechanism of this protective effect of PPIs in managing preeclampsia could be due to the reduction in the mRNA expression and secretion of antiangiogenic factors (sFlt1) and soluble endoglin (sEng) in placental endothelial cells, as these are the key component involved in the pathophysiology of preeclampsia [7,9,10]. This mechanistic association was supported by the findings of a recently published prospective cohort study where lower levels of sFLT-1 and sEng were noticed among pregnant PPI users with suspected preeclampsia [11]. PPIs are commonly used to treat gastroesophageal reflux disorder (GERD); however, in the last decade, the safety of PPIs has been a matter of scrutiny [12]. Our previous systematic reviews and meta-analyses found PPI use to be associated with several other non-pregnancy-related adverse health outcomes [13–16]. Nevertheless, PPIs are widely used by pregnant women due to their acceptable safety profiles and their availability as over-the-counter (OTC) drugs in many countries [17]. The evidence from cohort studies and a meta-analysis supported the PPI safety profiles among women who used PPIs during pregnancy and found no increased risk of congenital defects or preterm delivery [18,19].

Recently, several epidemiological studies examined the association of PPIs with preeclampsia risk [20–22]. A large cohort study from the US using the Truven Health MarketScan database found no association of PPIs with a decreased risk of preeclampsia or severe preterm preeclampsia [22]. Similar findings were reported by Choi et al. using the Korean Healthcare database [21]. However, a Swedish population register-based cohort study found reduced preterm and early preeclampsia risk in women who used PPIs in the third trimester [20]. These published studies presented conflicting evidence, and to date, no meta-analysis has been performed to explore this association, as confirmed through a preliminary search in multiple databases. Therefore, this systematic review and meta-analysis aimed to synthesize the evidence and assess the overall risk of preeclampsia in women using PPIs during pregnancy.

2. Materials and Methods

2.1. Protocol

The protocol for this systematic review was prospectively published as a preprint at medRxiv [23]. The principles laid down in the Cochrane Handbook of Systematic Review of Interventions and the JBI reviewers manual were utilized [24,25]. Preferred reporting items for systematic review and meta-analysis (PRISMA 2020) and meta-analysis of observational studies in epidemiology (MOOSE) reporting guidelines were followed [26,27]. Refer to Supplementary Table S1 for the detailed checklist.

2.2. Search Strategy

The literature search was conducted in each database from the inception date to 13 September 2021 to identify published and unpublished studies assessing preeclampsia risk in women receiving PPIs during pregnancy. The three-step search strategy was used; an initial limited search was conducted in MEDLINE (Ovid) and Embase (Ovid), using keywords and index terms related to PPIs and preeclampsia without restriction to any date or language; then, a detailed search was performed across all major databases by analyzing the text words and index terms used to describe the articles. We searched MEDLINE (Ovid), Embase (Ovid), Scopus, Web of Science Core Collection, Emcare (Ovand id), and CINAHL (EBSCO). The sources of grey literature were ProQuest Dissertations & Theses Global and clinical trials registers, ClinicalTrials.gov (accessed on 13 September 2021), and the WHO International Clinical Trials Registry Platform (ICTRP). Search strings were developed by a medical information specialist (AL). Lastly, bibliographies of the relevant articles were scanned manually for additional articles. The search strategies used for different databases were provided in Supplementary Table S2 with their respective hits.

2.3. Study Selection/Inclusion Criteria

Two reviewers independently reviewed the retrieved articles based on title and abstract screening, which was followed by second-level screening based on full-text articles. Covidence systematic review software was used for completing the article screening process [28].

Studies were eligible for inclusion if they met the inclusion criteria mentioned in Table 1:

Table 1. Eligibility criteria for the selection of articles.

Criterion	Inclusion Criteria	Exclusion Criteria
Population	Pregnant women at any stage of gestation	Non-pregnant women
Exposure	Exposure to any proton pump inhibitors • Omeprazole • Esomeprazole • Pantoprazole • Rabeprazole • Lansoprazole • Dexlansoprazole • Ilaprazole	Drugs other than proton pump inhibitors
Comparator	Nonexposure or exposure to H2RA antagonist	N/A
Outcomes	Studies reporting: • Preeclampsia risk at any stage of pregnancy • Preterm preeclampsia risk	Studies reporting any other outcomes: • Cost-effectiveness • HRQoL • Cost and resource use
Study design	Studies assessing preeclampsia risk, including: • Retrospective cohort • Prospective cohort • Case–control studies	Following was excluded: • Animal studies • In vitro studies • Literature reviews • Pharmacodynamic and pharmacokinetic studies
Time period	Studies published until September 2021	N/A

H2RA: Histamine 2 receptors antagonist; HRQoL: Health-related quality of life; N/A: Not applicable.

2.4. Data Extraction and Risk of Bias

Two reviewers independently extracted all the relevant data based on the study characteristics (author, publication year, data source, and study period); details on patient characteristics; exposure; comparator; ascertainment of PPI use; confirmation of outcome; effect estimates (unadjusted and adjusted risk); and conclusions. Any discrepancy during the data extraction process was resolved by discussion. There was no missing data, so none of the primary authors was contacted for any additional data.

The risk of bias in the included studies was evaluated using the Newcastle–Ottawa Scale (NOS) independently by two reviewers [29]. According to the NOS, a study can achieve a maximum of 4 points in the selection, 2 points in the comparability, and 3 points in the exposure (case–control studies) or outcome (cohort studies) domain of the scale. Studies were classified as having a high, moderate, or low risk of bias, depending on the adjustment for appropriate confounders and the adequacy of the exposure and outcome ascertainment and not based on a numerical score [30].

2.5. Certainty of Evidence

We used the Grading of Recommendations Assessment, Development and Evaluation (GRADE) methodology to assess the certainty of evidence [31]. The certainty assessment was judged as either high, moderate, low, or very low, based on the risk of bias, inconsistency, indirectness, imprecision, and publication bias.

2.6. Statistical Analysis

The primary outcome of interest was to assess the pooled relative risk of preeclampsia among women receiving PPIs during pregnancy. The risk ratio (RR) and odds ratio were used interchangeably, as PPI use and preeclampsia events were very rare [32]. Heterogeneity was determined based on Cochrane chi-square and I2 statistics [33]. The Cochrane chi-square value ($p < 0.10$) and I2 statistics $\geq 50\%$ represent important heterogeneity [33]. Since we anticipated heterogeneity in terms of the population characteristics and settings of the studies, we used the random effect model. A subgroup analysis was performed based on the trimester of pregnancy and preterm and term preeclampsia. The leave-one-out method was used to understand the impact of each study on the pooled effect size. Meta-regression and statistical evaluation of the publication bias using funnel plot approaches were not feasible due to the limited number of studies. Review Manager (RevMan) version 5.4.1 was used to perform the meta-analysis using the generic inverse variance method. Summary of the findings table was created using the GRADEpro GDT tool [34].

3. Results

3.1. Studies Characteristics

The database search yielded 600 articles; three studies [20–22] involving 4,877,565 pregnant women, of whom 119,017 were PPI users, were included in the meta-analysis. A list of articles excluded with exclusion reasons during the full-text screening phase are presented in Supplementary Table S3. Refer to the PRISMA chart (Figure 1) for the study inclusion process.

The design of the three studies was a retrospective cohort design, and they were published within the time frame of 2019–2021. All the eligible studies were published as a full text, except the study by Choi et al., published as a research letter. Included studies were conducted in the US, Sweden, and Korea. PPI exposure was defined as exposure to PPIs at any time during pregnancy or individually during the first, second, and third trimesters. Studies ascertained the PPI exposure through prescription records or claims data, and the outcome of preeclampsia was confirmed based on the International Classification of Diseases (ICD) code—9th or 10th edition. Refer to Table 2 for a detailed description of the included study characteristics.

3.2. Quality Assessment and Certainty of Evidence

The risk of bias in the three included studies was low. All the included studies selected the patients and control from the same databases and adjusted for several possible confounding factors. The details of this assessment are presented in Table 3. The certainty of the evidence on the risk of preeclampsia and preterm preeclampsia among women receiving PPIs during pregnancy was low to very low, as per the GRADE rating system (Table 4a,b). Of note, the absolute effects were trivial or very small.

3.3. Meta-Analysis (Preeclampsia Risk)

The risk of preeclampsia among pregnant women who received PPIs anytime during pregnancy was statistically significantly increased (Figure 2a) with a pooled RR of 1.27 (95% CI: 1.23–1.31), $p < 0.00001$ in an adjusted analysis (adjusted for several possible confounding factors).

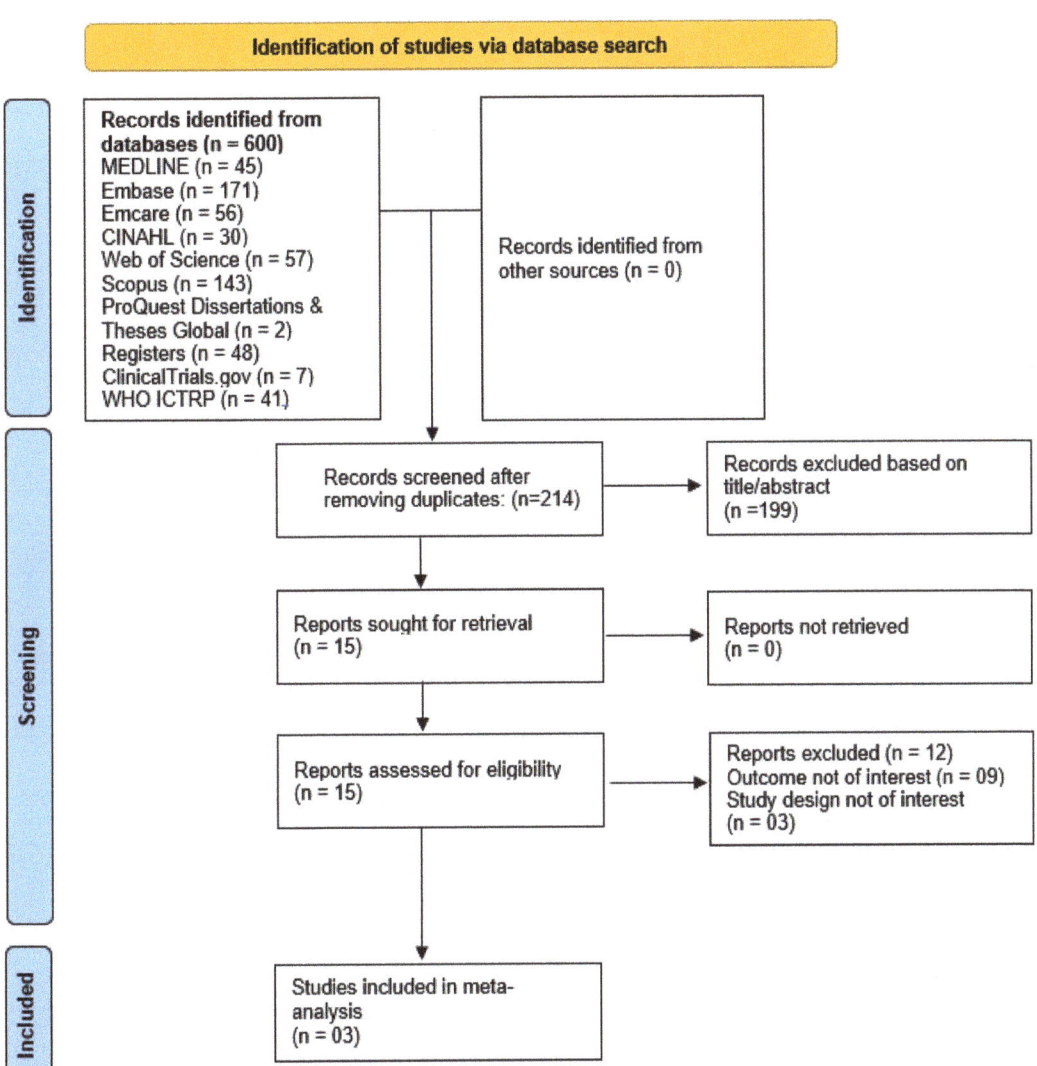

Figure 1. PRISMA flowchart showing the study inclusion process.

The subgroup analysis revealed a statistically significantly higher risk of preeclampsia in pregnant women receiving PPIs in each of the three trimesters (Figure 2b). All the analyses were adjusted for maternal age, chronic kidney disease, autoimmune disease, multiple gestation, pregestational diabetes, chronic hypertension, nulliparity, and multiple pregnancies.

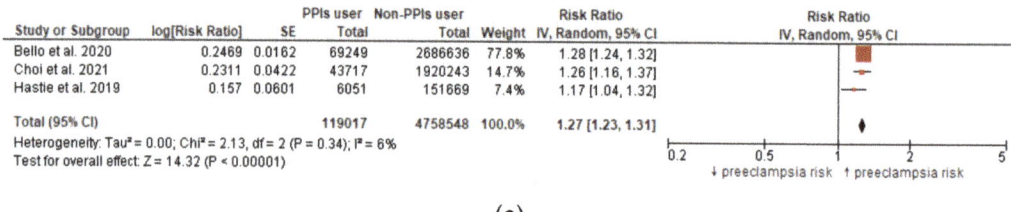

(a)

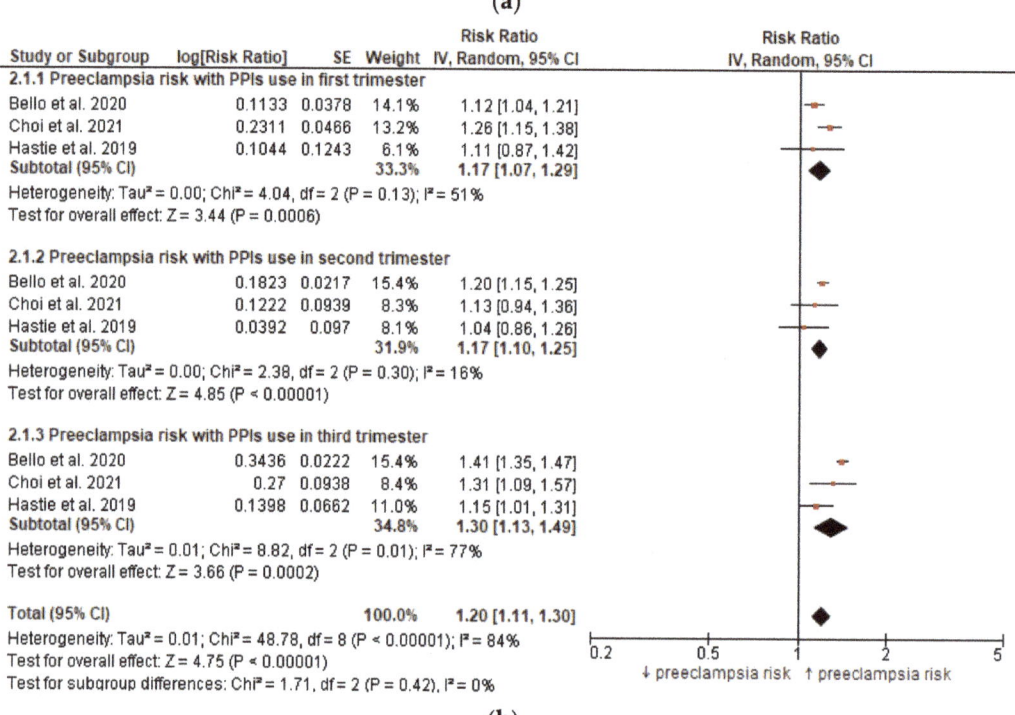

(b)

Figure 2. (a) Preeclampsia risk in women exposed to PPIs anytime during pregnancy. (b) Preeclampsia risk in women exposed to PPIs in different trimesters of pregnancy.

3.4. Meta-Analysis (Preterm Preeclampsia Risk)

Two studies reported data for the preterm preeclampsia risk among pregnant women receiving PPIs anytime during pregnancy, and the pooled estimate (Figure 3a) revealed a nonsignificant association ($p = 0.83$).

The subgroup analysis based on the use of PPIs in various trimesters and the risk of preterm preeclampsia (Figure 3b) revealed a significantly higher risk in the second trimester, with a pooled relative risk of 1.32 (95% CI: 1.19–1.46), $p < 0.00001$. However, the association was nonsignificant in the first or third trimesters.

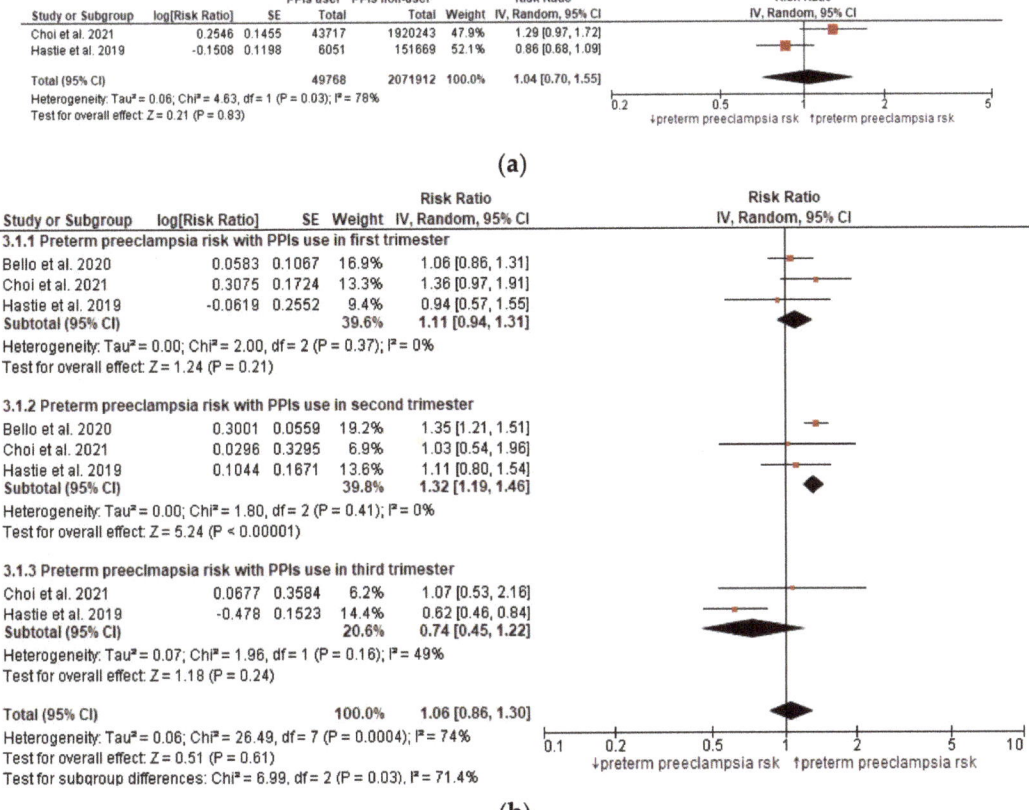

Figure 3. (a) Preterm preeclampsia risk in women exposed to PPIs anytime during pregnancy. (b) Preterm preeclampsia risk in women exposed to PPIs in different trimesters of pregnancy.

3.5. Sensitivity Analysis

A sensitivity analysis was performed by excluding each study one by one (leave-one-out) from the pooled analysis. None of the studies had any significant influence on the pooled effect size. The RR for preeclampsia was identical to the main results.

Table 2. Characteristics of the included studies.

Author, Year & Country	Study Design, Setting	Study Duration	Database/Source	Participants	Exposure	Comparator	Outcomes	Cohort Size	Definition of PPI Exposure	Ascertainment of PPI Use	Assessment of Outcome	Effect Estimates Unadjusted	Effect Estimates Adjusted	Adjusted for	Conclusion
Bello et al., 2020, US [22]	Cohort study	2008 to 2014	Truven Health MarketScan database	Women receiving PPIs during pregnancy in the Truven Health MarketScan Database	PPI user (Esomeprazole, lansoprazole, omeprazole, pantoprazole, dexlansoprazole, and rabeprazole)	No exposure to PPIs	Diagnosis of preeclampsia	Total: 2,755,885 PPI user: 69,249 Non-PPI user: 2,686,636	PPI exposure any time during pregnancy or individually during the 1st, 2nd, and 3rd trimesters	Outpatient pharmaceutical claims data	Idiopathic PD diagnosis confirmed by based on the presence of International Classification of Diseases, Ninth Edition, Clinical Modification (ICD-9-CM) diagnosis codes for mild (642.4.x), severe (642.5.x), or superimposed (642.7.x) preeclampsia or eclampsia (642.6.x).	Preeclampsia Any time PPI use: 1.42 (1.38, 1.46) 1st trimester PPI use: 1.20 (1.11, 1.30) 2nd trimester PPI use: 1.34 (1.28, 1.41) 3rd trimester PPI use: 1.56 (1.50, 1.63) Preterm severe preeclampsia (1.41, 1.77) Eclampsia 1st trimester PPI use: 1.15 (0.93, 1.43) 2nd trimester PPI use: 1.58	Preeclampsia Any time PPI use: 1.28 (1.24, 1.32) 1st trimester PPI use: 1.12 (1.04, 1.22) 2nd trimester PPI use: 1.20 (1.15, 1.26) 3rd trimester PPI use: 1.41 (1.35, 1.47) Preterm severe preeclampsia 1.35 (1.21, 1.52) Eclampsia 1st trimester PPI use: 1.06 (0.86, 1.32) 2nd trimester PPI use:	Maternal age, and the five clinical characteristics (chronic kidney disease, autoimmune disease, multiple gestation, Pregestational diabetes, and chronic hypertension)	PPI prescription during pregnancy was not associated with decreased risk for preeclampsia
Choi et al., 2021, Korea [21]	Cohort study	2011 to 2017	Health Insurance Review and Assessment database	Women receiving PPIs during pregnancy in Korea's healthcare database	Use of any PPI, including omeprazole, esomeprazole, pantoprazole, rabeprazole, lansoprazole, dexlansoprazole, or ilaprazole at any point across gestation	(1). Non-PPI user, and (2). H2RA user	Diagnosis of preeclampsia	Total: 1,963,960 PPI user: 43,717 Non-PPI user: 1,920,243	≥1 PPI prescription in 4 windows: any time during pregnancy, first, second, and third trimester	Database (based on drug chemical code, prescription supply, dosage, and others)	ICD-10 diagnostic code	Preeclampsia Any time PPI use: 1.55 (1.44–1.68) 1st trimester PPI use: 1.56 (1.42, 1.72) 2nd trimester PPI use: 1.43 (1.19, 1.72) 3rd trimester PPI use: 1.69 (1.42, 2.03) Preterm preeclampsia Any time PPI use: 1.55 (1.18–2.04) 1st trimester PPI use: 1.62 (1.17–2.24) 2nd trimester PPI use: 1.31 (0.68–2.52) 3rd trimester PPI use: 1.37 (0.68–2.74)	Preeclampsia Any time PPI use: 1.26 (1.16–1.36) 1st trimester PPI use: 1.26 (1.15, 1.39) 2nd trimester PPI use: 1.13 (0.94, 1.35) 3rd trimester PPI use: 1.31 (1.09, 1.56) Preterm preeclampsia Any time PPI use: 1.29 (0.97–1.71) 1st trimester PPI use: 1.36 (0.97–1.89) 2nd trimester PPI use: 1.03 (0.54–1.99) 3rd trimester PPI use: 1.07 (0.53–2.14)	Maternal age and insurance type, multiparity, multiple gestation, CCI, indications for acid suppressive medications, including gastroesophageal reflux disease, heartburn, ulcer (e.g., various ulcers and GTD), maternal medical conditions (e.g., asthma, anxiety, diabetes, depression, and chronic hypertension), inflammatory diseases, headache, renal disease, thyroid disorder, concurrent medications, and proxies of health care utilization	PPI use during pregnancy was not associated with a reduced risk of preeclampsia

Table 2. Cont.

Author, Year & Country	Study Design, Setting	Study Duration	Database/Source	Participants	Exposure	Comparator	Outcomes	Cohort Size	Definition of PPI Exposure	Ascertainment of PPI Use	Assessment of Outcome	Effect Estimates Unadjusted	Effect Estimates Adjusted	Adjusted for	Conclusion
Hastie et al., 2019, Sweden [20]	Cohort study	2013 to 2017	Swedish pregnancy register	Women receiving PPIs during pregnancy in Swedish pregnancy register	Use of any PPI, including omeprazole, esomeprazole, pantoprazole, rabeprazole, or lansoprazole at any point across gestation	Non-PPI users	Diagnosis of preeclampsia	Total: 157,720 PPI user: 6051 Non-PPI user: 151,669	PPI use was categorized by use ever during pregnancy, first trimester (0–12 weeks of gestation), second trimester (13–27 weeks), and third trimester (from 28 weeks of gestation onward).	Based on the prescription record maintained in Swedish pregnancy register	Preeclampsia was identified by the diagnosis codes O14 or O15 according to International Classification of Diseases, Tenth Revision coding. (n = 7258)	Preeclampsia Any time PPI use: 1.17 (1.02–1.35) 1st trimester PPI use: 1.20 (0.95, 1.52) 2nd trimester PPI use: 1.15 (0.97, 1.36) 3rd trimester PPI use: 1.21 (1.07, 1.37) Preterm preeclampsia Any time PPI use: 0.90 (0.73–1.13) 1st trimester PPI use: 0.95 (0.59, 1.49) 2nd trimester PPI use: 1.13(0.83–1.54) 3rd trimester PPI use: 0.66 (0.40–1.07)	Preeclampsia Any time PPI use: 1.17 (1.04–1.32) 1st trimester PPI use: 1.11 (0.87–1.42) 2nd trimester PPI use: 1.04 (0.86–1.25) 3rd trimester PPI use: 1.15 (1.01–1.32) Preterm preeclampsia Any time PPI use: 0.86 (0.68–1.09) 1st trimester PPI use: 0.94 (0.57–1.54) 2nd trimester PPI use: 1.11(0.80–1.54) 3rd trimester PPI use: 0.62 (0.16–0.84)	Propensity matched (maternal age, body mass index, year of delivery, country of birth, smoking status, educational level, occupation, use of assisted reproduction, and the presence of pregestational disorders	PPIs have a potential role in preventing preterm preeclampsia

CCI: Charlson comorbidity index; H2RA: histamine 2 receptor antagonists; PPI: proton pump inhibitor; ZES: Zollinger-Ellison syndrome.

Table 3. Quality assessment of the included studies.

Cohort Studies	Selection				Comparability	Outcome			
Study author	Representation of the exposed cohort	Selection of the non-exposed cohort	Ascertainment of exposure	Demonstration that outcome of interest was not present at the start of the study	Comparability of cohorts on the basis of design or analysis	Assessment of outcome	Was follow-up long enough for outcomes to occur	Accuracy of follow-up of cohorts	Overall risk of bias
Bello, 2020, US [22]	*	*	*	*	**	*	*	*	Low
Choi, 2021, Korea [21]	*	*	*	*	**	*	*	*	Low
Hastie, 2019, Sweden [20]	*	*	*	*	**	*	*	*	Low

* = this symbol represents the number of stars given to each category according to the star-based scoring systems employed to assess the risk of bias of each study as detailed in the Section 2.4 in the main text.

Table 4. (a) Summary of the findings table showing the certainty of the evidence for preeclampsia risk in women exposed to PPIs (anytime during pregnancy) compared to non-PPIs. (b) Summary of the findings table showing the certainty of the evidence for preterm preeclampsia risk in women exposed to PPIs (anytime during pregnancy) compared to non-PPIs.

№ of Studies	Study Design	Certainty Assessment					№ of Patients		Effect		Certainty
		Risk of Bias	Inconsistency	Indirectness	Imprecision	Other Considerations	Preeclampsia during AnyTime PPIs Use	Placebo	Relative (95% CI)	Absolute (95% CI)	
							Preeclampsia risk				
3	observational studies	not serious	not serious	not serious	not serious	none	1294/119,017 (1.1%)	31,204/4,758,548 (0.7%)	RR 1.27 (1.23 to 1.31)	2 more per 1000 (from 2 more to 2 more)	⊕⊕○○ Low

№ of Studies	Study Design	Certainty assessment					№ of patients		Effect		Certainty
		Risk of Bias	Inconsistency	Indirectness	Imprecision	Other Considerations	Preterm preeclampsia during Anytime PPIs Use	Placebo	Relative (95% CI)	Absolute (95% CI)	
							Preterm preeclampsia risk				
2	observational studies	not serious	serious [a]	not serious	not serious	none	129/49,768 (0.3%)	3626/2,071,912 (0.2%)	RR 1.04 (0.70–1.55)	0 fewer per 1000 (from 1 fewer to 1 more)	⊕○○○ VERY Low

(a) Patients: Preeclampsia risk in pregnant women exposed to PPIs compared to non-PPIs. Risk factor: PPI. Comparisons: Non-PPI user. CI: Confidence interval; RR: Risk ratio. GRADE Working Group grades of evidence: Low certainty: The true effect might be markedly different from the estimated effect. (b) Patients: Preterm preeclampsia risk in pregnant women exposed to PPIs compared to non-PPIs. Risk factor: PPI. Comparisons: Non-PPI user. CI: Confidence interval; RR: Risk ratio. Explanations: [a] High heterogeneity was observed with an I^2 value of 78%. GRADE Working Group grades of evidence: Very low certainty. The true effect is probably markedly different from the estimated effect.

4. Discussion

This is the first systematic review and meta-analysis to investigate the risk of preeclampsia and preterm preeclampsia among women receiving PPIs during pregnancy. We found a significantly higher risk of preeclampsia in pregnant women exposed to PPIs anytime during pregnancy or during each specific trimester, although this risk was trivial or very small in absolute terms. PPI use was also associated with a significant increase in the risk of preterm preeclampsia only in the second trimester.

The certainty in the estimates was low, which suggests the need for randomized trials that evaluate patient important outcomes, as very few trials exist or are ongoing. One trial has demonstrated no prolongation in the gestation period with esomeprazole in women with preterm preeclampsia [35]. In addition, that trial showed no significant change in the relevant biomarkers levels (sFlt1, sEng, and placental growth factor) and maternal, fetal, or neonatal outcomes [35]. Similarly, a recently published randomized, double-blinded placebo-controlled trial by Abbas et al. [36] also confirmed no significant change in the antiangiogenic markers in women with early onset preeclampsia who received 40 mg of esomeprazole daily. This trial also found a nonsignificant effect of esomeprazole on the length of pregnancy and maternal and fetal complications [36]. Several trials are currently underway to assess the efficacy of PPIs, either alone or in combination with agents such as metformin or sildenafil for the management of preeclampsia. Table 5 provides a detailed list of the relevant ongoing trials.

The strength of the current systematic review was the exhaustive search for all the eligible published and unpublished studies from multiple literature sources, including gray literature, enabling a large sample size to estimate the risk of both preeclampsia and preterm preeclampsia based on the use of PPIs in different gestation ages.

However, a few important limitations need to be considered. First, the included studies did not specifically ascertain medication adherence, and the assessment of PPI exposure was based on the claims data and prescription records. Further, the availability of PPIs as OTC drugs in two of the included studies may lead to an inaccurate assessment of their exposure and, thus, raise the possibility of confounding [37]. Second, only one study adjusted the findings for the body mass index (BMI), although the BMI is known to be associated with preeclampsia [38]. Lastly, a small number of studies and the observational nature of the included studies and confounding by indication should be considered while interpreting the findings.

Table 5. List of ongoing clinical trials.

Trial Number	Trial Name or Title	Methods	Participants	Interventions	Outcomes	Start Date	Recruitment Status	Link to Trials
NCT03717740	Esomeprazole for the Prevention of Preeclampsia	Randomized double-blinded placebo-controlled intervention trial	Pregnant women presenting prior to 17 + 0 weeks' gestation with moderate to high risk of preeclampsia	Esomeprazole single dose of 40 mg orally once a day from 12+ and 17 weeks of pregnancy until 34 weeks of pregnancy	Primary Outcome Measures: Number of Participants With early onset Preeclampsia Secondary Outcome Measures: • Prevention of preeclampsia between 37 and 41 • The number of cases of Fetal Growth Restriction • The number of cases of preterm birth	1 December 2018	Recruiting	https://clinicaltrials.gov/ct2/show/NCT03717740 (accessed on 4 October 2021)
NCT03717701	Metformin and Esomeprazole in Treatment of Early Onset Preeclampsia	Randomized double-blinded placebo-controlled intervention trial	Pregnant women presenting at a Gestational age between 28 + 0 weeks and 32 + 0 weeks presented with preterm preeclampsia	Metformin 1000 mg orally once a day; Esomeprazole 40 mg orally once a day	Primary Outcome Measures: Prolongation of gestation measured from the time of enrollment to the time of delivery. Secondary Outcome Measures: • Severe morbidity • The change in serum level of sFlt-1 and endoglin • Any side effects	1 December 2018	Recruiting	https://clinicaltrials.gov/ct2/show/NCT03717701 (accessed on 4 October 2021)
NCT03724838	Esomeprazole With Sildenafil Citrate in Women With Early-onset Preeclampsia	Randomized, double-blind, placebo-controlled trial	Pregnant women presenting at a Gestational age between 28 + 0 weeks and 32 + 0 weeks presented with preterm preeclampsia	Patients will take esomeprazole single dose of 40 mg orally once a day; Patients will take Sildenafil Citrate 40 mg every 8 h; other comparators	Primary outcome measures: Prolongation of gestation measured from the time of enrollment to the time of delivery Secondary outcome measures: • Severe morbidity • Side effects • The change in serum level of sFlt-1 and endoglin	1 December 2018	Recruiting	https://clinicaltrials.gov/ct2/show/NCT03724838 (accessed on 4 October 2021)
EUCTR2018-000263-28-NL or Netherland Trial Register L7718	Potential effect of proton-pump inhibitor on angiogenic markers in preeclampsia: a pilot study	Randomised controlled trial	Women with (≥18 years) with a singleton pregnancy diagnosed with PE with a gestational age of ≥20 weeks and <34 weeks	Omeprazole	Primary outcome measures: The difference in sFlt-1 levels in women who have received PPI, in comparison to women who have not received PPI, at different time points. Secondary outcome measures: • The change in serum levels of PlGF, sEndoglin, ET-1 and CT-proET-1 levels between PPI and non-PPI group at different time points (before and after administration) • The change in cord blood levels of sFlt-1, PlGF, sEndoglin, ET-1 and CT-proET-1 at time of delivery between PPI and non-PPI group.	17 December 2018	Ongoing	https://www.clinicaltrialsregister.eu/ctr-search/trial/2018-000263-28/NL (accessed on 4 October 2021) https://www.trialregister.nl/trial/7718 (accessed on 4 October 2021)
IRCT2017082333680N2	The evaluation of esomeprazole efficacy in treatment of early onset pre-eclampsia	Randomized, single-blind, placebo-controlled trial	Pregnant women with hypertensive Pregnancy and the gestational age between 26 to 32 weeks with single-crowned pregnancy	The intervention group received 12 mg betamethasone in two doses every 24 h plus prescribed 40 mg esomeprazole daily. The control group received 12 mg Betamethasone in two doses every 24 h plus prescribed 40 mg placebo daily.	Primary outcome measure: Duration of admission to delivery Secondary outcome measure: • Frequency of maternal and fetal complications in patients with preeclampsia • Biomarker level of tyrosine kinase and endoglycine	18 April 2017	Ongoing	https://en.irct.ir/trial/25917 (accessed on 4 October 2021)

Table 5. Cont.

Trial Number	Trial Name or Title	Methods	Participants	Interventions	Outcomes	Start Date	Recruitment Status	Link to Trials
ChiCTR1900026972	A randomized controlled trial for efficacy of esomeprazole in the treatment of early-onset preeclampsia	Randomized controlled trial	Pregnant women with gestational age between 26 + 0 weeks and 33+ 6 weeks; Diagnosis of pre-eclampsia, gestational hypertension	Forty milligrams of esomeprazole+ Standard treatment vs. control group	Primary outcome measure: Duration of admission to delivery Secondary outcome measures: The change in levels of sFlt-1, and sEndoglin	1 January 2020	Recruiting	https://www.chictr.org.cn/showprojen.aspx?proj=44939 (accessed on 4 October 2021)
ACTRN12618000690257	A Prospective, Pre-ecLampsia/Eclampsia Prevention Intervention	Multi-centre, double blind, randomised, placebo-controlled trial	Nulliparous women with singleton pregnancy (12–20 weeks)	Forty milligrams of oral esomeprazole tablets once daily	Primary outcome measure: Incidence of preeclampsia Secondary outcome measure: • Incidence of term preeclampsia • Gestation of pregnancy at delivery • fetal/neonatal complications/adverse outcomes • Exploratory measurement of preeclampsia-related maternal biomarkers (sFLT-1, sEng, PlGF, ET-1 and VCAM-1) • Others	31 October 2018	Recruiting	https://www.anzctr.org.au/Trial/Registration/TrialReview.aspx?id=374798 (accessed on 4 October 2021)
ACTRN12618001753224	Can esomeprazole improve outcomes in women at high risk of pre-eclampsia? The ESPRESSO Study	Multi-centre, double blind, placebo-controlled superiority trial.	Pregnant women screened at 11 + 0 to 13 + 6 weeks gestation and at high risk (>1%) of pre-eclampsia	Esomeprazole 40 mg oral tablet once a day prior to 16 weeks gestation and continuing until delivery of pregnancy. Aspirin 150 mg oral tablet at night commencing prior to 16 weeks gestation and continuing until 36 weeks gestation as a background therapy	Primary outcome measures: Mean arterial pressure, measured by 24-h ambulatory blood pressure at 36 weeks of gestation Secondary outcome measures: • Circulating sFlt-1, sEN, PLGF, sFlt-1/PLGF ratio concentrations at 36 weeks of gestation • Weight of the baby, apgar score, neonatal hospital discharge	18 April 2019	Recruiting	https://www.anzctr.org.au/Trial/Registration/TrialReview.aspx?id=375343 (accessed on 4 October 2021)

5. Conclusions

PPIs use may be associated with a trivial increase in the risk of preeclampsia in pregnant women. There is no evidence supporting that PPI use decreases the risk of preeclampsia or preterm preeclampsia. We recommend that future epidemiological studies consider all possible confounding factors, including the BMI. Furthermore, future population-based studies should ascertain the risk of preeclampsia and preterm preeclampsia separately by including a sufficiently large number of (preeclampsia and preterm preeclampsia) cases. The ongoing clinical trials of PPIs are expected to shed light on this important clinical question.

Supplementary Materials: The following are available online at https://www.mdpi.com/article/10.3390/jcm11164675/s1: Supplementary Table S1: PRISMA and MOOSE checklists. Table S2: Complete search strategy. Table S3: List of articles excluded with reasons during the full-text screening.

Author Contributions: Conceptualization, S.H.; methodology, S.H. and M.H.M.; meta-analysis, S.H.; investigation, S.H.; resources, S.H. and M.K.; data curation, S.H. and A.S.; writing—original draft preparation, S.H.; writing—review and editing, S.H., A.S., J.K., B.A., M.H.M., A.S.J., A.L. and M.K.; visualization, S.H.; supervision, S.H.; project administration, S.H.; and funding acquisition, M.K. All authors have read and agreed to the published version of the manuscript.

Funding: S.H. was supported by the Operational Programme Research, Development and Education–Project, Postdoc2MUNI (No. CZ.02.2.69/0.0/0.0/18_053/0016952). J.K. and M.K. were supported by the INTER-EXCELLENCE grant number LTC20031—"Towards an International Network for Evidence-based Research in Clinical Health Research in the Czech Republic".

Institutional Review Board Statement: Ethical review and approval were waived for this study due to its observational nature and its use of publicly accessible data.

Informed Consent Statement: Not applicable.

Data Availability Statement: The data that support the findings of this study are available from the corresponding author upon reasonable request.

Conflicts of Interest: The authors declare no conflict of interest.

References

1. Wang, W.; Xie, X.; Yuan, T.; Wang, Y.; Zhao, F.; Zhou, Z.; Zhang, H. Epidemiological trends of maternal hypertensive disorders of pregnancy at the global, regional, and national levels: A population-based study. *BMC Pregnancy Childbirth* **2021**, *21*, 364. [CrossRef] [PubMed]
2. Mayrink, J.; Souza, R.; Feitosa, F.E.; Filho, E.A.R.; Leite, D.; Vettorazzi, J.; Calderon, I.; Sousa, M.H.; Costa, M.L.; Preterm SAMBA study group; et al. Incidence and risk factors for Preeclampsia in a cohort of healthy nulliparous pregnant women: A nested case-control study. *Sci. Rep.* **2019**, *9*, 9517. [CrossRef] [PubMed]
3. García-Basteiro, A.L.; Quintó, L.; Macete, E.; Bardají, A.; González, R.; Nhacolo, A.; Sigauque, B.; Sacoor, C.; Rupérez, M.; Sicuri, E.; et al. Infant mortality and morbidity associated with preterm and small-for-gestational-age births in Southern Mozambique: A retrospective cohort study. *PLoS ONE* **2017**, *12*, e0172533. [CrossRef] [PubMed]
4. Crump, C.; Sundquist, J.; Sundquist, K. Preterm delivery and long term mortality in women: National cohort and co-sibling study. *BMJ* **2020**, *370*, m2533. [CrossRef] [PubMed]
5. D'Onofrio, B.M.; Class, Q.A.; Rickert, M.E.; Larsson, H.; Långström, N.; Lichtenstein, P. Preterm birth and mortality and morbidity: A population-based quasi-experimental study. *JAMA Psychiatry* **2013**, *70*, 1231–1240. [CrossRef] [PubMed]
6. Hannan, N.J.; Kaitu'u-Lino, T.U.; Tuohey, L.; Brownfoot, F.; Tong, S.; Onda, K. Proton Pump Inhibitors Induce Heme-Oxygenase-1 and Decrease sFlt1 and sEng Production in Primary Placental and Endothelial Cells: A Novel Candidate Therapeutic for Preeclampsia. In *Reproductive Sciences*; Sage Publications Inc.: Thousand Oaks, CA, USA, 2014.
7. Onda, K.; Hannan, N.; Beard, S. [6-OR]: Proton pump inhibitors for treatment of preeclampsia. *Pregnancy Hypertens. Int. J. Women's Cardiovasc. Health* **2015**, *5*, 3.
8. Onda, K.; Tong, S.; Beard, S.; Binder, N.; Muto, M.; Senadheera, S.N.; Parry, L.; Dilworth, M.; Renshall, L.; Brownfoot, F.; et al. Proton Pump Inhibitors Decrease Soluble fms-Like Tyrosine Kinase-1 and Soluble Endoglin Secretion, Decrease Hypertension, and Rescue Endothelial Dysfunction. *Hypertension* **2017**, *69*, 457–468. [CrossRef]
9. Tong, S.; Tu'uhevaha, J.; Hastie, R.; Brownfoot, F.; Cluver, C.; Hannan, N. Pravastatin, proton pump inhibitors, metformin, micronutrients and biologics: New horizons for the prevention or treatment of preeclampsia. *Am. J. Obstet. Gynecol.* **2020**, *226*, S1157–S1170. [CrossRef]

10. Binder, N.K.; Brownfoot, F.C.; Beard, S.; Cannon, P.; Nguyen, T.V.; Tong, S.; Kaitu'U-Lino, T.J.; Hannan, N.J. Esomeprazole and sulfasalazine in combination additively reduce sFlt-1 secretion and diminish endothelial dysfunction: Potential for a combination treatment for preeclampsia. *Pregnancy Hypertens. Health* **2020**, *22*, 86–92. [CrossRef]
11. Saleh, L.; Samantar, R.; Garrelds, I.M.; Meiracker, A.H.V.D.; Visser, W.; Danser, A.J. Low Soluble Fms-Like Tyrosine Kinase-1, Endoglin, and Endothelin-1 Levels in Women with Confirmed or Suspected Preeclampsia Using Proton Pump Inhibitors. *Hypertension* **2017**, *70*, 594–600. [CrossRef]
12. Des Varannes, S.B.; Coron, E.; Galmiche, J.-P. Short and long-term PPI treatment for GERD. Do we need more-potent anti-secretory drugs? *Best Pract. Res. Clin. Gastroenterol.* **2010**, *24*, 905–921. [CrossRef] [PubMed]
13. Hussain, S.; Siddiqui, A.N.; Habib, A.; Hussain, S.; Najmi, A.K. Proton pump inhibitors' use and risk of hip fracture: A systematic review and meta-analysis. *Rheumatol. Int.* **2018**, *38*, 1999–2014. [CrossRef] [PubMed]
14. Hussain, S.; Singh, A.; Habib, A.; Najmi, A.K. Proton pump inhibitors use and risk of chronic kidney disease: Evidence-based meta-analysis of observational studies. *Clin. Epidemiol. Glob. Health* **2019**, *7*, 46–52. [CrossRef]
15. Hussain, S.; Singh, A.; Zameer, S.; Jamali, M.C.; Baxi, H.; Rahman, S.O.; Alam, M.; Altamish, M.; Singh, A.K.; Anil, D.; et al. No association between proton pump inhibitor use and risk of dementia: Evidence from a meta-analysis. *J. Gastroenterol. Hepatol.* **2020**, *35*, 19–28. [CrossRef]
16. Singh, A.; Hussain, S.; Jha, R.; Jayraj, A.S.; Klugar, M.; Antony, B. Proton pump inhibitor use and the risk of hepatocellular carcinoma: A systematic review of pharmacoepidemiological data. *J. Evid. Based Med.* **2021**, *14*, 278–280. [CrossRef]
17. Johnson, D.A.; Katz, P.O.; Armstrong, D.; Cohen, H.; Delaney, B.C.; Howden, C.W.; Katelaris, P.; Tutuian, R.I.; Castell, D.O. The Safety of Appropriate Use of Over-the-Counter Proton Pump Inhibitors: An Evidence-Based Review and Delphi Consensus. *Drugs* **2017**, *77*, 547–561. [CrossRef]
18. Pasternak, B.; Hviid, A. Use of Proton-Pump Inhibitors in Early Pregnancy and the Risk of Birth Defects. *N. Engl. J. Med.* **2010**, *363*, 2114–2123. [CrossRef]
19. Li, C.M.; Zhernakova, A.; Engstrand, L.; Wijmenga, C.; Brusselaers, N. Systematic review with meta-analysis: The risks of proton pump inhibitors during pregnancy. *Aliment. Pharmacol. Ther.* **2020**, *51*, 410–420. [CrossRef]
20. Hastie, R.; Bergman, L.; Cluver, C.A.; Wikman, A.; Hannan, N.J.; Walker, S.P.; Wikström, A.; Tong, S.; Hesselman, S. Proton Pump Inhibitors and Preeclampsia Risk Among 157 720 Women: A Swedish Population Register–Based Cohort Study. *Hypertension* **2019**, *73*, 1097–1103. [CrossRef]
21. Choi, A.; Noh, Y.; Park, S.-H.; Choe, S.-A.; Shin, J.-Y. Exploration of Proton Pump Inhibitors Use During Pregnancy and Preeclampsia. *JAMA Netw. Open* **2021**, *4*, e2124339. [CrossRef]
22. Bello, N.A.; Huang, Y.; Syeda, S.K.; Wright, J.D.; D'Alton, M.E.; Friedman, A.M. Receipt of Proton-Pump Inhibitors during Pregnancy and Risk for Preeclampsia. *Am. J. Perinatol.* **2020**, *38*, 1519–1525. [CrossRef]
23. Hussain, S.; Singh, A.; Antony, B.; Klugarová, J.; Klugar, M. Proton pump inhibitors use and risk of preeclampsia. *medRxiv* **2021**. [CrossRef]
24. Aromataris, E.; Munn, Z. (Eds.) *JBI Manual for Evidence Synthesis*; JBI: Adelaide, Australia, 2020.
25. Higgins, J.; Thomas, J. *Cochrane Handbook for Systematic Reviews of Interventions*, 2nd ed.; John Wiley and Sons, Ltd.: Chichester, UK, 2019; pp. 143–176.
26. Page, M.J.; McKenzie, J.E.; Bossuyt, P.M.; Boutron, I.; Hoffmann, T.C.; Mulrow, C.D.; Shamseer, L.; Tetzlaff, J.M.; Akl, E.A.; Brennan, S.E.; et al. The PRISMA 2020 statement: An updated guideline for reporting systematic reviews. *BMJ* **2021**, *88*, 105906.
27. Stroup, D.F.; Berlin, J.A.; Morton, S.C.; Olkin, I.; Williamson, G.D.; Rennie, D.; Moher, D.; Becker, B.J.; Sipe, T.A.; Thacker, S.B. Meta-analysis of observational studies in epidemiology: A proposal for reporting. Meta-analysis Of Observational Studies in Epidemiology (MOOSE) group. *JAMA* **2008**, *283*, 2008–2012. [CrossRef] [PubMed]
28. Hussain, S.; Singh, A.; Antony BS, E.; Kulgarova, J.; Licenik, R.; Klugar, M. Association of acute kidney injury with the risk of dementia: A meta-analysis protocol. *medRxiv* **2021**. [CrossRef]
29. Wells, G.A.; Shea, B.; O'Connell, D.; Peterson, J.; Welch, V.; Losos, M.; Tugwell, P. The Newcastle-Ottawa Scale (NOS) for Assessing the Quality of Nonrandomised Studies in Meta-Analyses. 2000. Available online: https://www.ohri.ca//programs/clinical_epidemiology/oxford.asp (accessed on 4 October 2021).
30. Viswanathan, M.; Patnode, C.D.; Berkman, N.D.; Bass, E.; Chang, S.; Hartling, L.; Murad, M.H.; Treadwell, J.R.; Kane, R.L. Recommendations for assessing the risk of bias in systematic reviews of health-care interventions. *J. Clin. Epidemiol.* **2018**, *97*, 26–34. [CrossRef]
31. Group, G.W. Grading quality of evidence and strength of recommendations. *BMJ* **2004**, *328*, 1490.
32. Kwok, C.S.; Jeevanantham, V.; Dawn, B.; Loke, Y.K. No consistent evidence of differential cardiovascular risk amongst proton-pump inhibitors when used with clopidogrel: Meta-analysis. *Int. J. Cardiol.* **2013**, *167*, 965–974. [CrossRef]
33. Singh, A.; Hussain, S.; Najmi, A.K. Number of studies, heterogeneity, generalisability, and the choice of method for meta-analysis. *J. Neurol. Sci.* **2017**, *381*, 347. [CrossRef]
34. McMaster University. Evidence Prime. GRADEpro GDT: GRADEpro Guideline Development Tool [Software]. 2022. Available online: gradepro.org (accessed on 4 October 2021).
35. Cluver, C.A.; Hannan, N.J.; van Papendorp, E.; Hiscock, R.; Beard, S.; Mol, B.W.; Theron, G.B.; Hall, D.R.; Decloedt, E.H.; Stander, M.; et al. Esomeprazole to treat women with preterm preeclampsia: A randomized placebo controlled trial. *Am. J. Obstet. Gynecol.* **2018**, *219*, 388.e1–388.e17. [CrossRef]

36. Abbas, A.M.; Othman, Y.M.; Abdallah, M.M.; Ellah, N.H.A.; Azim, H.G.A.; Shaamash, A.H. Effect of esomeprazole on maternal serum soluble fms-like tyrosine kinase-1 and endoglin in patients with early-onset preeclampsia. *Proc. Obstet. Gynecol.* **2021**, *99*, 1–14. [CrossRef]
37. Ramu, B.; Mohan, P.; Rajasekaran, M.S.; Jayanthi, V. Prevalence and risk factors for gastroesophageal reflux in pregnancy. *Indian J. Gastroenterol.* **2010**, *30*, 144–147. [CrossRef] [PubMed]
38. Poorolajal, J.; Jenabi, E. The association between body mass index and preeclampsia: A meta-analysis. *J. Matern. Neonatal Med.* **2016**, *29*, 3670–3676. [CrossRef] [PubMed]

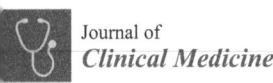

Review

Preeclampsia and Fetal Growth Restriction as Risk Factors of Future Maternal Cardiovascular Disease—A Review

Sylwia Sławek-Szmyt [1,*], Katarzyna Kawka-Paciorkowska [2], Aleksandra Ciepłucha [1], Maciej Lesiak [1] and Mariola Ropacka-Lesiak [2]

1. 1st Department of Cardiology, Poznan University of Medical Sciences, 61-848 Poznan, Poland
2. Department of Perinatology and Gynecology, Poznan University of Medical Sciences, 60-535 Poznan, Poland
* Correspondence: sylwia.slawek@skpp.edu.pl; Tel.: +48-854-9146

Abstract: Cardiovascular diseases (CVDs) remain the leading cause of death in women worldwide. Although traditional risk factors increase later-life CVD, pregnancy-associated complications additionally influence future CVD risk in women. Adverse pregnancy outcomes, including preeclampsia and fetal growth restriction (FGR), are interrelated disorders caused by placental dysfunction, maternal cardiovascular maladaptation to pregnancy, and maternal abnormalities such as endothelial dysfunction, inflammation, hypercoagulability, and vasospasm. The pathophysiologic pathways of some pregnancy complications and CVDs might be linked. This review aimed to highlight the associations between specific adverse pregnancy outcomes and future CVD and emphasize the importance of considering pregnancy history in assessing a woman's CVD risk. Moreover, we wanted to underline the role of maternal cardiovascular maladaptation in the development of specific pregnancy complications such as FGR.

Keywords: cardiovascular disease; pregnancy complications; fetal growth restriction; preeclampsia; maternal morbidity

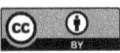

1. Introduction

Cardiovascular diseases (CVDs) are the leading cause of women's mortality globally, accounting for approximately one of every three female deaths [1]. The population-adjusted risk of CVDs-related death is significantly higher for women compared to men, 21% versus 15%, respectively [2]. Despite the significant decline in CVDs-related death in the last few decades, the mortality for women has decreased much slower than for men [3]. The underlying risk factors are frequently present many years before the clinical presentation of CVDs. Moreover, there has been growing evidence that women with a history of certain pregnancy complications are at increased risk of developing CVDs in the future [4,5]. These adverse pregnancy outcomes (APOs) include fetal growth disorders, gestational hypertension, or preeclampsia (See Table 1) [6].

Pregnancy acts as a maternal stress test, and the development of obstetric complications plays a potential role in a woman's susceptibility to future CVDs. The etiologic pathways of pregnancy complications and CVDs might also be linked (e.g., metabolic syndrome, vascular dysfunction, or inflammation) [7]. The importance of these associations has been raised by the current guidelines, which now recommend a pregnancy history as a part of the routine evaluation of cardiovascular risk in women [8,9].

It is increasingly apparent that the effects of the maternal cardiovascular system maladaptation changes the predisposition to CVDs development after pregnancy. We aimed to systematically evaluate and quantify the evidence on the relationship between specific APOs' and maternal risk of future cardiovascular disease. However, other factors, such as diabetes, renal impairment, or other dysmetabolic conditions will not be included in the analysis.

Table 1. Definitions of adverse pregnancy outcomes (APOs).

Type of APO	Definition
Gestational hypertension	De novo hypertension that develops after 20 weeks of pregnancy: - systolic blood pressure equal to or higher than 140 mmHg AND/OR - diastolic pressure equal to or higher than 90 mmHg on two separate occasions in a patient who was previously normotensive without proteinuria or other end-organ involvement [6].
Preeclampsia	De novo hypertension that develops after 20 weeks of pregnancy AND: 1. Proteinuria ($\geq$300 mg/24-h of 0.3 g/g by urine protein: creatinine ratio or +1 by urine dipstick), OR 2. In the absence of proteinuria: - serum creatinine $\geq$ 90 µmol/L - alkaline or aspartate transaminase > 40 IU/L - platelet count < 150 000/µL - neurological complications (including altered mental status, blindness, stroke, severe headaches, clonus, and persistent visual scotomata) - uteroplacental dysfunction (including fetal growth disorder, abnormal umbilical artery Doppler waveform analysis or stillbirth) [10,11].
Fetal growth restriction (a) Early-onset (diagnosed before 32 weeks of gestation):	1. Fetal abdominal circumference below the 3rd percentile for gestational age OR 2. Estimated fetal weight below the 3rd percentile for gestational age, OR 3. The absence of end-diastolic flow of the umbilical artery on Doppler, AND - estimated fetal weight, or waist circumference below the 10th percentile for gestational age, AND - the pulsatility index of the uterine, and/or umbilical arteries above the 95th percentile for gestational age [12].
(b) Late-onset (diagnosed at or after 32 weeks of gestation):	1. Fetal abdominal circumference below the 3rd percentile for gestational age, OR 2. Estimated fetal weight below the 3rd percentile for gestational age, AND the combination of at least two of the following parameters: - estimated fetal weight or fetal abdominal circumference below the 10th percentile for gestational age, - the reduction in more than two quartiles in the growth curve - the cerebroplacental association below the 5th for gestational age - the pulsatility index of the umbilical artery above the 95th percentile for gestational age [12].
Gestational diabetes mellitus	One or more of the following criteria met at any time of pregnancy: - fasting plasma glucose 5.1–6.9 mmol/L (92–125 mg/dL) - 1-h plasma glucose $\geq$ 10.0 mmol/L (180 mg/dL) following a 75 g oral glucose load [13].

2. Preeclampsia

Preeclampsia is a pregnancy-specific disorder with an estimated incidence of 2–8% of all gestations associated with high maternal, fetal, and neonatal morbidity and mortality worldwide [14–16]. A detailed definition of preeclampsia is provided in Table 1. There is growing evidence of long-term cardiovascular sequelae in women who had preeclampsia during pregnancy [17,18].

2.1. Preeclampsia and Maternal Cardiovascular Risk

Several studies have shown the relationship between preeclampsia and future maternal CVDs [19–23]. The CHAMPS (Cardiovascular Health After Maternal Placental Syndromes) study indicated a more than a 2-fold increased risk of CVD (defined as hospital admission or revascularization for coronary artery, cerebrovascular, or peripheral artery disease at least 90 days after the delivery discharge date) in women affected by preeclampsia with absent traditional CVD risk factors (HR: 2.1; 95% CI: 1.8–2.4), and approximately 12-fold increased risk of CVD in women with a history of preeclampsia and metabolic syndrome (hazard ratio [HR]: 11.7; 95% confidence interval [CI]: 4.9–28.3) as compared to women with neither [19]. Apart from the pregnancy-specific factors and age, other risk factors are shared by preeclampsia and CVDs, but a direct causative relationship has not yet been determined. Lin et al., in a study performed on a Taiwanese cohort, demonstrated an increased risk of major adverse cardiovascular events including myocardial infarction, cardiogenic shock, heart failure, stroke, malignant dysrhythmia, or any other condition requiring percutaneous cardiac intervention, coronary artery bypass, an implantable cardiac defibrillator, or thrombolysis within three years of a preeclamptic pregnancy (HR: 12.6; 95% CI: 2.4–66.3) [20]. Kestenbaum et al., showed more than a 3-fold increase in cardiovascular events (hospitalizations due to MI, stroke, or percutaneous coronary artery interventions) (HR: 3.3; 95% CI: 1.7–6.5) and a higher number of thromboembolic events (HR: 2.3; 95% CI: 1.3 to 4.2) among women with previous severe preeclampsia during a mean follow-up of approximately eight years [22]. Furthermore, a Norwegian population-based cohort study with a median 13-year follow-up found an increased risk of CVD-related death defined as coronary artery disease, disease of the pulmonary circulation, or other diseases affecting the heart in women with a history of preeclampsia during pregnancy (RR: 1.65, 95% CI: 1.01–2.70), but the risk of CVD-related death was markedly higher in women with preeclampsia and preterm delivery (RR: 8.12, 95% CI: 4.31–15.33) as compared to women with a history of uncomplicated pregnancy [23]. The results of the British CALIBER (Cardiovascular Research using Linked Bespoke Studies and Electronic Health Records) study were similar, along with the reported overall first-time cardiovascular event incidence of 2.77% in the first nine years after a delivery complicated by preeclampsia in contrast to a 1.4% rate in women after an uncomplicated pregnancy [24].

Recent metanalysis reported that even after adjusting for potential confounders including age, body mass index, and diabetes mellitus, preeclampsia was related to increased risk of heart failure (RR: 1.6, 95% CI: 0.73–3.5), stroke (RR: 1.18; 95% CI, 0.95–1.46), coronary artery disease (RR: 1.46; 95% CI: 0.95–2.25), and death because of coronary artery disease (RR: 2.10; 95% CI, 1.25–3.51) or cardiovascular disease (RR: 2.21; 95% CI, 1.83–2.66), more than ten years after a pregnancy affected by preeclampsia. However, the increase in the risk for heart failure, stroke, and CVD-related death was even higher during the first decade after a pregnancy complicated with preeclampsia [25].

Notably, another large cohort study indicated an elevated risk of CVD-related death in women with a history of preeclampsia (HR: 2.14; 95% CI: 1.29–3.57), with a further significant risk acceleration if preeclampsia occurred before 34 weeks of gestation (HR: 9.54; 95% CI: 4.5–20.26) [26]. Moreover, Riise et al., reported a further increase in the CVD risk defined by coronary artery disease, after the recurrence of preeclampsia (HR 2.20; 95% CI: 0.91–5.32 in recurrent preeclampsia and HR 1.95; 95% CI: 1.31–2.91 for a single pre-eclampsia pregnancy), compared with uncomplicated pregnancies. When preeclampsia was combined with FGR or preterm birth, the risk was markedly higher (HR 4.66; 95% CI: 2.31–9.37 in recurrent preeclampsia as in comparison to one episode of preeclampsia; HR 2.81; 95% CI: 1.70–4.61) [27]. Other studies also support these results [RR 2.40; 95% CI: 2.15–2.68] [28–30]. Details are presented in Table 2. A higher frequency of heart failure (HR 4.2; 95% CI: 2.9–6.1) and cerebrovascular disease (HR 3.0; 95% CI: 1.70–4.61) among women with recurrent preeclampsia compared to women with unaffected pregnancy has also been reported [31].

Table 2. Selected published studies of preeclampsia and future risk of cardiovascular disease.

Study/First Author (Reference)	Design	Population Size	Follow-Up (Period, Years)	Outcome Measure	Risk of Outcome Measures HR (95% CI)
Ray [20]	Retrospective	1,030,000	-	CVD	2.1 (1.8–2.4)
Lin [21]	Registry	1,132,064	>3 years	Any MACE	12.6 (2.4–66.3)
				MI	13.0 (4.6–6.3)
				Heart failure	8.3 (4.2–16.4)
				Stroke	14.5 (1.3–165.1)
				MACE-related death	2.3 (1.6–3.1)

Table 2. Cont.

Study/First Author (Reference)	Design	Population Size	Follow-Up (Period, Years)	Outcome Measure	Risk of Outcome Measures HR (95% CI)
Kestenbaum [22]	Retrospective	31,239	-	CV events Thromboembolic events	2.2 (1.3–3.6) (mild pre-eclampsia) and 3.3 (1.7–6.5) (severe pre-eclampsia) 2.3 (1.3–4.2) (severe pre-eclampsia)
Irgens [23]	Registry	626,272	0 to 25 years (median 13 years)	CVD-related death	1.65, (1.01–2.70)—with preeclampsia 8.12 (4.31–15.33) with preeclampsia and preterm birth
Mongraw-Chaffin [26]	Retrospective	14,403	Median 37 years	CVD-related death	2.14 (1.29–3.57) 9.54 (4.50–20.26) if onset of preeclampsia before 34 weeks' gestation
Auger [32]	Registry	1,108,581	0–25.2 years (Median 15.5 years)	CAD HF Cerebrovascular disease	3.3 (2.1–5.2) 4.2 (2.9–6.1) 3.0 (2.3–4.1)—with recurrent preeclampsia
CALIBER [24]	Registry	1,300,000	-	CAD Stroke Heart failure, Hypertension CVD-related death	1.67 (1.54–1.81) 1.9 (1.53–2.35) 2.13 (1.64–2.76) 4.47 (4.32–4.62) 2.12 (1.49–2.99)
Wikstrom [33]	Registry	403,555	15 years	CAD	1.6 (1.3–2.0) with GHA 1.9 (1.6–2.2) with mild preeclampsia 2.8 (CI 2.2–3.7) with severe pre-eclampsia
Smith [34]	Registry	129,920	15–19 years	CAD-related death	1.7 (0.9–3.3)
Lykke [35]	Registry	782,287	14.6 years	CVD-related death	2.08 (1.63–2.64)
Kessous [36]	Registry	96,370	10 years	CVD: hospitalization for CAD, stroke, peripheral vascular disease, hyperlipidemia, angina, hypertension, atherosclerosis, MI, heart failure, pulmonary heart disease, cardiac arrest, cardiac catheterization, or cardiovascular stress test	1.7 (1.6–1.9)
Crillo [37]	Registry	14,062	40 years	CAD-related death	3.6 (1.04–12.19)
Hannaford [38]	Prospective	23,000	Not available	Hypertension CAD Angina Venous thromboembolism	2.35 (2.08–2.65) 1.65 (1.26–2.16) 1.53 (1.09–2.15) 1.62 (1.09–2.41)

Table 2. Cont.

Study/First Author (Reference)	Design	Population Size	Follow-Up (Period, Years)	Outcome Measure	Risk of Outcome Measures HR (95% CI)
McDonald [39]	Metanalysis	2,375,751	Not available	CVD-related death Stroke Peripheral artery disease	2.29 (1.73–3.04) 2.03 (1.54–2.67) 1.87 (0.94–3.73)
Wu [25]	Metanalysis	6,400,000	Not available	CAD CAD-related death Heart failure stroke CVD-related death	1.46 (0.95–2.25) 2.1 (1.25–3.51) 1.6 (0.73–3.5) 1.18 (0.95–1.46) 2.21 (1.83–2.66)

Abbreviations: CAD, coronary artery disease; CV, cerebrovascular; CVD, cardiovascular disease; HF, heart failure; MACE, major adverse cardiovascular event; MI, myocardial infarction.

2.2. Potential Mechanisms Linking Preeclampsia and Development of Future Maternal Cardiovascular Diseases

A few potential explanations for the association between preeclampsia and CVD are discussed. It has been proposed that preeclampsia may contribute as a predictor of cardiovascular events through distinct pathways [25]. On the other hand, the link between future CVD and preeclampsia may in part be due to shared risk factors between these entities. An unfavorable cardiovascular risk profile characterized by dyslipidemia, insulin resistance, diabetes, obesity, or endothelial dysfunction, heightened inflammatory responses, and hypercoagulable states frequent in preeclamptic women may result in an increased risk of CVD [14,25,40]. Another theory, which may be related to the above-mentioned, includes permanent vascular changes with excessive endothelial dysfunction that mediate the risk for future CVD [41].

Preeclampsia is characterized by pathological remodeling of the placental vessels, which is considered the main cause of uteroplacental ischemia. Spiral arteries do not undergo a physiological transformation and retain thick walls with a narrow lumen. The unsuccessful remodeling of spiral arteries results in high-velocity maternal blood flow at the intervillous space (approximately of 1–2 m/s) with a high spurt destroying the villi and forming thrombus-lined echogenic cystic lesions which can also be released to maternal circulation [42]. Furthermore, remodeling failure results in a repeated cycle of placental ischemia/reperfusion and leads to endothelial dysfunction, increases in the formation of reactive oxygen species (ROS) and the release of inflammatory cytokines and antiangiogenic factors, and maternal immune cell imbalance [43]. ROS decreases the bioavailability of proangiogenic factors such as nitric oxide which can result in impaired vasodilation, and angiogenesis, and increases the bioavailability of antiangiogenic factors such as soluble fms-like tyrosine kinase 1 (sFlt-1) soluble Endoglin (sEng) [44]. sFlt-1 is linked with defective angiogenesis and endothelial dysfunction by binding vascular endothelial growth factor and placental growth factor, while sEng which is a cell-surface co-receptor of transforming growth factor β (TGF β) initiates the proliferation and migration of endothelial cells [42]. It is believed that these antiangiogenic biomarkers strongly contribute to endothelial damage during the preeclamptic pregnancy, but do not remain significantly elevated after the delivery. It is hypothesized that the vascular damage sustained during the preeclamptic pregnancy persists and contributes to its own cascade in the CVD development in these patients [41]. Moreover, ROS disrupts maternal endothelial function by releasing cell-free fetal DNA and extracellular vesicles such as exomes into the maternal circulation [42].

Endothelial dysfunction is associated with inflammation and in consequence atherosclerosis [43]. The lipid deposition in the walls of the uterine spiral arteries resembles the early stages of atherosclerosis [45]. During early atherogenesis, low-density lipoprotein delivers cholesterol to the activated macrophages, which scavenge lipids. In an inflammatory milieu, the cholesterol cannot be recycled back into the circulation to the liver instead, it is trapped in the macrophages due to impaired reverse cholesterol transport in inflammation [46].

Acute atherosis in spiral arteries is represented by subendothelial lipid-filled foam cells enriched by CD68-positive macrophages, arterial wall fibrinoid necrosis, and perivascular lymphocytic infiltration [46,47]. It is also postulated that T regulatory cells (Tregs) protect against the development of atherosclerosis by downregulating effector T cell responses, despite their main role in maternal immunoregulation. However, the Tregs differentiation is stimulated by TGF β. As the above-mentioned TGF β is modulated by sEng, so it seems that high concentrations of sEng could locally inhibit the generation of Tregs cells and thereby promote acute atherosis [46].

The novel hypothesis links cellular fetal microchimerism (cFMC) with acute atherosis and the future development of CVD [48]. cFMC arises when cells of fetal origin are released into maternal blood and tissues during pregnancy [48]. These cells are known to possess stem cell-like properties, with the potential to differentiate into endothelial cells, smooth muscle cells, or leukocytes, and may persist in maternal circulation for decades [49]. Recent studies reported that cFMCs are more frequent in pregnancies complicated by preeclampsia or severe FGR than in healthy pregnancies [50,51]. It is hypothesized that in the dysfunctional placenta, fetal cells transfer more freely into the maternal bloodstream and induce a maternal anti-fetal immune response towards the fetal cells expressing foreign HLA surface peptides. If fetal cells persist in the circulation or are engrafted in maternal endothelial cells, they could induce further inflammation, especially in vessel walls, and initiate the development of inflammatory arterial lesions, particularly as acute atherosis [48].

Another possible mechanism involved in endothelial dysfunction seen in both atherosclerosis and preeclampsia is abnormal endothelial to mesenchymal transition (EndMT) [43]. EndMT is a normal, complex, dynamic, and reversible process during pregnancy in which epithelial cells lose polarity and adhesiveness, change to a mesenchymal phenotype, and acquire increased mobility [52]. Abnormal EndMT is observed in preeclampsia and is frequent in atherosclerotic lesions and plays a role in plaque progression and calcification [43].

It is hypothesized that in preeclamptic women, the endothelial integrity is not fully restored and remains more sensitized to stress-related or inflammatory stimuli as observed in atherosclerosis [43]. It was recently reported that women with placental malperfusion lesions had an adverse cardiovascular profile comprised of microvascular rarefaction with abnormalities in circulating endothelial and antiangiogenic factors, higher blood pressure, and more atherogenic lipids years after delivery [53]. Drost et al., showed that women with a history of preeclampsia have higher levels of SE-selectin and pregnancy-associated plasma protein A(PAPPA) compared to women with healthy pregnancies a decade after PE, after adjustment for traditional CVD risk factors [54]. SE-selectin is a marker of endothelial dysfunction, while PAPPA is a metalloproteinase associated with the presence of vulnerable atherosclerotic plaques and myocardial infarction [54,55]. Metalloproteinases may be the link between placental alterations in pregnancy and CVD in later life, supporting the hypothesis that vascular alterations in preeclampsia lead to persistent vascular damage and early development of atherosclerosis [54]. It is also postulated that comorbidities (e.g., gestational diabetes) may worsen the clinical course of preeclampsia by sharing similar placental vascular alterations that synergistically increase the risk of future CVD [56,57].

It is also hypothesized that several common genetic or epigenetic mechanisms may predispose to both acute atherosis and atherosclerosis and future CVDs [58]. It was found that women with a polymorphism of the regulator of the G protein signaling (RGS2) gene are at a higher risk of both preeclampsia and acute atherosis [59]. Reduced expression of RGS2 has also been linked to arterial hypertension [58].

Furthermore, subclinical markers of CVD, such as coronary artery calcium score (CACS), are also significantly higher in women with a previous pregnancy complicated by preeclampsia even after adjustment for age, blood pressure, and body mass index [22,23,60–62]. Moreover, 47% of women with prior preeclampsia had coronary atherosclerotic plaques on coronary computed tomography angiography and 4.3% had significant stenosis [63]. Formerly preeclamptic women develop coronary artery calcifications on average five years earlier from the age of 45 years onwards than women with prior normotensive pregnancy [64]. It was hypothesized that the body may not recover from the changes in the vascular and metabolic systems associated with preeclampsia and may demonstrate in later life with future cardiovascular events [64]. Similarly, previous studies demonstrated an increase in carotid intima-media thickness, a marker of subclinical atherosclerosis augmentation index in women with previous preeclampsia compared to age- and parity-matched controls [65].

Recent studies have shown that extracellular vesicles (EVs) are essential mediators in preeclampsia-related maternal CVDs [66,67]. EVs are membrane-bound particles consisting of bioactive proteins, lipids, DNA, mRNA, and microRNA (miR) that participate in cell-to-cell communication [66]. Placenta-derived EVs interact with the maternal immune system resulting in vascular inflammation and endothelial injury [66]. Several miRNAs in the placenta or blood of women with preeclampsia have been reported to be upregulated or downregulated compared with healthy pregnant women [67]. In particular, has-miRNA-134 overexpression is hypothesized to be involved in the inhibition of trophoblast cell infiltration by targeting integrin beta-1. has-miRNA-134 has also been associated with atherosclerosis, particularly acute myocardial infarction [67]. has-miRNA-23a-3p overexpression has been demonstrated to be involved in the pathophysiology of myocardial infarction and heart failure [68]. has-miRNA-23a-3p upregulation has been reported in the pathophysiology of myocardial infarction and heart failure and vascular calcification [68]. The up-regulation of has-miRNA-499a-5p has been linked with hypertension, preeclampsia, and FGR [69].

Physiological heart hypertrophy, which occurs during pregnancy in response to volume overload and hormonal stimuli, enables the heart to fulfill its function without significant long-term detrimental effects on cardiac function [66,70]. Higher vulnerability of ischemia-reperfusion injury during pregnancy complicated by preeclampsia is associated with increased ROS generation and decreased threshold for triggering the mitochondrial permeability transition pore opening. Pregnancy also has an impact on the number and content of EVs affecting the function of the heart. Placenta-derived EVs may impact ischemia-related injury due to a higher generation of ROS and activation of apoptosis during pregnancy [40]. Recently, Powell et al., demonstrated that EVs from preeclamptic women contribute to arterial tone regulation. They documented that ex vivo exposure of isolated mouse mesenteric arteries to EVs purified from the plasma of pregnant women with preeclampsia led to constriction in response to intraluminal pressure and resistance to methacholine-stimulated relaxation [71]. Furthermore, it is also suggested that EVs-exosomes from preeclampsia contribute to the dissemination of endothelial damage by sequestering the free vascular endothelial growth factor (VEGF) in the maternal circulation [72–78].

Moreover, gravidas with preeclampsia have significantly lower levels of angiotensin II compared to normal pregnancy, and these women have exacerbated vascular responses to angiotensin II in later life which also contributes to impaired microvascular function [74,75]. Interestingly, the expression of neprilysin is significantly increased in preeclampsia [76]. Neprilysin is released into the maternal circulation bound to placenta-derived EVs [66]. Increased levels of neprilysin might contribute to the persistence of hypertension and cardiac remodeling after pregnancy. A few studies based on animal models found the important role of the upregulated endothelin-1-mediated signaling in reduced endothelium-dependent dilation in preeclampsia [41,77].

Another possible mechanism linking preeclampsia with future CVD is increased sympathetic activity [44]. It has been reported that maladaptive baroreceptor responses are associated with persistently reduced plasma volume in women after a pregnancy complicated with preeclampsia opposite to normal sympathetic activity in women with uncomplicated pregnancies who return to euvolemia [44,78].

The mechanisms underlying the development of heart failure in women with prior preeclampsia remain poorly understood. It was previously suggested that preeclampsia might be a part of a pathway that leads to impairments in cardiac function [79]. Miralles et al., reported that preeclampsia might have long-term effects on the maternal cardiovascular system independently of any predisposing conditions. They used the STOX1 (the first gene identified in human families with preeclampsia via positional cloning) mouse model of preeclampsia and showed the expression of this gene in the disruption of cytotrophoblast function, associated with a marked imbalance between nitrosative and oxidative stresses within the placenta. They observed left ventricular hypertrophy, fibrotic cardiomyocytes, kidney glomerulitis, and modified transcriptome profile of the endothelial cells in female mice with preeclampsia as compared to normotensive controls [80]. Transcriptomic analysis indicated the deregulation of 165 genes in the heart, mainly linked with cardiac hypertrophy, and of 1149 genes in purified endothelial cells, associated with inflammation and cellular stress [80].

Women with pregnancies affected by preeclampsia have evidence of biventricular diastolic dysfunction and impaired systolic strain despite preservation of global systolic function assessed by ejection fraction [81]. During a hypertensive pregnancy, a significant increase in ventricular mass and relative ventricular wall thickness is also observed, indicating that the disproportion between wall thickens and the increase in ventricular volume [82]. Additionally, preeclampsia might cause structural and functional vascular changes that, along with cardiac remodeling, may result in microcirculatory shortfall [83]. Several previous studies indicated that in 25% to 72% of these women, the above-mentioned cardiac adaptations persist and do not revert during the postpartum period, causing a higher vulnerability to develop cardiovascular disease in later life [84–86]. A recent metanalysis showed a higher left ventricular mass index in women with prior preeclampsia with a mean difference of 4.25 g/m2 (95% CI, 2.08–6.42) [87]. On the contrary, others reported either no increase in left ventricular mass or a reversion to a pre-pregnancy state [81,85,88–90].

Most studies demonstrated a reduction in global strain in all principal directions (radial, circumferential, longitudinal), whereas few studies with relatively low samples did not indicate a significant difference [81,85,91,92]. In comparison with the no preeclampsia population, they also demonstrated a lower E/A ratio and a higher E/e' ratio with a mean difference of -0.08 (95% CI, -0.15, -0.01) and 0.84 (95% CI, 0.41, 1.27), respectively [87]. Therefore, subtle contractional dysfunction may already occur without loss of ejection fraction in formerly preeclamptic women, indicating global strain as a sensitive parameter for early detection of cardiac function abnormalities [85].

3. Fetal Growth Restriction

Fetal growth restriction (FGR) is a condition of placental etiology with characteristics of inappropriate maternal cardiovascular system adaptation during pregnancy. In this APO, the fetus does not reach its biological growth potential due to impaired placental function, which may result from a variety of factors [93]. It is estimated that FGR complicates up to 10% of pregnancies and is one of the leading causes of infant morbidity and mortality [93,94]. The etiology of FGR is complex and can be caused by maternal (hypertension, diabetes, cardiopulmonary disease, anemia, malnutrition, smoking, drug use), fetal causes (genetic factors, congenital malformations, fetal infection, multiple pregnancies), and placental causes (placental insufficiency, placental infarction, placental mosaicism) [94]. FGR has been classified based on gestational age at prenatal ultrasound diagnosis as early-onset—diagnosed before 32 weeks of gestation and late-onset—diagnosed at or after 32 weeks of gestation [93,95]. The recent international Delphi consensus proposed an algorithm-based definition of FGR, which combine information on multiple fetal growth indicators in a deterministic manner [12]. Details are presented in Table 1.

The etiology of FGR differs depending on whether we consider early or late-onset fetal growth restriction. In early-onset FGR, two possible mechanisms concerning placental abnormalities and maternal cardiovascular system adaptation explain why this disorder occurs [16]. Moreover, early-onset FGR is frequently associated with preeclampsia (60–70%). On the other hand, the late-onset FGR is suggested to unmask a preexisting sub-clinical maternal cardiac dysfunction [96].

3.1. Fetal Growth Restriction and Maternal Cardiovascular Risk

Previous studies indicated that women with a pregnancy complicated by FGR risk developing CVDs in later life. FGR, similarly to CVDs, is characterized by chronic inflammation and oxidative stress [97]. Conditions such as obesity, hyperlipidemia, insulin resistance, and hypertension are linked with FGR and CVDs [98,99]. Recently, Bijl et al., demonstrated that women with a pregnancy complicated by early-onset FGR had unfavorable short-term cardiometabolic profiles with frequent obesity and low high-density lipoprotein- cholesterol levels (<1.29 mmol/L) in comparison with a control group [100]. Borna et al., reported that delivery of a low-birth-weight child, a surrogate marker of FGR increases the risk of future coronary artery disease approximately 6.5- fold. This association is independent of cigarette smoking, hypertension, hyperlipidemia, diabetes mellitus, age, body mass index (BMI), and waist circumference [98]. On the other hand, the results of the HUNT (Nord-Trøndelag Health) study indicated that pregnancy complications including preterm gestational age, led to only minor improvements in 10-year CVD risk prediction for parous women, as estimated by changes in model discrimination and reclassification [7]. It was also reported that pregnancy complication history does not add to CVD risk stratification for women aged fifty years and older. However, at younger ages, pregnancy complication history is known to predict the development of conventional CVD risk factors and may improve clinical risk prediction before the age of fifty years [101].

3.2. Potential Mechanisms Linking Fetal Growth Restriction and Development of Future Maternal Cardiovascular Diseases

Although preeclampsia and FGR are different entities, they present as interrelated disorders and share similar pathogenesis of inadequate placentation, inflammation, and maternal vascular dysfunction [102]. It is postulated that FGR is a result of poor trophoblastic invasion leading to defective spiral artery remodeling and, consequently, increased maternal peripheral vascular resistance and cardiac afterload [46,103,104]. However, it is also hypothesized that altered cardiovascular function characterized by low maternal cardiac output (CO) and high systemic vascular resistance (SVR) can exist before pregnancy and cause inappropriate placental perfusion and hence trophoblast impairment [96,105,106]. The interplay between the SVR and CO causes a secondary increase in preload and greater contractility of the left ventricle (LV) and consequently increase in LV mass [5]. Recent studies demonstrated that women with pregnancies complicated with normotensive FGR have a persistent myocardial impairment [98,107]. Melchiorre et al., reported that two-thirds of women with pregnancies complicated by FGR had poorer diastolic reserve with impaired myocardial relaxation, and a third had overt diastolic chamber dysfunction despite a preserved geometry and ejection fraction as assessed 12 weeks after delivery [107]. Orabona et al., showed subclinical LV impairment in systodiastolic function with concentric remodeling and smaller LV volumes, a slight alteration in right ventricular systolic function, and left atrial strain, similarly to women with former preeclampsia [99]. During normal pregnancy, eccentric cardiac remodeling typically occurs. Currently, it is believed that concentric remodeling is strongly linked with cardiac fibrosis and has considerable prognostic value in the development of CVDs [108,109]. It was found that most patients with pregnancies complicated by FGR have abnormal LV strain values. The plausible underlying mechanism may be related to chronic inflammation and oxidative stress, which impair production and/or activation of intracellular mediators and result in myocardial stiffening and interstitial connective tissue deposition leading to overt diastolic dysfunction and relative ischemia [99]. However, due to the lack of longitudinal studies, it is not yet elucidated whether FGR causes permanent cardiovascular alterations or whether these women have preexisting impairments contributing to complicated pregnancies.

The reduced CO and Increased SVR "re a'sociated with the activation of the renin-angiotensin-aldosterone system. Previous studies indicated dysregulated angiotensin-processing enzyme and neprilysin expression with the vasoconstrictor pathway predominance [110].

Vascular dysfunction signs in FGR include a small placenta, decidual arteriopathy, placental infarcts with loss of functional placental parenchyma, and abnormalities of the placental villous tree, involving distal villous hypoplasia [96]. Similarly to preeclampsia, repeated ischemia/reperfusion events are associated with increased levels of antiangiogenic sFlt-1 and suppressed secretion of proangiogenic placenta growth factor (PlGF) [111]. It is believed that the sFlt-1/PlGF ratio corresponds to the severity of placental vascular dysfunction [112]. Inadequate trophoblastic invasion with the persistence of smooth muscle in the vessel walls and vascular damage results in acute atherosis and fibrinoid necrosis of vessels [113,114]. Moreover, cFMCs are also detected in pregnancies complicated by severe FRF combined with impaired placental perfusion [48]. Moreover, patients with previous FGR had a more severe degree of endothelial dysfunction than those with previous preeclampsia [115].

Notably, it was proven that maternal genes might modulate fetal growth by altering the intrauterine environment and uterine blood flow or by directly inheriting genes that regulate fetal growth changing. An increased risk of coronary artery disease and FGR is associated with mutations in genes encoding G proteins, glucokinase, angiotensinogen, and coagulation factors [116–119].

Placenta-derived eVs are involved in maternal immunotolerance towards the fetal allograft, inflammation, and angiogenesis. The fraction of circulating placenta-derived eVs is reduced in FGR, likely because of the impaired placental trophoblast activity, and may act as fetal growth markers [120,121]. A few studies indicated upregulation of specific eVs containing miRNAs including miR-499a-5p, and miR-1-3p, miR-127-3p, and miR-519a, and downregulation of others, particularly miR-210, miR-518b as a common feature of placental insufficiencies including FGR [122–124]. Among dysregulated miRNAs in CVD, miR-499-5p and miR-127-3p are highly overexpressed in heart failure and myocardial infarction [125,126]. miR-210 is a well-known hypoxia miRNA, which is upregulated in normal cells exposed to hypoxia in various diseases. In CVD, miR-210 is thought to protect the cardiovascular system from potentially lethal injury by inhibiting cell apoptosis and promoting angiogenesis, thus potentially guiding to revascularization [127]. However, the potential links between these miRNAs on maternal cardiovascular system dysfunction remain unclear. Thus, more studies are required to investigate whether epigenetic factors and the expression of miRNAs are predictive in evaluating the association between FGR and lifespan risk of CVDs.

It is postulated that FGR following maternal chronic bacterial infections is strongly related to a higher risk for atherosclerosis. Moreover, atherosclerotic plaques contain bacterial DNA, and it seems reasonable that an infectious trigger underlies the development of acute atherosis as well [48]. Exposure of human primary trophoblast to bacterial lipopolysaccharide leads to tumor necrosis factor α (TNFα) upregulation and macrophage accumulation in these cells [43]. TNFα is a strong inflammatory cytokine that is also upregulated in atherosclerosis. It was also demonstrated that in patients with FGR, the inflammatory response is stronger and remains stronger over time when compared to women with uncomplicated pregnancies [128]. Thus, TNFα seems to be a key player in several shared pathologic mechanisms of both FGR and atherosclerosis [43].

4. Summary

Adverse pregnancy outcomes such as FGR and preeclampsia are strongly related to long-term maternal CVDs risk. These pregnancy complications likely share common pathophysiologic pathways and are related to similar predisposing factors in women. Nonetheless, the intermediary mechanisms responsible for this association have not been sufficiently elucidated. Since pregnancy occurs early in a woman's life, typically before the onset of clinically evident CVDs, it serves as a unique opportunity to evaluate a woman's later life CVDs risk and introduce meaningful risk-reduction strategies. Future studies should address the issue of a structured screening for CVDs and the impact of timely preventive intervention in improving cardiovascular health in women with pregnancies affected by APOs.

Author Contributions: Conceptualization, S.S.-S., M.L. and M.R.-L.; writing, S.S.-S. and K.K.-P.; review and editing, A.C., M.L. and M.R.-L.; supervision, M.L. and M.R.-L. All authors have read and agreed to the published version of the manuscript.

Funding: This research received no external funding.

Institutional Review Board Statement: Not applicable.

Informed Consent Statement: Not applicable.

Data Availability Statement: Not applicable.

Conflicts of Interest: The authors declare no conflict of interest.

References

1. Collaborators GCoD. Global, regional, and national age-sex specific mortality for 264 causes of death, 1980–2016: A systematic analysis for the Global Burden of Disease Study 2016. *Lancet* **2017**, *390*, 1151–1210. [CrossRef]
2. Yusuf, S.; Hawken, S.; Ôunpuu, S.; Dans, T.; Avezum, A.; Lanas, F.; McQueen, M.; Budaj, A.; Pais, P.; Varigos, J.; et al. Effect of potentially modifiable risk factors associated with myocardial infarction in 52 countries (the INTERHEART study): Case-control study. *Lancet* **2004**, *364*, 937–952. [CrossRef]
3. Mensah, G.A.; Wei, G.S.; Sorlie, P.D.; Fine, L.J.; Rosenberg, Y.; Kaufmann, P.G. Decline in Cardiovascular Mortality: Possible Causes and Implications. *Circ. Res.* **2017**, *120*, 366–380. [CrossRef] [PubMed]
4. Brown, H.L.; Smith, G.N. Pregnancy Complications, Cardiovascular Risk Factors, and Future Heart Disease. *Obs. Gynecol. Clin. North Am.* **2020**, *47*, 487–495. [CrossRef]
5. Hauspurg, A.; Ying, W.; Hubel, C.A.; Michos, E.D.; Ouyang, P. Adverse pregnancy outcomes and future maternal cardiovascular disease. *Clin. Cardiol.* **2018**, *41*, 239–246. [CrossRef]
6. Hypertension in pregnancy. Report of the American College of Obstetricians and Gynecologists' Task Force on Hypertension in Pregnancy. *Obstet. Gynecol.* **2013**, *122*, 1122–1131.
7. Markovitz, A.R.; Stuart, J.J.; Horn, J.; Williams, P.L.; Rimm, E.B.; Missmer, S.A.; Åsvold, B.O. Does pregnancy complication history im-prove cardiovascular disease risk prediction? Findings from the HUNT study in Norway. *Eur. Heart J.* **2019**, *40*, 1113–1120. [CrossRef]
8. Grundy, S.M.; Stone, N.J.; Bailey, A.L.; Beam, C.; Birtcher, K.K.; Blumenthal, R.S. 2018 AHA/ACC/AACVPR/AAPA/ABC/ACPM/ADA/AGS/APhA/ASPC/NLA/PCNA Guideline on the Management of Blood Cholesterol: A Report of the American College of Cardiology/American Heart Association Task Force on Clinical Practice Guidelines. *Circulation* **2019**, *139*, e1082–e1143.
9. Visseren, F.L.J.; Mach, F.; Smulders, Y.M.; Carballo, D.; Koskinas, K.; Bäck, M.; Benetos, A.; Biffi, A.; Boavida, J.-M.; Capodanno, D.; et al. 2021 ESC Guidelines on cardiovascular disease prevention in clinical practice. *Eur. Heart J.* **2021**, *42*, 3227–3337. [CrossRef]
10. Brown, M.A.; Magee, L.A.; Kenny, L.C.; Karumanchi, S.A.; McCarthy, F.P.; Saito, S.; Hall, D.R.; Warren, C.E.; Adoyi, G.; Ishaku, S. International Society for the Study of Hypertension in Pregnancy (ISSHP). The hypertensive disorders of pregnancy: ISSHP classification, diagnosis & management recommendations for international practice. *Pregnancy Hypertens.* **2018**, 291–310. [CrossRef]
11. ACOG Practice Bulletin No. 202: Gestational Hypertension and Preeclampsia. *Obstet. Gynecol.* **2019**, *133*, 1. [CrossRef]
12. Gordijn, S.J.; Beune, I.M.; Thilaganathan, B.; Papageorghiou, A.; Baschat, A.A.; Baker, P.N.; Silver, R.M.; Wynia, K.; Ganzevoort, W. Consensus definition of fetal growth restriction: A Delphi procedure. *Ultrasound Obstet. Gynecol.* **2016**, *48*, 333–339. [CrossRef] [PubMed]
13. World Health Organization. *Diagnostic Criteria and Classification of Hyperglycaemia Are First Detected in Pregnancy*; World Health Organization: Geneva, Switzerland, 2013. Available online: https://apps.who.int/iris/handle/10665/85975 (accessed on 11 September 2022).
14. Minhas, A.S.; Ying, W.; Ogunwole, S.M.; Miller, M.; Zakaria, S.; Vaught, A.J.; Hays, A.G.; Creanga, A.A.; Cedars, A.; Michos, E.D.; et al. The Association of Adverse Pregnancy Outcomes and Cardiovascular Disease: Current Knowledge and Future Directions. *Curr. Treat. Options Cardiovasc. Med.* **2020**, *22*, 61. [CrossRef] [PubMed]
15. Duley, L. The Global Impact of Pre-eclampsia and Eclampsia. *Semin. Perinatol.* **2009**, *33*, 130–137. [CrossRef] [PubMed]
16. Valdés, G. Preeclampsia and cardiovascular disease: Interconnected paths that enable detection of the subclinical stages of obstetric and cardiovascular diseases. *Integr. Blood Press. Control.* **2017**, *10*, 17–23. [CrossRef]
17. Oliver-Williams, C.; Johnson, J.D.; Vladutiu, C.J. Maternal Cardiovascular Disease After Pre-Eclampsia and Gestational Hypertension: A Narrative Review. *Am. J. Lifestyle Med.* **2022**. [CrossRef]

18. Poon, L.C.; Magee, L.A.; Verlohren, S.; Shennan, A.; von Dadelszen, P.; Sheiner, E. A literature review and best practice advice for second and third trimester risk stratification, monitoring, and management of pre-eclampsia: Compiled by the Pregnancy and Non-Communicable Diseases Committee of FIGO (the International Federation of Gynecology and Obstetrics). *Int. J. Gynaecol. Obstet.* **2021**, *154* (Suppl. 1), 3–31.
19. Lokki, A.I.; Daly, E.; Triebwasser, M.; Kurki, M.I.; Roberson, E.; Häppölä, P.; Auro, K.; Perola, M.; Heinonen, S.; Kajantie, E.; et al. Protective Low-Frequency Variants for Preeclampsia in the Fms Related Tyrosine Kinase 1 Gene in the Finnish Population. *Hypertension* **2017**, *70*, 365–371. [CrossRef]
20. Ray, J.G.; Vermeulen, M.J.; Schull, M.; Redelmeier, D.A. Cardiovascular health after maternal placental syndromes (CHAMPS): Population-based retrospective cohort study. *Lancet* **2005**, *366*, 1797–1803. [CrossRef]
21. Lin, Y.-S.; Tang, C.-H.; Yang, C.-Y.C.; Wu, L.-S.; Hung, S.-T.; Hwa, H.-L.; Chu, P.-H. Effect of Pre-Eclampsia–Eclampsia on Major Cardiovascular Events Among Peripartum Women in Taiwan. *Am. J. Cardiol.* **2011**, *107*, 325–330. [CrossRef]
22. Kestenbaum, B.; Seliger, S.L.; Easterling, T.R.; Gillen, D.L.; Critchlow, C.W.; Stehman-Breen, C.O.; Schwartz, S.M. Cardiovascular and thromboembolic events following hypertensive pregnancy. *Am. J. Kidney Dis.* **2003**, *42*, 982–989. [CrossRef] [PubMed]
23. Irgens, H.U.; Reisæter, L.; Irgens, L.M.; Lie, R.T.; Roberts, J.M. Long term mortality of mothers and fathers after pre-eclampsia: Population based cohort study Pre-eclampsia and cardiovascular disease later in life: Who is at risk? *BMJ* **2001**, *323*, 1213–1217. [CrossRef] [PubMed]
24. Leon, L.J.; McCarthy, F.P.; Direk, K.; Gonzalez-Izquierdo, A.; Prieto-Merino, D.; Casas, J.P. Preeclampsia and Cardiovascular Disease in a Large UK Pregnancy Cohort of Linked Electronic Health Records: A CALIBER Study. *Circulation* **2019**, *140*, 1050–1060. [CrossRef]
25. Wu, P.; Haththotuwa, R.; Kwok, C.S.; Babu, A.; Kotronias, R.A.; Rushton, C. Preeclampsia and Future Cardiovascular Health: A Systematic Review and Meta-Analysis. *Circ. Cardiovasc. Qual. Outcomes* **2017**, *10*, e003497. [CrossRef] [PubMed]
26. Mongraw-Chaffin, M.L.; Cirillo, P.M.; Cohn, B.A. Preeclampsia and cardiovascular disease death: Prospective evidence from the child health and development studies cohort. *Hypertension* **2010**, *56*, 166–171. [CrossRef]
27. Riise, H.K.R.; Sulo, G.; Tell, G.S.; Igland, J.; Nygård, O.; Vollset, S.E.; Iversen, A.; Austgulen, R.; Daltveit, A.K. Incident Coronary Heart Disease After Preeclampsia: Role of Reduced Fetal Growth, Preterm Delivery, and Parity. *J. Am. Hear. Assoc.* **2017**, *6*, e004158. [CrossRef]
28. Kovacs, A.F.; Lang, O.; Turiak, L.; Acs, A.; Kohidai, L.; Fekete, N.; Alasztics, B.; Meszaros, T.; Buzas, E.I.; Rigo, J., Jr.; et al. The impact of circulating preeclampsia-associated extracellular vesicles on the migratory activity and phenotype of THP-1 monocytic cells. *Sci. Rep.* **2018**, *8*, 5426. [CrossRef]
29. Motawi, T.M.; Sabry, D.; Maurice, N.W.; Rizk, S.M. Role of mesenchymal stem cells exosomes derived microRNAs; miR-136, miR-494 and miR-495 in pre-eclampsia diagnosis and evaluation. *Arch. Biochem. Biophys.* **2018**, *659*, 13–21. [CrossRef]
30. Hromadnikova, I.; Dvorakova, L.; Kotlabova, K.; Krofta, L. The Prediction of Gestational Hypertension, Preeclampsia and Fetal Growth Restriction via the First Trimester Screening of Plasma Exosomal C19MC microRNAs. *Int. J. Mol. Sci.* **2019**, *20*, 2972. [CrossRef]
31. Berends, A.L.; de Groot, C.J.; Sijbrands, E.J.; Sie, M.P.; Benneheij, S.H.; Pal, R. Shared constitutional risks for maternal vascular-related pregnancy complications and future cardiovascular disease. *Hypertension* **2008**, *51*, 1034–1041. [CrossRef]
32. Auger, N.; Fraser, W.D.; Schnitzer, M.; Leduc, L.; Healy-Profitós, J.; Paradis, G. Recurrent pre-eclampsia and subsequent cardiovascular risk. *Heart* **2017**, *103*, 235–243. [CrossRef] [PubMed]
33. Wikstrom, A.-K.; Haglund, B.; Olovsson, M.; Lindeberg, S.N. The risk of maternal ischaemic heart disease after gestational hypertensive disease. *BJOG Int. J. Obstet. Gynaecol.* **2005**, *112*, 1486–1491. [CrossRef] [PubMed]
34. Smith, G.C.; Pell, J.P.; Walsh, D. Pregnancy complications and maternal risk of ischaemic heart disease: A retrospective cohort study of 129 290 births. *Lancet* **2001**, *357*, 2002–2006. [CrossRef]
35. Lykke, J.A.; Langhoff-Roos, J.; Lockwood, C.J.; Triche, E.W.; Paidas, M.J. Mortality of mothers from cardiovascular and non-cardiovascular causes following pregnancy complications in first delivery. *Paediatr. Périnat. Epidemiol.* **2010**, *24*, 323–330. [CrossRef] [PubMed]
36. Kessous, R.; Shoham-Vardi, I.; Pariente, G.; Sergienko, R.; Sheiner, E. Long-term maternal atherosclerotic morbidity in women with pre-eclampsia. *Heart* **2015**, *101*, 442–446. [CrossRef]
37. Cirillo, P.M.; Cohn, B.A. Pregnancy complications and cardiovascular disease death: 50-year follow-up of the Child Health and Development Studies pregnancy cohort. *Circulation* **2015**, *132*, 1234–1242. [CrossRef]
38. Hannaford, P.; Ferry, S.; Hirsch, S. Cardiovascular sequelae of toxaemia of pregnancy. *Heart* **1997**, *77*, 154–158. [CrossRef]
39. McDonald, S.D.; Malinowski, A.; Zhou, Q.; Yusuf, S.; Devereaux, P.J. Cardiovascular sequelae of preeclampsia/eclampsia: A systematic review and meta-analyses. *Am. Hear. J.* **2008**, *156*, 918–930. [CrossRef]
40. Li, J.; Umar, S.; Iorga, A.; Youn, J.-Y.; Wang, Y.; Regitz-Zagrosek, V.; Cai, H.; Eghbali, M. Cardiac vulnerability to ischemia/reperfusion injury drastically increases in late pregnancy. *Basic Res. Cardiol.* **2012**, *107*, 504–518. [CrossRef]
41. Stanhewicz, A. Residual vascular dysfunction in women with a history of preeclampsia. *Am. J. Physiol. Integr. Comp. Physiol.* **2018**, *315*, R1062–R1071. [CrossRef]
42. Odukoya, S.A.; Moodley, J.; Naicker, T. Current Updates on Pre-eclampsia: Maternal and Foetal Cardiovascular Diseases Predilection, Science or Myth? Future cardiovascular disease risks in mother and child following pre-eclampsia. *Curr. Hypertens. Rep.* **2021**, *23*, 16. [CrossRef] [PubMed]

43. de Jager, S.C.A.; Meeuwsen, J.A.L.; van Pijpen, F.M.; Zoet, G.A.; Barendrecht, A.D.; Franx, A.; Pasterkamp, G.; van Rijn, B.B.; Goumans, M.J.; den Ruijter, H.M. Preeclampsia and coronary plaque erosion: Manifestations of endothelial dysfunction resulting in cardi-ovascular events in women. *Eur. J. Pharmacol.* **2017**, *816*, 129–137. [CrossRef] [PubMed]
44. Turbeville, H.R.; Sasser, J.M. Preeclampsia beyond pregnancy: Long-term consequences for mother and child. *Am. J. Physiol. Physiol.* **2020**, *318*, F1315–F1326. [CrossRef]
45. Staff, A.C.; Dechend, R.; Pijnenborg, R. Learning from the placenta: Acute atherosis and vascular remodeling in preeclampsia—Novel aspects for atherosclerosis and future cardiovascular health. *Hypertension* **2010**, *56*, 1026–1034. [CrossRef] [PubMed]
46. Staff, A.; Dechend, R.; Redman, C. Review: Preeclampsia, acute atherosis of the spiral arteries and future cardiovascular disease: Two new hypotheses. *Placenta* **2012**, *34*, S73–S78. [CrossRef]
47. Kim, J.-Y.; Kim, Y.M. Acute Atherosis of the Uterine Spiral Arteries: Clinicopathologic Implications. *J. Pathol. Transl. Med.* **2015**, *49*, 462–471. [CrossRef]
48. Pitz Jacobsen, D.; Fjeldstad, H.E.; Johnsen, G.M.; Fosheim, I.K.; Moe, K.; Alnæs-Katjavivi, P.; Dechend, R.; Sugulle, M.; Staff, A.C. Acute Atherosis Lesions at the Fetal-Maternal Border: Current Knowledge and Implications for Maternal Cardiovascular Health. *Front. Immunol.* **2021**, *12*, 791606. [CrossRef] [PubMed]
49. Kara, R.J.; Bolli, P.; Karakikes, I.; Matsunaga, I.; Tripodi, J.; Tanweer, O.; Altman, P.; Shachter, N.S.; Nakano, A.; Najfeld, V.; et al. Fetal Cells Traffic to Injured Maternal Myocardium and Undergo Cardiac Differentiation. *Circ. Res.* **2012**, *110*, 82–93. [CrossRef]
50. Gammill, H.S.; Aydelotte, T.M.; Guthrie, K.A.; Nkwopara, E.C.; Nelson, J.L. Cellular Fetal Microchimerism in Preeclampsia. *Hypertension* **2013**, *62*, 1062–1067. [CrossRef]
51. Al-Mufti, R.; Lees, C.; Albaiges, G.; Hambley, H.; Nicolaides, K. Fetal cells in maternal blood of pregnancies with severe fetal growth restriction. *Hum. Reprod.* **2000**, *15*, 218–221. [CrossRef]
52. Du, L.; Kuang, L.; He, F.; Tang, W.; Sun, W.; Chen, D. Mesenchymal-to-epithelial transition in the placental tissues of patients with preeclampsia. *Hypertens. Res.* **2016**, *40*, 67–72. [CrossRef] [PubMed]
53. Catov, J.M.; Muldoon, M.F.; Gandley, R.E.; Brands, J.; Hauspurg, A.; Hubel, C.A.; Tuft, M.; Schmella, M.; Tang, G.; Parks, W.T. Maternal Vascular Lesions in the Placenta Predict Vascular Impairments a Decade After Delivery. *Hypertension* **2022**, *79*, 424–434. [CrossRef] [PubMed]
54. Drost, J.T.; Maas, A.H.; Holewijn, S.; Joosten, L.A.; van Eyck, J.; van der Schouw, Y.T.; de Graaf, J. Novel cardiovascular biomarkers in women with a history of early preeclampsia. *Atherosclerosis* **2014**, *237*, 117–122. [CrossRef] [PubMed]
55. Krishnamoorthy, S.; Khoo, C.W.; Lim, H.S.; Lane, D.A.; Pignatelli, P.; Basili, S.; Violi, F.; Lip, G.Y. Prognostic role of plasma von Wil-lebrand factor and soluble E-selectin levels for future cardiovascular events in a 'real-world' community cohort of patients with atrial fibrillation. *Eur. J. Clin. Investig.* **2013**, *43*, 1032–1038. [CrossRef]
56. Skjaerven, R.; Wilcox, A.; Klungsøyr, K.; Irgens, L.M.; Vikse, B.E.; Vatten, L.J.; Lie, R.T. Cardiovascular mortality after pre-eclampsia in one child mothers: Prospective, population based cohort study. *BMJ* **2012**, *345*, e7677. [CrossRef]
57. Maffei, S.; Guiducci, L.; Cugusi, L.; Cadeddu, C.; Deidda, M.; Gallina, S.; Sciomer, S.; Gastaldelli, A.; Kaski, J.C. Working Group on "Gender difference in cardiovascular disease" of the Italian Society of Cardiology. Women-specific predictors of cardiovascular disease risk-new paradigms. *Int. J. Cardiol.* **2019**, *286*, 190–197. [CrossRef]
58. Staff, A.C.; Johnsen, G.M.; Dechend, R.; Redman, C.W.G. Preeclampsia and uteroplacental acute atherosis: Immune and inflammatory factors. *J. Reprod Immunol.* **2014**, *101–102*, 120–126. [CrossRef]
59. Kvehaugen, A.S.; Melien, Ø.; Holmen, O.L.; Laivuori, H.; Øian, P.; Andersgaard, A.B.; Dechend, R.; Staff, A.C. Single Nucleotide Polymorphisms in G Protein Signaling Pathway Genes in Preeclampsia. *Hypertension* **2013**, *61*, 655–661. [CrossRef]
60. White, W.M.; Mielke, M.; Araoz, P.A.; Lahr, B.D.; Bailey, K.R.; Jayachandran, M.; Miller, V.M.; Garovic, V.D. A history of preeclampsia is associated with a risk for coronary artery calcification 3 decades later. *Am. J. Obstet. Gynecol.* **2016**, *214*, 519.e1–519.e8. [CrossRef]
61. Zoet, G.A.; Benschop, L.; Boersma, E.; Budde, R.P.; Fauser, B.C.; Van Der Graaf, Y.; De Groot, C.J.; Maas, A.H.; Van Lennep, J.E.R.; Steegers, E.A.; et al. Prevalence of Subclinical Coronary Artery Disease Assessed by Coronary Computed Tomography Angiography in 45- to 55-Year-Old Women With a History of Preeclampsia. *Circulation* **2018**, *137*, 877–879. [CrossRef]
62. Beckman, J.P.; Camp, J.J.; Lahr, B.D.; Bailey, K.R.; Kearns, A.E.; Garovic, V.D. Pregnancy history, coronary artery calcification and bone mineral density in menopausal women. *Climacteric* **2018**, *21*, 53–59. [CrossRef] [PubMed]
63. Benschop, L.; Brouwers, L.; Zoet, G.A.; Meun, C.; Boersma, E.; Budde, R.P.; Fauser, B.C.; de Groot, C.M.; van der Schouw, Y.T.; Maas, A.H.; et al. Early Onset of Coronary Artery Calcification in Women With Previous Preeclampsia. *Circ. Cardiovasc. Imaging* **2020**, *13*, e010340. [CrossRef] [PubMed]
64. Ahmed, R.; Dunford, J.; Mehran, R.; Robson, S.; Kunadian, V. Pre-eclampsia and future cardiovascular risk among women: A review. *J. Am. Coll. Cardiol.* **2014**, *63*, 1815–1822. [CrossRef] [PubMed]
65. Aykas, F.; Solak, Y.; Erden, A.; Bulut, K.; Dogan, S.; Sarli, B.; Acmaz, G.; Afsar, B.; Siriopol, D.; Covic, A.; et al. Persistence of cardiovascular risk factors in women with previous preeclampsia: A long-term follow-up study. *J. Investig. Med.* **2015**, *63*, 641–645. [CrossRef] [PubMed]
66. Schuster, J.; Cheng, S.; Padbury, J.; Sharma, S. Placental extracellular vesicles and pre-eclampsia. *Am. J. Reprod. Immunol.* **2020**, *85*, e13297. [CrossRef]
67. Murugesan, S.; Saravanakumar, L.; Powell, M.F.; Rajasekaran, N.S.; Kannappan, R.; Berkowitz, D.E. Role of exosomal microRNA signatures: An emerging factor in preeclampsia-mediated cardiovascular disease. *Placenta* **2020**, *103*, 226–231. [CrossRef]

68. Lin, Z.; Murtaza, I.; Wang, K.; Jiao, J.; Gao, J.; Li, P.-F. miR-23a functions downstream of NFATc3 to regulate cardiac hypertrophy. *Proc. Natl. Acad. Sci. USA* **2009**, *106*, 12103–12108. [CrossRef]
69. Hromadnikova, I.; Kotlabova, K.; Hympanova, L.; Krofta, L. Cardiovascular and cerebrovascular disease associated mi-croRNAs are dysregulated in placental tissues affected with gestational hypertension, preeclampsia and intrauterine growth restriction. *PLoS ONE* **2015**, *10*, e0138383. [CrossRef]
70. Pillay, P.; Maharaj, N.; Moodley, J.; Mackraj, I. Placental exosomes and pre-eclampsia: Maternal circulating levels in normal pregnancies and, early and late onset pre-eclamptic pregnancies. *Placenta* **2016**, *46*, 18–25. [CrossRef]
71. Powell, J.S.; Gandley, R.E.; Lackner, E.; Dolinish, A.; Ouyang, Y.; Powers, R.W.; Morelli, A.E.; Hubel, C.A.; Sadovsky, Y. Small extra-cellular vesicles from plasma of women with preeclampsia increase myogenic tone and decrease endothelium-dependent relaxation of mouse mesenteric arteries. *Pregnancy Hypertens.* **2022**, *28*, 66–73. [CrossRef]
72. Tong, M.; Chen, Q.; James, J.L.; Stone, P.R.; Chamley, L.W. Micro- and Nano-vesicles from First Trimester Human Placentae Carry Flt-1 and Levels Are Increased in Severe Preeclampsia. *Front. Endocrinol.* **2017**, *8*, 174. [CrossRef] [PubMed]
73. Ghafourian, M.; Mahdavi, R.; Jonoush, Z.A.; Sadeghi, M.; Ghadiri, N.; Farzaneh, M.; Salehi, A.M. The implications of exosomes in pregnancy: Emerging as new diagnostic markers and therapeutics targets. *Cell Commun. Signal.* **2022**, *20*, 51. [CrossRef] [PubMed]
74. Stanhewicz, A.E.; Jandu, S.; Santhanam, L.; Alexander, L.M. Increased Angiotensin II Sensitivity Contributes to Microvascular Dysfunction in Women Who Have Had Preeclampsia. *Hypertension* **2017**, *70*, 382–389. [CrossRef] [PubMed]
75. Saxena, A.R.; Karumanchi, S.A.; Brown, N.J.; Royle, C.M.; McElrath, T.F.; Seely, E.W. Increased Sensitivity to Angiotensin II Is Present Postpartum in Women With a History of Hypertensive Pregnancy. *Hypertension* **2010**, *55*, 1239–1245. [CrossRef] [PubMed]
76. Gill, M.; Motta-Mejia, C.; Kandzija, N.; Cooke, W.; Zhang, W.; Cerdeira, A.S.; Bastie, C.; Redman, C.; Vatish, M. Placental Syncytiotrophoblast-Derived Extracellular Vesicles Carry Active NEP (Neprilysin) and Are Increased in Preeclampsia. *Hypertension* **2019**, *73*, 1112–1119. [CrossRef]
77. Alexander, B.T.; Rinewalt, A.N.; Cockrell, K.L.; Massey, M.B.; Bennett, W.A.; Granger, J.P. Endothelin type a receptor blockade at-tenuates the hypertension in response to chronic reductions in uterine perfusion pressure. *Hypertension* **2001**, *37 Pt 2*, 485–489. [CrossRef]
78. Fischer, T.; Schobel, H.P.; Frank, H.; Andreae, M.; Schneider, K.T.M.; Heusser, K. Pregnancy-induced sympathetic overactivity: A precursor of preeclampsia*. *Eur. J. Clin. Investig.* **2004**, *34*, 443–448. [CrossRef]
79. Bello, N.; Rendon, I.S.H.; Arany, Z. The relationship between pre-eclampsia and peripartum cardiomyopathy: A systematic review and meta-analysis. *J. Am. Coll. Cardiol.* **2013**, *62*, 1715–1723. [CrossRef]
80. Miralles, F.; Collinot, H.; Boumerdassi, Y.; Ducat, A.; Duché, A.; Renault, G.; Marchiol, C.; Lagoutte, I.; Bertholle, C.; Andrieu, M.; et al. Long-term cardiovascular disorders in the STOX1 mouse model of preeclampsia. *Sci. Rep.* **2019**, *9*, 14179. [CrossRef]
81. Borna, S.; Neamatipoor, E.; Radman, N. Risk of coronary artery disease in women with history of pregnancies complicated by preeclampsia and LBW. *J. Matern. Neonatal. Med.* **2011**, *25*, 1114–1116. [CrossRef]
82. De Haas, S.; Ghossein-Doha, C.; Geerts, L.; van Kuijk, S.M.J.; van Drongelen, J.; Spaanderman, M.E.A. Cardiac remodeling in normotensive pregnancy and in pregnancy complicated by hypertension: Systematic review and meta-analysis. *Ultrasound Obs. Gynecol.* **2017**, *50*, 683–696. [CrossRef] [PubMed]
83. Barr, L.C.; Liblik, K.; Johri, A.M.; Smith, G.N. Maternal Cardiovascular Function Following a Pregnancy Complicated by Preeclampsia. *Am. J. Perinatol.* **2020**, *39*, 1055–1064. [CrossRef] [PubMed]
84. Melchiorre, K.; Sutherland, G.R.; Liberati, M.; Thilaganathan, B. Preeclampsia Is Associated With Persistent Postpartum Cardiovascular Impairment. *Hypertension* **2011**, *58*, 709–715. [CrossRef] [PubMed]
85. Brandt, Y.; Ghossein-Doha, C.; Gerretsen, S.C.; Spaanderman, M.E.A.; Kooi, M.E. Noninvasive Cardiac Imaging in Formerly Preeclamptic Women for Early Detection of Subclinical Myocardial Abnormalities: A 2022 Update. *Biomolecules* **2022**, *12*, 415. [CrossRef] [PubMed]
86. DeMartelly, V.A.; Dreixler, J.; Tung, A.; Mueller, A.; Heimberger, S.; Fazal, A.A. Long-Term Postpartum Cardiac Function and Its Association With Preeclampsia. *J. Am. Heart Assoc.* **2021**, *10*, e018526. [CrossRef]
87. Reddy, M.; Wright, L.; Rolnik, D.L.; Li, W.; Mol, B.W.; La Gerche, A.; da SilvaCosta, F.; Wallace, E.; Palmer, K. Evaluation of Cardiac Function in Women With a History of Preeclampsia: A Systematic Review and Meta-Analysis. *J. Am. Hear. Assoc.* **2019**, *8*, e013545. [CrossRef]
88. Al-Nashi, M.; Eriksson, M.J.; Östlund, E.; Bremme, K.; Kahan, T. Cardiac structure and function, and ventricular-arterial interaction 11 years following a pregnancy with preeclampsia. *J. Am. Soc. Hypertens.* **2016**, *10*, 297–306. [CrossRef]
89. Clemmensen, T.S.; Christensen, M.; Kronborg, C.J.S.; Knudsen, U.B.; Løgstrup, B.B. Long-term follow-up of women with early onset pre-eclampsia shows subclinical impairment of the left ventricular function by two-dimensional speckle tracking echo-cardiography. *Pregnancy Hypertens.* **2018**, *14*, 9–14. [CrossRef]
90. Ghossein-Doha, C.; Spaanderman, M.E.; Al Doulah, R.; Van Kuijk, S.M.; Peeters, L.L. Maternal cardiac adaptation to subse-quent pregnancy in formerly pre-eclamptic women according to recurrence of pre-eclampsia. *Ultrasound Obs. Gynecol.* **2016**, *47*, 96–103. [CrossRef]
91. Levine, L.D.; Lewey, J.; Koelper, N.; Downes, K.L.; Arany, Z.; Elovitz, M.A. Persistent cardiac dysfunction on echocar-diography in African American women with severe preeclampsia. *Pregnancy Hypertens.* **2019**, *17*, 127–132. [CrossRef]
92. Orabona, R.; Vizzardi, E.; Sciatti, E.; Prefumo, F.; Bonadei, I.; Valcamonico, A.; Metra, M.; Frusca, T. Maternal cardiac function after HELLP syndrome: An echocardiography study. *Ultrasound Obstet. Gynecol.* **2017**, *50*, 507–513. [CrossRef] [PubMed]

93. Martins, J.G.; Biggio, J.R.; Abuhamad, A.; pubs@smfm.org SfM-FMSEa. Society for Maternal-Fetal Medicine. Consult Series #52: Diagnosis and management of fetal growth restriction: (Replaces Clinical Guideline Number 3, April 2012). *Am. J. Obstet. Gynecol.* **2020**, *223*, B2–B17. [PubMed]
94. Jaddoe, V.W.V.; De Jonge, L.L.; Hofman, A.; Franco, O.; Steegers, E.A.P.; Gaillard, R. First trimester fetal growth restriction and cardiovascular risk factors in school age children: Population based cohort study. *BMJ* **2014**, *348*, g14. [CrossRef] [PubMed]
95. Figueras, F.; Caradeux, J.; Crispi, F.; Eixarch, E.; Peguero, A.; Gratacos, E. Diagnosis and surveillance of late-onset fetal growth restriction. *Am. J. Obstet. Gynecol.* **2018**, *218*, S790–S802.e1. [CrossRef] [PubMed]
96. Mecacci, F.; Avagliano, L.; Lisi, F.; Clemenza, S.; Serena, C.; Vannuccini, S. Fetal Growth Restriction: Does an Integrated Maternal Hemodynamic-Placental Model Fit Better? *Reprod Sci.* **2021**, *28*, 2422–2435. [CrossRef] [PubMed]
97. Sia, W.W.; Pertman, S.M.; Yan, R.M.; Tsuyuki, R.T. Are Preeclampsia and Adverse Obstetrical Outcomes Predictors of Cardiovascular Disease? *A Case-Control Study of Women With Heart Disease. J. Obstet. Gynaecol. Can.* **2019**, *12*, 1760–1767. [CrossRef]
98. Neiger, R. Long-Term Effects of Pregnancy Complications on Maternal Health: A Review. *J Clin Med.* **2017**, *6*, 76. [CrossRef]
99. Orabona, R.; Mohseni, Z.; Sciatti, E.; Mulder, E.G.; Prefumo, F.; Lorusso, R. Maternal myocardial dysfunction after normotensive fetal growth restriction compared with hypertensive pregnancies: A speckle-tracking study. *J. Hypertens.* **2020**, *38*, 1955–1963. [CrossRef]
100. Bijl, R.C.; Cornette, J.M.; Vasak, B.; Franx, A.; Lely, A.T.; Bots, M.L.; van Rijn, B.B.; Koster, M.P. Cardiometabolic Profiles in Women with a History of Hypertensive and Normotensive Fetal Growth Restriction. *J. Womens Health* **2022**, *31*, 63–70. [CrossRef]
101. Timpka, S.; Fraser, A.; Schyman, T.; Stuart, J.J.; Åsvold, B.O.; Mogren, I.; Franks, P.W.; Rich-Edwards, J.W. The value of pregnancy complication history for 10-year cardiovascular disease risk prediction in middle-aged women. *Eur. J. Epidemiol.* **2018**, *33*, 1003–1010. [CrossRef]
102. Lane-Cordova, A.D.; Khan, S.S.; Grobman, W.A.; Greenland, P.; Shah, S.J. Long-Term Cardiovascular Risks Associated With Adverse Pregnancy Outcomes: JACC Review Topic of the Week. *J. Am. Coll. Cardiol.* **2019**, *73*, 2106–2116. [CrossRef] [PubMed]
103. Burton, G.J.; Jauniaux, E. Pathophysiology of placental-derived fetal growth restriction. *Am. J. Obstet. Gynecol.* **2018**, *218*, S745–S761. [CrossRef] [PubMed]
104. Bamfo, J.E.; Kametas, N.A.; Chambers, J.B.; Nicolaides, K.H. Maternal cardiac function in fetal growth-restricted and non-growth-restricted small-for-gestational age pregnancies. *Ultrasound Obs. Gynecol.* **2007**, *29*, 51–57. [CrossRef]
105. Tay, J.; Masini, G.; McEniery, C.M.; Giussani, D.A.; Shaw, C.J.; Wilkinson, I.B. Uterine and fetal placental Doppler indices are associated with maternal cardiovascular function. *Am. J. Obstet. Gynecol.* **2019**, *220*, 96.e1–96.e8. [CrossRef] [PubMed]
106. Foo, F.L.; Mahendru, A.A.; Masini, G.; Fraser, A.; Cacciatore, S.; MacIntyre, D.A.; McEniery, C.M.; Wilkinson, I.B.; Bennett, P.R.; Lees, C.C. Association Between Prepregnancy Cardiovascular Function and Subsequent Preeclampsia or Fetal Growth Restriction. *Hypertension* **2018**, *72*, 442–450. [CrossRef] [PubMed]
107. Melchiorre, K.; Sutherland, G.R.; Liberati, M.; Thilaganathan, B. Maternal cardiovascular impairment in pregnancies com-plicated by severe fetal growth restriction. *Hypertension* **2012**, *60*, 437–443. [CrossRef]
108. Mohseni, Z.; Spaanderman, M.E.A.; Oben, J.; Calore, M.; Derksen, E.; Al-Nasiry, S.; De Windt, L.J.; Ghossein-Doha, C. Cardiac remodeling and pre-eclampsia: An overview of microRNA expression patterns. *Ultrasound Obstet. Gynecol.* **2017**, *52*, 310–317. [CrossRef]
109. Muiesan, M.L.; Salvetti, M.; Monteduro, C.; Bonzi, B.; Paini, A.; Viola, S.; Poisa, P.; Rizzoni, D.; Castellano, M.; Agabiti-Rosei, E. Left Ventricular Concentric Geometry During Treatment Adversely Affects Cardiovascular Prognosis in Hypertensive Patients. *Hypertension* **2004**, *43*, 731–738. [CrossRef]
110. Delforce, S.; Lumbers, E.R.; Ellery, S.J.; Murthi, P.; Pringle, K.G. Dysregulation of the placental renin–angiotensin system in human fetal growth restriction. *Reproduction* **2019**, *158*, 237–245. [CrossRef]
111. Benton, S.J.; McCowan, L.M.; Heazell, A.E.; Grynspan, D.; Hutcheon, J.A.; Senger, C.; Burke, O.; Chan, Y.; Harding, J.E.; Yockell-Lelièvre, J.; et al. Placental growth factor as a marker of fetal growth restriction caused by placental dysfunction. *Placenta* **2016**, *42*, 1–8. [CrossRef]
112. Korzeniewski, S.J.; Romero, R.; Chaiworapongsa, T. Maternal plasma angiogenic index-1 (placental growth fac-tor/soluble vascular endothelial growth factor receptor-1) is a biomarker for the burden of placental lesions consistent with uteroplacental underperfusion: A longitudinal case-cohort study. *Am. J. Obstet. Gynecol.* **2016**, *214*, 629.e1–629.e17. [CrossRef]
113. Labarrere, C.; Alonso, J.; Manni, J.; Domenichini, E.; Althabe, O. Immunohistochemical Findings in Acute Atherosis Associated With Intrauterine Growth Retardation. *Am. J. Reprod. Immunol. Microbiol.* **1985**, *7*, 149–155. [CrossRef] [PubMed]
114. Sehgal, A.; Murthi, P.; Dahlstrom, J.E. Vascular changes in fetal growth restriction: Clinical relevance and future therapeutics. *J. Perinatol.* **2018**, *39*, 366–374. [CrossRef] [PubMed]
115. Yinon, Y.; Kingdom, J.C.; Odutayo, A.; Moineddin, R.; Drewlo, S.; Lai, V.; Cherney, D.Z.; Hladunewich, M.A. Vascular dysfunction in women with a history of preeclampsia and intrauterine growth restriction: Insights into future vascular risk. *Circulation* **2010**, *122*, 1846–1853. [CrossRef]
116. Hocher, B.; Slowinski, T.; Stolze, T.; Pleschka, A.; Neumayer, H.H.; Halle, H. Association of maternal G protein beta3 subunit 825T allele with low birthweight. *Lancet* **2000**, *355*, 1241–1242. [CrossRef]
117. Hattersley, A.T.; Beards, F.; Ballantyne, E.; Appleton, M.; Harvey, R.; Ellard, S. Mutations in the glucokinase gene of the fetus result in reduced birth weight. *Nat. Genet.* **1998**, *19*, 268–270. [CrossRef] [PubMed]

118. Zhang, X.Q.; Varner, M.; Dizon-Townson, D.; Song, F.; Ward, K. A Molecular Variant of Angiotensinogen Is Associated with Idiopathic Intrauterine Growth Restriction. *Obstet. Gynecol.* **2003**, *101*, 237–242. [CrossRef]
119. Kupferminc, M.J.; Eldor, A.; Steinman, N.; Many, A.; Bar-Am, A.; Jaffa, A.; Fait, G.; Lessing, J.B. Increased Frequency of Genetic Thrombophilia in Women with Complications of Pregnancy. *N. Engl. J. Med.* **1999**, *340*, 9–13. [CrossRef]
120. Miranda, J.; Paules, C.; Nair, S.; Lai, A.; Palma, C.; Scholz-Romero, K.; Rice, G.E.; Gratacos, E.; Crispi, F.; Salomon, C. Placental exosomes profile in maternal and fetal circulation in intrauterine growth restriction—Liquid biopsies to monitoring fetal growth. *Placenta* **2018**, *64*, 34–43. [CrossRef]
121. Awamleh, Z.; Gloor, G.B.; Han, V.K.M. Placental microRNAs in pregnancies with early onset intrauterine growth restriction and preeclampsia: Potential impact on gene expression and pathophysiology. *BMC Med. Genom.* **2019**, *12*, 91. [CrossRef]
122. Hromadnikova, I.; Kotlabova, K.; Dvorakova, L.; Krofta, L. Maternal Cardiovascular Risk Assessment 3-to-11 Years Postpartum in Relation to Previous Occurrence of Pregnancy-Related Complications. *J. Clin. Med.* **2019**, *8*, 544. [CrossRef]
123. Rodosthenous, R.S.; Burris, H.; Sanders, A.P.; Just, A.C.; Dereix, A.E.; Svensson, K.; Solano, M.; Téllez-Rojo, M.M.; Wright, R.; Baccarelli, A.A. Second trimester extracellular microRNAs in maternal blood and fetal growth: An exploratory study. *Epigenetics* **2017**, *12*, 804–810. [CrossRef] [PubMed]
124. Hoskins, I.A.; Hemming, V.G.; Johnson, T.R.; Winkel, C.A. Effects of alterations of zinc-to-phosphorus ratios and meconium content on Group B Streptococcus growth in human amniotic fluid in vitro. *Am. J. Obstet. Gynecol.* **1987**, *157*, 770–773. [CrossRef]
125. Yuan, R.; Zhang, X.; Fang, Y.; Nie, Y.; Cai, S.; Chen, Y.; Mo, D. mir-127-3p inhibits the proliferation of myocytes by targeting KMT5a. *Biochem. Biophys. Res. Commun.* **2018**, *503*, 970–976. [CrossRef] [PubMed]
126. Moreira-Costa, L.; Barros, A.S.; Lourenço, A.P.; Leite-Moreira, A.F.; Nogueira-Ferreira, R.; Thongboonkerd, V.; Vitorino, R. Exo-some-Derived Mediators as Potential Biomarkers for Cardiovascular Diseases: A Network Approach. *Proteomes* **2021**, *9*, 8. [CrossRef] [PubMed]
127. Guan, Y.; Song, X.; Sun, W.; Wang, Y.; Liu, B. Effect of Hypoxia-Induced MicroRNA-210 Expression on Cardiovascular Disease and the Underlying Mechanism. *Oxidative Med. Cell. Longev.* **2019**, *2019*, 4727283. [CrossRef]
128. Azizieh, F.Y.; Raghupathy, R.G. Tumor Necrosis Factor-α and Pregnancy Complications: A Prospective Study. *Med Princ. Pr.* **2014**, *24*, 165–170. [CrossRef]

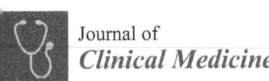

Journal of
Clinical Medicine

Article

The Impact of Coexisting Gestational Diabetes Mellitus on the Course of Preeclampsia

Katarzyna Pankiewicz [1,*], Ewa Szczerba [2], Anna Fijałkowska [2], Janusz Sierdziński [3], Tadeusz Issat [1] and Tomasz Mikołaj Maciejewski [1]

[1] Department of Obstetrics and Gynecology, Institute of Mother and Child in Warsaw, 01-211 Warsaw, Poland
[2] Department of Cardiology, Institute of Mother and Child in Warsaw, 01-211 Warsaw, Poland
[3] Department of Medical Informatics and Telemedicine, Medical University of Warsaw, Litewska 14/16, 00-581 Warsaw, Poland
* Correspondence: katarzynahak@wp.pl; Tel.: +48-22-3277044

Abstract: A strict correlation between gestational diabetes mellitus (GDM) and preeclampsia (PE) has been shown in previous studies. This case-control observational study evaluates the influence of concomitant GDM on the severity of PE. Ninety-nine patients were included: thirty-eight with PE without GDM (group 1), fourteen with PE and concomitant GDM (group 2), and forty-seven with uncomplicated pregnancies (group 3). Adverse maternal/fetal and neonatal outcomes were registered. Patients underwent blood sample analysis of serum PlGF, sFlt-1, creatinine levels, and platelet count (PLT). The incidence of preterm birth, FGR, HELLP syndrome, and NICU admission was significantly higher in group 1 in comparison to groups 2 and 3, whereas RDS was diagnosed most often in group 2 in comparison to groups 1 and 3. All studied biochemical parameters differed between the control group and both PE groups; however, there were no differences between patients with PE with and without GDM. The presented study indicates that the coexistence of GDM may mitigate the course of PE. The lack of differences between patients with PE with and without GDM in serum levels of studied biomarkers may also confirm its usefulness in the diagnosis and management of PE in patients with coexisting GDM.

Keywords: gestational diabetes mellitus; preeclampsia; soluble fms-like tyrosine kinase 1; placental growth factor

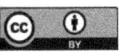

1. Introduction

Preeclampsia (PE) complicates about 3–8% of pregnancies, whereas gestational diabetes mellitus (GDM) complicates about 8.7–14% of pregnancies [1–3]. PE is defined according to The International Society for the Study of Hypertension in Pregnancy (ISSHP) as the presence of a new-onset hypertension after 20 weeks' gestation accompanied by proteinuria or evidence of maternal acute kidney injury, liver dysfunction, neurological features, hemolysis or thrombocytopenia, or fetal growth restriction (FGR) [4]. PE is a multifaceted disorder; however, an inadequate trophoblast invasion of maternal spiral arteries with subsequent maternal global endothelial dysfunction is seen as the main mechanism involved in the development of this disease [5]. During PE, maternal symptoms are a consequence of the imbalance between circulating angiogenic factors, i.a., vascular endothelial growth factor (VEGF), and placental growth factor (PlGF); and antiangiogenic factors, i.a., soluble fms-like tyrosine kinase 1 (sFlt-1) and soluble endoglin (sEng) [6]. Moreover, these biomarkers can be used in the screening and diagnosis of PE [7–10].

GDM is defined according to the International Diabetes Federation (IDF) as spontaneous hyperglycemia developing during pregnancy [11]. It is mostly the result of impaired glucose tolerance due to pancreatic β-cell dysfunction on a background of chronic insulin resistance. During normal gestation, women are able to counteract peripheral insulin resistance with a significant increase of their basal and nutrient-stimulated insulin secretion from pancreatic b cells. When women are not able to intensify insulin secretion, GDM occurs [12]. It is widely known that GDM is a risk factor for developing PE during pregnancy, and many studies have shown a strict correlation between these two diseases [13–15]. Additionally, both diseases may have serious long-term consequences for the mother and fetus, such as a significantly increased risk of developing hypertension, heart failure, stroke, end-stage chronic kidney disease (CKD), and diabetes mellitus later (DM) in life [16–21].

The risk of developing PE in patients with GDM has been, up to date, widely studied [22–25]. PE and GDM share several risk factors, such as advanced maternal age, nulliparity, multiple pregnancy, ethnicity, and pregestational obesity. Although both diseases also share some pathophysiological pathways (e.g., sterile inflammation), the main mechanisms take place in the placenta and present completely differently—proangiogenic state in GDM, and antiangiogenic state in PE [21]. This is a reason to suspect that the influence of GDM on the course of PE may be significant, causing a shift in the imbalance between proangiogenic and antiangiogenic factors derived from the placenta. On the other hand, there is also a possibility that the usefulness of the PE biomarkers PlGF and sFlt-1 in the diagnosis and prediction of pregnancy complications during PE might not be maintained on the same level in patients with both PE and GDM.

To our best knowledge, there is only one study referring to the impact of GDM on the course of pregnancy complicated by hypertensive disorders indicating an increased risk of adverse pregnancy outcomes in women with both gestational hypertension (GH) and GDM [26]. There is also another study comparing PE biomarkers in patients with PE alone, PE+GDM, GDM alone, and healthy controls demonstrating that sFlt-1 overproduction is also related to PE in GDM pregnancies, even though it is characterized by a less severe endothelial dysfunction [21].

The aim of this study was to evaluate the influence of concomitant GDM on the severity of PE and its complications (maternal and neonatal adverse outcomes), and the usefulness of PE biomarkers in patients with both PE and GDM. Both diseases are currently the most taxing and common problems in antenatal care, especially PE, being responsible for about 16–18% of maternal perinatal deaths and up to 40% of fetal and neonatal deaths [1]. Thus, after realizing the translational potential of this study, the better understanding of the coexistence of both diseases may lead to significant improvements in antenatal care.

2. Materials and Methods

2.1. Study Population and Protocol

In this case-control observational prospective study, adult women (>18 years of age) in singleton pregnancies admitted to the Department of Gynecology and Obstetrics, Institute of Mother and Child in Warsaw between November 2013–April 2018, with the diagnosis of preeclampsia with and without concomitant GDM were included. The results obtained in preeclamptic patients with and without GDM were compared to those obtained in healthy pregnant volunteers. PE was defined according to the 2011 European Society of Cardiology (ESC) Guidelines [27], whereas GDM was defined according to the IDF 2011 Guidelines [28]. The exclusion criteria for all groups included: gestational age < 22 weeks, multiple pregnancies, history of CKD, antiphospholipid syndrome, congenital and acquired heart defects, congenital or acquired coagulopathies (hemorrhagic diathesis or thrombophilia), pregestational diabetes, and symptoms of infectious diseases (including suspected chorioamnionitis). All patients underwent blood sample biochemical analysis—measurements of serum PlGF, sFlt-1, and creatinine levels, as well as platelet count (PLT). The following adverse maternal/fetal outcomes were evaluated: preterm birth, HELLP syndrome, FGR, oligohydramnion, and placental abruption. Additionally, the following adverse neonatal outcomes were registered: admission to neonatal intensive care unit (NICU), respiratory distress syndrome (RDS), necrotic enterocolitis (NEC), intraventricular hemorrhage grade III and IV (IVH III and IV), sepsis, bronchopulmonary dysplasia (BPD), and neonatal death. HELLP syndrome was defined as elevated liver enzymes (ASPAT > 70 U/L), hemolysis (LDH > 600 U/L), and low platelets (<100,000/mL). FGR was defined as an estimated intrauterine weight below the 10th percentile after gestational age had been confirmed by a first-trimester ultrasound. Oligohydramnion was diagnosed when the amniotic fluid index (AFI) was below the 5th percentile for the gestational age.

The study was approved by the Local Bioethics Committee at the Institute of Mother and Child, and written informed consent was obtained from all participants. The study was performed in accordance with the guidelines described in the Declaration of Helsinki [29].

2.2. Blood Sample Preparation and Analysis

Whole blood samples were collected on the day of enrollment to the study, then were centrifuged at 25 °C for 20 min at 2000× g, and obtained sera were stored at −80 °C until further analysis. Serum sFlt-1 and PlGF levels were assessed using fully automated immunoassays (Elecsys® sFlt-1 and Elecsys® PlGF, Roche Diagnostics, Germany), and then the sFlt-1/PlGF ratio was calculated. Serum creatinine levels were assessed using automated kinetic colorimetric assay based on the Jaffé method in an alkaline solution, with picrate (Creatinine Jaffé Gen.2®, Roche Diagnostics, Germany). The estimated glomerular filtration rate (eGFR) was calculated using the Chronic Kidney Disease Epidemiology Collaboration (CKD-EPI) equation (gender- and race-specific): GFR = 141 × min $(Scr/\kappa, 1)^{-0.329}$ × max $(Scr/0.7, 1)^{-1.209}$ × 0.993^{age} × 1.018, where Scr is a serum creatinine level. The gold standard in GFR estimation is 24 h urine creatinine clearance, but it can be troublesome in different circumstances. The authors are aware that none of the available GFR formulas were fully validated in pregnancy; however, it is only additional information in this study, and the authors treat it with caution.

2.3. Statistical Analysis

The survey was conducted on the basis of strictly prepared forms. The dataset was collected in a relational database. The collected research material was analyzed using SAS 9.4 statistical software (SAS Institute Inc., 100 SAS Campus Drive, Cary, NC 27513-2414, USA). Continuous variables are expressed as the mean +/− SD and median, with a sample representativeness of 95% CI. Discrete variables are presented as numbers or letters, and categorical variables are marked accordingly. Statistical analysis describing the interrelationships between the examined variables, as well as comparisons between patients groups, were performed using the Mann–Whitney U test, Chisq test, and ANOVA Kruskal–Wallis. The value of $p < 0.05$ was taken as the significance level of the above-mentioned analyses.

3. Results

Ninety-nine patients were included in the study: thirty-eight with PE without GDM (group 1), fourteen with PE and concomitant GDM (group 2), and forty-seven with uncomplicated pregnancies (group 3). In the analyzed time period, our department carried out about 1700 deliveries, and among them, about 20–22 patients were diagnosed with PE, including about 4–5 women with PE and GDM. Hence, the vast majority of the PE population hospitalized in our clinic was enrolled (a few patients did not agree to participate in the study and could not be included).

Among patients with PE and GDM, 11 (78.57%) women were treated with diet alone (GDMG1), and 3 (21.43%) were treated with insulin (GDMG2). The demographic and clinical characteristics of the study participants are presented in Table 1. One of the most important differences between the groups was the mode of delivery—the rate of cesarean section was highest in group 2 in comparison to group 1 and 3.

Table 1. Demographic and clinical characteristic of study participants.

	Group 1 (n = 38) PE without GDM	Group 2 (n = 14) PE with GDM	Group 3 (n = 47) Control Group	Chi^2	p Value
Maternal age (years)	31.53 ± 5.68	34.93 ± 3.29	30.4 ± 4.9	N/A	†
Gestational age at study enrollment (weeks)	33.58 ± 2.85	33.57 ± 4.33	36.49 ± 2.24	N/A	††
Gestational age at delivery (weeks)	34.97 ± 2.95	34.64 ± 4.38	38.53 ± 1.73	N/A	‡
Nulliparity	27 (71.05%)	7 (50.0%)	24 (51.06%)	3.96	0.48
Maternal Medical history:					
Hypothyroidism and other concomitant disease *	14 (36.84%)	8 (57.14%)	13 (27.7%)	4.16	0.125
Obesity	12 (31.58%)	7 (50.0%)	11 (23.4%)	3.66	0.16
Delivery mode:					
Cesarean section	31 (81.58%)	13 (92.86%)	12 (25.53%)	35.61	<0.001
Vaginal birth	7 (18.42%)	1 (7.14%)	35 (74.47%)	33.32	<0.001

† Kruskal–Wallis test p value gr. 1 vs. 2 = 0.066, gr. 1 vs. 3 = 0.99, gr. 2 vs. 3 = 0.007; †† Kruskal–Wallis test p value gr. 1 vs. 2 = 1.00, gr. 1 vs. 3 < 0.01, gr. 2 vs. 3 = 0.027; ‡ Kruskal–Wallis test p value gr. 1 vs. 2 = 1.00, gr. 1 vs. 3 < 0.01, gr. 2 vs. 3 < 0.01. * other concomitant diseases in patients included in the study were: asthma, sarcoidosis, ulcerative colitis, juvenile arthritis, rheumatoid arthritis; these data were collected from patients' medical history and not from personal examination; thus, diagnostic criteria could differ between individuals; PE, preeclampsia; GDM, gestational diabetes mellitus; Chi^2, chi-squared test; N/A, not applicable.

3.1. Maternal/Fetal Outcomes

The incidence of preterm birth was highest in group 1, with 25 (65.79%) cases, whereas in group 2, it was 6 (42.86%) cases, and 4 (8.51%) in group 3. All these differences were statistically significant (Chi^2 = 30.56, $p < 0.001$; Figure 1). Similarly, FGR was diagnosed most often in group 1: 18 (47.37%) patients, in comparison to 2 (14.29%) cases in group 2, and 1 (2.13%) patient in the control group (Chi^2 = 26.2, $p < 0.001$). HELLP syndrome occurred in seven (18.42%) patients with PE without GDM, and there was no case of this complication in other groups (Chi^2 = 12.09, $p = 0.002$). There was no difference between groups in the incidence of oligohydramnion (Chi^2 = 0.92, $p = 0.63$). Considering the intensiveness of antihypertensive treatment, there was a significant difference between group 1 and 2. Monotherapy was effective in 14 (36.84%) patients in group 1, and 7 (50%) women in group 2 (Chi^2 = 25.15, $p < 0.001$), whereas polytherapy with two or more drugs was necessary in 24 (63.16%) patients in group 1, and 7 (50%) patients in group 2 (Chi^2 = 41.62, $p < 0.001$). All preeclamptic patients (with and without GDM) received methyldopa as a first-choice treatment. When it was insufficient for appropriate blood pressure control, patients were treated with either beta blockers (labetalol or metoprolol) or calcium antagonists (amlodipine or nifedipine). In group 1, 23 (60.5%) patients received a beta blocker, and 11 (28.9%) received a calcium antagonist, whereas in group 2, 7 (50%; Chi^2 = 0.46, $p = 0.5$) women were treated with beta blockers, and 4 (28.6%; Chi^2 = 0.0007, $p = 0.98$) with calcium antagonists. There was also a need for magnesium sulfate (MgSO$_4$) infusion in six (15.79%) patients with PE alone, and in three (21.43%; Chi^2= 0.2273, $p = 0.63$) patients with PE and GDM.

3.2. Neonatal Outcomes

There were significant between-group differences in neonatal outcomes. The mean birthweight was significantly higher in the control group (3273.5 ± 491.56 g; median 3300 g, 95% CI 3129.184–3417.84 g) than in the PE groups, both without and with GDM (2239.2 ± 762.58 g, median 2220 g, 95% CI 1988.56–2489.86 g; $p < 0.001$; and 2523.6 ± 1079.3 g, median 2485 g, 95% CI 1900.4–3146,74 g; $p = 0.043$, respectively). However, there was no difference in the mean birthweight between group 1 and 2 ($p = 0.461$). The first-minute Apgar score was significantly higher in the control group than in group 1 (9.64 vs. 8.76; $p = 0.028$), but there were no differences between all groups in the fifth-minute Apgar score. Among all 99 newborns included in the study, one died (in group 2). The admission to NICU was necessary in eight (21.05%) babies in group 1, and two (14.29%) newborns in group 2, whereas none of the children born in the control group needed NICU admission. These differences were statistically significant (Chi^2 = 10.57, p = 0.005). Among other neonatal complications, RDS was diagnosed most often in group 2: five (35.71%) cases in comparison to six (15.79%) cases in group 1, and one (2.13%) case in the control group (Chi^2 = 12.20, p = 0.002). Neonatal outcomes are presented in detail in Table 2.

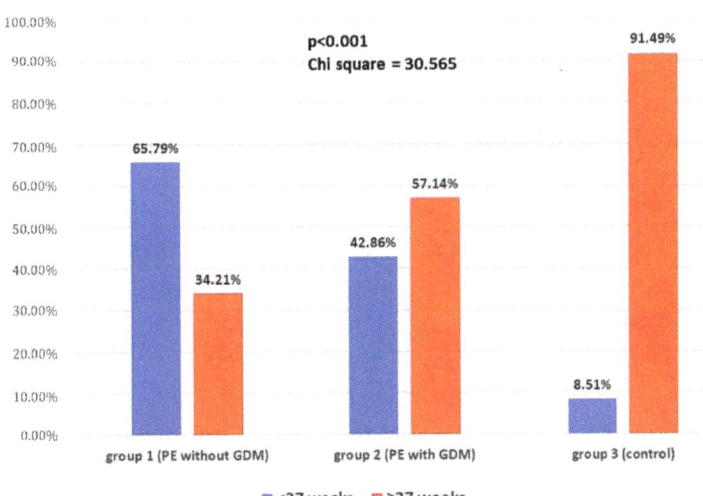

Figure 1. The incidence of preterm delivery in the study groups.

Table 2. Neonatal outcomes.

	Group 1 (n = 38) PE without GDM	Group 2 (n = 14) PE with GDM	Group 3 (n = 47) Control Group	Chi^2	p
Birthweight (g)	2239.2 ± 762.58	2523.6 ± 1079.3	3273.5 ± 491.56	N/A	†
First-minute Apgar score	8.76 ± 1.62	8.29 ± 2.49	9.64 ± 0.965	N/A	††
Fifth-minute Apgar score	9.54 ± 0.77	9.29 ± 1.38	9.89 ± 0.43	N/A	‡
Neonatal complicationsDeath	0	1 (7.14%)	0	6.13	0.047
Admission to NICU	8 (21.05%)	2 (14.29%)	0	10.57	0.005
RDS	6 (15.79%)	5 (35.71%)	1 (2.13%)	12.20	0.002
IVH III/IV	1 (2.63%)	0	0	1.62	0.445
NEC	2 (5.26%)	0	0	3.28	0.194
sepsis	3 (7.89%)	0	0	4.97	0.084
BPD	2 (5.26%)	0	0	3.28	0.194
without any complication	30 (78.95%)	8 (57.14%)	46 (97.87%)	15.59	<0.001

† Kruskal–Wallis test p value gr. 1 vs. 2 = 0.461, gr. 1 vs. 3 = < 0.001, gr. 2 vs. 3 = 0.043; †† Kruskal–Wallis test p value gr. 1 vs. 2 = 1.0, gr. 1 vs. 3 = 0.028, gr. 2 vs. 3 = 0.052; ‡ Kruskal–Wallis test p value gr. 1 vs. 2 = 1.0, gr. 1 vs. 3 = 0.14, gr. 2 vs. 3 = 0.29; PE, preeclampsia; GDM, gestational diabetes mellitus; NICU, neonatal intensive care unit; RDS, respiratory distress syndrome; IVH III/IV, intraventricular hemorrhage grade III or IV; NEC, necrotic enterocolitis; BPD, bronchopulmonary dysplasia; Chi^2, chi-squared test; N/A, not applicable.

3.3. Biochemical Parameters

In all studied biochemical parameters and ratios, i.e., serum PlGF, sFlt-1, and creatinine levels, eGFR and PLT differed between the control group and both PE groups; however, there were no differences in all these parameters between patients with PE with and without GDM. These results are presented in Table 3.

Table 3. Biochemical parameters (median value of each parameter with SD).

	Group 1 (PE without GDM)	Group 2 (PE with GDM)	Group 3 (Control)	p Value (Kruskal–Wallis Test)		
				Gr. 1 vs. 2	Gr. 1 vs. 3	Gr. 2 vs. 3
sFlt-1 (pg/mL)	12054.0 ± 6757.45 (95% CI 10842.65–15284.88)	10109.5 ± 5265.4 (95% CI 7966.46–14046.8)	3556.0 ± 2218.7 (95% CI 3160.69–4463.56)	1.00	<0.001	<0.001
PlGF (pg/mL)	54.75 ± 75.33 (95% CI 50.46–109.98)	68.70 ± 53.38 (95% CI 52.47–114.1)	192.9 ± 404.7 (95% CI 209.66–447.32)	1.00	<0.001	<0.001
sFlt-1/PlGF	209.27 ± 253.88 (95% CI 189.73–356.63)	162.7 ± 327.37 (95% CI 66.9–444.9)	15.7 ± 22.24 (95% CI 16.97–30.02)	1.00	<0.001	<0.001
PLT	189.5 ± 58.88 (95% CI 174.88–213.59)	159.0 ± 79.6 (95% CI 136.7–228.7)	217.0 ± 49.69 (95% CI 211.54–240.72)	0.868	0.022	0.008
Creatinine (μmo/L)	55.0 ± 12.71 (95% CI 53.03–61.63)	61.0 ± 15.88 (95% CI 53.05–71.38)	49.0 ± 7.09 (95% CI 45.17–50.04)	1.00	<0.01	0.001
eGFR (mL/min/1.73^2)	119.8 ± 15.92 (95% CI 110.03–120.81)	112.05 ± 18.85 (95% CI 95.78–117.55)	124.6 ± 8.24 (95% CI 123.74–129.4)	0.487	0.004	<0.001

PE, preeclampsia; GDM, gestational diabetes mellitus; sFlt-1, soluble fms-like tyrosine kinase; PlGF, placental growth factor; PLT, platelet count per mm^3; eGFR, estimated glomerular filtration rate.

4. Discussion

The present study aimed to assess the possible impact of GDM coexistence on the course and severity of PE. We demonstrated that women with PE and GDM were less likely to give birth prematurely and to develop FGR and HELLP syndrome, and required less intensive antihypertensive treatment than women with PE, but without GDM. The cesarean section rate was, in turn, significantly higher in women with both diseases than with PE alone. Newborns from mothers with PE and GDM less frequently required admission to the NICU; however, they were more likely to develop RDS than newborns from mothers with PE without GDM.

Available studies demonstrated a strong association between diabetes and PE, i.e., both pregestational and GDM were confirmed as risk factors for developing PE. PE is diagnosed in 15–20% of pregnant women with type 1 diabetes and in 10–14% of pregnant women with type 2 diabetes in comparison to 2–8% of women without diabetes [30,31]. In a study based on the German Perinatal Quality Registry including 647,392 patients, the risk of developing PE was increased in patients with GDM, even after adjustment by age, nationality, job status, smoking, parity, multiple pregnancy, pre-pregnancy weight, and gestational weight gain (OR 1.29, 95% CI 1.19–1.41) [13]. Moreover, other birth registry studies, performed in Sweden and Canada, confirmed GDM as an independent risk factor for PE [14,32]. Additionally, women with PE in their first pregnancy have an increased risk of GDM in the second pregnancy in comparison to patients with neither of these two diseases in their first pregnancy (OR 1.2, 95% CI 1.1–1.3) [22]. The association of GDM and PE may be related to the common risk factors shared by both diseases, such as advanced maternal age, nulliparity, multiple pregnancies, obesity, and Black race. However, many maladaptations to pregnancy present in both diseases have been also identified. They include insulin resistance, endothelial dysfunction, angiogenic imbalance, and oxidative stress [15,33,34]. Recent studies demonstrated that other signaling pathways may also be involved in the pathophysiology of PE in GDM patients, e.g., kisspeptin-1 and its receptor [35]. The genetic background makes it possible to underline the association between GDM and PE as well— to date, ACE gene I/D polymorphism and miRNA146A rs2910164 (G/C) polymorphism have been confirmed as being related to an increased incidence of PE in women with GDM [25,36].

Both PE and GDM are related to an increased risk of adverse perinatal outcomes, and, thus, are important global public health concerns. Nunes et al. investigated the influence of PE, advanced maternal age, and maternal obesity on neonatal outcomes in patients with GDM. They found that among these three factors, only the coexistence of PE showed an association with adverse neonatal outcomes, such as neonatal morbidity, low and very low birthweight, and preterm delivery [24]. To our knowledge, there is only one study comparing perinatal outcomes in patients with hypertensive disorders of pregnancy (HDP) with and without GDM. Preterm delivery rates in this study were more than threefold greater in the HDP and GDM group and HDP-alone group in comparison to healthy controls, with an adjusted OR of 4.84 (95% CI 4.34–5.4) and 3.92 (95% CI 3.65–4.21), respectively. Additionally, the rate of small-for-gestational-age (SGA) babies was greater in patients with HDP with and without GDM in comparison to the control group, with an adjusted OR of 6.57 (95% CI 5.56–7.75) and 5.81 (95% CI 5.15–6.55), respectively. The incidence of adverse outcomes increased further in women with PE and eclampsia [26]. Our results contradict these results, because in our research, the incidence of preterm birth and FGR was lower in patients with PE and coexisting GDM than in women with PE alone. Our results indicate the less severe course of PE in women with concomitant GDM, as evidenced also by a lower incidence of NICU admissions among neonates from mothers with PE and GDM than in PE alone. On the other hand, there was an increased rate of RDS among babies from mothers suffering from both PE and GDM, but there is a vast body of evidence that GDM alone is associated with an increased risk of neonatal RDS [37], because maternal hyperglycemia delays fetal lung maturation [38].

Another important finding of the presented study is that the cesarean section rate was highest in patients with both PE and GDM, and this is consistent with earlier studies, including the above-mentioned research performed by Lin et al. [26]. GDM is a common risk of ending delivery with C-section, which is also associated with fetal macrosomia observed among women with GDM [39,40].

As mentioned at the beginning, the main mechanism of developing PE is thought to be an imbalance between angiogenic and antiangiogenic factors leading to maternal global endothelial dysfunction. In our study, we compared the serum levels of the most important angio- and antiangiogenic biomarkers, i.e., PlGF and sFlt-1, in patients with PE with and without coexisting GDM. As expected, significant differences were found between women with PE (both with and without GDM) and healthy pregnant women. Nevertheless, there were no statistically significant differences between patients with PE and GDM and PE alone. We suggest that such a result may indicate no impact of GDM on the usefulness of these biomarkers in clinical practice to predict PE and related adverse outcomes. Similar to our study, Nuzzo et al. found that the serum sFlt-1 level was significantly increased and serum PlGF was significantly decreased in patients with PE alone and PE with GDM in comparison to women with GDM alone and healthy controls. However, they also demonstrated higher values of sFlt-1/PlGF ratio in patients with PE alone than in PE and GDM. Clinical parameters, such as the incidence of pathological umbilical Doppler, low Apgar score, and NICU admission, were, in this study, increased in women with PE alone in comparison with PE-GDM patients, suggesting the possible influence of GDM on the course of PE, which is consistent with our study as well [41]. Cohen et al. presented elevated serum levels of sFlt-1 and reduced serum levels of PlGF in patients with pregestational diabetes who developed PE, just as women without diabetes have been shown to have in PE [42]. Kapustin et al. investigated the placental expression of PlGF and endoglin in patients with PE and GDM, and found that PlGF expression was undermost in PE. In GDM treated with insulin, PlGF expression was also reduced in comparison to GDM patients treated only with diet, indicating that placental PlGF expression in GDM is also altered and dependent on the control of the glycemia level during pregnancy [43]. There is evidence that in women with obesity, GDM may modify the association between PlGF in early pregnancy and PE [44]. Nonetheless, in our study, there was no difference between the incidence of obesity in all studied groups; thus, there is no risk of bias in this point.

Less is known about the mechanism that could be a reason of the possible phenomenon that GDM might alleviate the course of PE. However, in a recently published study, Kul et al. investigated the prevalence of coronary microvascular dysfunction (CMD) in women with combined PE and GDM. They found that in patients with GDM, additional PE on top of GDM was associated with a significant increased risk of CMD, even after adjusting for other covariates, but for patients with PE, the presence of GDM did not confer an additional risk after multivariate analysis [21]. The authors of this study suggest two possible explanations. First, is that PE has a direct and immediate effect on vasculature independent from hypertension, whereas the influence of disturbed glucose metabolism is time-dependent [21]. The second thing might be the level of immune activation, which is one of the central parts in the pathogenesis of PE, as well as endothelial dysfunction and CMD, whereas in GDM, the evidence for the role of inflammation in the pathophysiology of the disease is less robust [45,46]. Pro-inflammatory cytokines secreted in adipose tissue in GDM (such as TNFα, IL-1β, IL-6) impair insulin signaling and inhibit insulin release from β-cells; however, this relationship is complex and not straightforward, because there are studies reporting that GDM placentae secrete fewer pro-inflammatory cytokines than healthy placentae [12]. The difference in the immune response in PE and GDM should also be considered as one of the important mechanisms participating in the described PE and GDM coexistence phenomenon.

The potential mitigation of the severity of PE by the coexisting GDM has its justification in the pathophysiology of both diseases. PE is well-documented as an antiangiogenic state with general vasoconstriction and reduced placental perfusion. GDM is, in turn, considered as a pro-angiogenic state, and diabetic placentas exhibit enhanced vascularization in comparison to placentas from uncomplicated pregnancies. These results appear to be related to the reduced expression of Flt-1, and the increased activity of VEGF receptor 2 (KDR) [47]. The change in the placental VEGF/VEGF receptor expression ratio in hyperglycemia may favor angiogenesis in placental tissue, and could explain the hypercapillarization of villi seen in diabetic patients [48]. In our study, it is reflected in the incidence of FGR that was higher in PE patients without GDM. Increased placental weight and a decreased percentage of pathological uterine/umbilical Doppler in PE-GDM patients in comparison to PE alone in the above-mentioned study performed by Nuzzo et al. can also provide evidence of the possible placental adaptation attempt [41].

Another possibility is the potential impact of differences in the metabolic profiles of patients with and without GDM, and the incidence of metabolic syndrome (MetS) among them. MetS is a cluster of cardiovascular disease risk factors, including obesity, atherogenic dyslipidemia, raised blood pressure, insulin resistance, and pro-inflammatory states; although, there are several definitions and cut-points to describe and characterize MetS [49,50]. Women with MetS are at an increased risk of both PE and GDM [51,52]. Moreover, Grieger et al. demonstrated that more than half of women who had MetS in early pregnancy developed a pregnancy complication, in comparison to just over a third of women who did not have MetS [51]. We have no data about the components of MetS in our cohort; however, we can hypothesize that the results in patients with PE and GDM may arise more from metabolic abnormalities than from enhanced endothelial dysfunction, as in "pure" PE, because of different pathophysiological pathways, similar to the difference between early- and late-onset PE. The risk factors for cardiovascular disorders and PE are very similar, and it still remains unclear whether PE is an individual risk factor for future cardiovascular events or an early marker of women with high-risk profiles for cardiovascular disease, where the pregnancy can only be a trigger for cardiovascular alterations that manifest in the development of PE [20,53]. This leaves a lot of room for further research to explain these dependencies.

The main limitation of this study is the relatively small number of cases; thus, further analyses are required to confirm our data. The lack of a group of patients with GDM alone may also be considered as a limitation, because it could provide more important information. However, the authors recognized both diseases as having completely different pathophysiology and perinatal/neonatal outcomes (e.g., FGR vs. macrosomia), and focused on PE and the possible effect of coexisting GDM on the course of it. Moreover, the research discussed earlier in this paper presented different outcomes: in the GDM-alone group, the patients came closer to the control group than to PE patients [24,41].

The strength of the study is its prospective design and the high group homogeneity obtained, i.a., by applying narrow inclusion criteria (proteinuria as a necessary component), and the exclusion of multiple pregnancies, pregestational diabetes, and preexisting hypertension. In our opinion, proteinuria as a necessary component is an advantage, because it increases group homogeneity and helps avoiding bias related to the differences between many individual components of new PE definition (such as liver dysfunction, neurological features, thrombocytopenia, or FGR). There are only few data concerning the relationship between these components with the severity of the imbalance between angio- and antiangiogenic factors [6,54–56]; our previous study may serve as an example, where we demonstrated that in preeclamptic patients, renal function parameters correlate with serum sFlt-1 levels and sFlt/PlGF-1 ratio [57].

The strength of the study is also its translational potential—improving the knowledge of the pathomechanisms underlying the coexistence of PE and GDM, especially the molecular basis of the possible alleviating effect of GDM on the course of PE, which may lead to elaborating tailored, successful preventive and therapeutic strategies for women at a high risk of developing PE and its severe complications.

5. Conclusions

The presented study demonstrated that the incidence of adverse perinatal outcomes, such as preterm birth, FGR, HELLP syndrome, and neonatal admission to NICU, was significantly lower among women with PE and GDM in comparison to patients with PE alone, indicating that the coexistence of GDM may mitigate the course of PE. Additionally, there was no difference between patients with PE with and without GDM in the serum levels of biomarkers, such as sFlt-1 and PlGF, as well as in sFlt-1/PlGF ratio, confirming no influence of GDM on its usefulness in the diagnosis and management of PE.

Author Contributions: Conceptualization, K.P., A.F. and T.M.M.; methodology, K.P., A.F. and T.M.M.; formal analysis, K.P., J.S. and T.I.; investigation, K.P. and E.S.; data curation, K.P., E.S. and J.S.; writing—original draft preparation, K.P.; writing—review and editing, A.F., T.I. and T.M.M. All authors have read and agreed to the published version of the manuscript.

Funding: Ministry of Science and Higher Education, financed with subsidy from the state budget to the Institute of Mother and Child.

Institutional Review Board Statement: The study was conducted in accordance with the Declaration of Helsinki, and approved by the Local Ethics Committee of the Institute of Mother and Child (protocol no., 27/2013; date of approval, 17 October 2013).

Informed Consent Statement: Informed consent was obtained from all subjects involved in the study.

Data Availability Statement: Not applicable.

Conflicts of Interest: The authors declare no conflict of interest.

References

1. Ananth, C.V.; Lavery, J.A.; Friedman, A.M.; Wapner, R.J.; Wright, J.D. Serious Maternal Complications in Relation to Severe Pre-Eclampsia: A Retrospective Cohort Study of the Impact of Hospital Volume. *BJOG Int. J. Obstet. Gynaecol.* **2017**, *124*, 1246–1253. [CrossRef] [PubMed]
2. Eades, C.E.; Cameron, D.M.; Evans, J.M.M. Prevalence of Gestational Diabetes Mellitus in Europe: A Meta-Analysis. *Diabetes Res. Clin. Pract.* **2017**, *129*, 173–181. [CrossRef] [PubMed]
3. DeSisto, C.L.; Kim, S.Y.; Sharma, A.J. Prevalence Estimates of Gestational Diabetes Mellitus in the United States, Pregnancy Risk Assessment Monitoring System (PRAMS), 2007–2010. *Prev. Chronic Dis.* **2014**, *11*, E104. [CrossRef] [PubMed]
4. Brown, M.A.; Magee, L.A.; Kenny, L.C.; Karumanchi, S.A.; McCarthy, F.P.; Saito, S.; Hall, D.R.; Warren, C.E.; Adoyi, G.; Ishaku, S.; et al. The Hypertensive Disorders of Pregnancy: ISSHP Classification, Diagnosis & Management Recommendations for International Practice. *Pregnancy Hypertens.* **2018**, *13*, 291–310. [CrossRef]
5. Pankiewicz, K.; Fijałkowska, A.; Issat, T.; Maciejewski, T.M. Insight into the Key Points of Preeclampsia Pathophysiology: Uterine Artery Remodeling and the Role of MicroRNAs. *Int. J. Mol. Sci.* **2021**, *22*, 3132. [CrossRef]
6. Rana, S.; Burke, S.D.; Karumanchi, S.A. Imbalances in circulating angiogenic factors in the pathophysiology of preeclampsia and related disorders. *Am. J. Obstet. Gynecol.* **2022**, *226*, S1019–S1034. [CrossRef]

7. Tan, M.Y.; Syngelaki, A.; Poon, L.C.; Rolnik, D.L.; O'Gorman, N.; Delgado, J.L.; Akolekar, R.; Konstantinidou, L.; Tsavdaridou, M.; Galeva, S.; et al. Screening for Pre-Eclampsia by Maternal Factors and Biomarkers at 11–13 Weeks' Gestation. *Ultrasound Obstet. Gynecol.* **2018**, *52*, 186–195. [CrossRef]
8. Akolekar, R.; de Cruz, J.; Foidart, J.-M.; Munaut, C.; Nicolaides, K.H. Maternal Plasma Soluble Fms-like Tyrosine Kinase-1 and Free Vascular Endothelial Growth Factor at 11 to 13 Weeks of Gestation in Preeclampsia. *Prenat. Diagn.* **2010**, *30*, 191–197. [CrossRef]
9. Akolekar, R.; Zaragoza, E.; Poon, L.C.Y.; Pepes, S.; Nicolaides, K.H. Maternal Serum Placental Growth Factor at 11 + 0 to 13 + 6 Weeks of Gestation in the Prediction of Pre-Eclampsia. *Ultrasound Obstet. Gynecol.* **2008**, *32*, 732–739. [CrossRef]
10. Rana, S.; Powe, C.E.; Salahuddin, S.; Verlohren, S.; Perschel, F.H.; Levine, R.J.; Lim, K.-H.; Wenger, J.B.; Thadhani, R.; Karumanchi, S.A. Angiogenic Factors and the Risk of Adverse Outcomes in Women with Suspected Preeclampsia. *Circulation* **2012**, *125*, 911–919. [CrossRef]
11. Yuen, L.; Saeedi, P.; Riaz, M.; Karuranga, S.; Divakar, H.; Levitt, N.; Yang, X.; Simmons, D. Projections of the Prevalence of Hyperglycaemia in Pregnancy in 2019 and beyond: Results from the International Diabetes Federation Diabetes Atlas, 9th Edition. *Diabetes Res. Clin. Pract.* **2019**, *157*, 107841. [CrossRef] [PubMed]
12. Plows, J.F.; Stanley, J.L.; Baker, P.N.; Reynolds, C.M.; Vickers, M.H. The Pathophysiology of Gestational Diabetes Mellitus. *Int. J. Mol. Sci.* **2018**, *19*, 3342. [CrossRef] [PubMed]
13. Schneider, S.; Freerksen, N.; Röhrig, S.; Hoeft, B.; Maul, H. Gestational Diabetes and Preeclampsia—Similar Risk Factor Profiles? *Early Hum. Dev.* **2012**, *88*, 179–184. [CrossRef] [PubMed]
14. Ostlund, I.; Haglund, B.; Hanson, U. Gestational Diabetes and Preeclampsia. *Eur. J. Obstet. Gynecol. Reprod. Biol.* **2004**, *113*, 12–16. [CrossRef]
15. Weissgerber, T.L.; Mudd, L.M. Preeclampsia and Diabetes. *Curr. Diabetes Rep.* **2015**, *15*, 9. [CrossRef]
16. Melchiorre, K.; Sutherland, G.R.; Liberati, M.; Thilaganathan, B. Preeclampsia Is Associated with Persistent Postpartum Cardiovascular Impairment. *Hypertension* **2011**, *58*, 709–715. [CrossRef]
17. Irgens, H.U.; Reisaeter, L.; Irgens, L.M.; Lie, R.T. Long Term Mortality of Mothers and Fathers after Pre-Eclampsia: Population Based Cohort Study. *BMJ* **2001**, *323*, 1213–1217. [CrossRef]
18. Wu, P.; Haththotuwa, R.; Kwok, C.S.; Babu, A.; Kotronias, R.A.; Rushton, C.; Zaman, A.; Fryer, A.A.; Kadam, U.; Chew-Graham, C.A.; et al. Preeclampsia and Future Cardiovascular Health: A Systematic Review and Meta-Analysis. *Circ. Cardiovasc. Qual. Outcomes* **2017**, *10*, e003497. [CrossRef]
19. Wu, C.-C.; Chen, S.-H.; Ho, C.-H.; Liang, F.-W.; Chu, C.-C.; Wang, H.-Y.; Lu, Y.-H. End-Stage Renal Disease after Hypertensive Disorders in Pregnancy. *Am. J. Obstet. Gynecol.* **2014**, *210*, e1–e8. [CrossRef]
20. Pankiewicz, K.; Szczerba, E.; Maciejewski, T.; Fijałkowska, A. Non-Obstetric Complications in Preeclampsia. *Menopause Rev.* **2019**, *18*, 99–109. [CrossRef]
21. Kul, Ş.; Güvenç, T.S.; Baycan, Ö.F.; Çelik, F.B.; Çalışkan, Z.; Çetin Güvenç, R.; Çiftçi, F.C.; Caliskan, M. Combined Past Preeclampsia and Gestational Diabetes Is Associated with a Very High Frequency of Coronary Microvascular Dysfunction. *Microvasc. Res.* **2021**, *134*, 104104. [CrossRef] [PubMed]
22. Lee, J.; Ouh, Y.-T.; Ahn, K.H.; Hong, S.C.; Oh, M.-J.; Kim, H.-J.; Cho, G.J. Preeclampsia: A Risk Factor for Gestational Diabetes Mellitus in Subsequent Pregnancy. *PLoS ONE* **2017**, *12*, e0178150. [CrossRef] [PubMed]
23. Mistry, S.K.; Das Gupta, R.; Alam, S.; Kaur, K.; Shamim, A.A.; Puthussery, S. Gestational Diabetes Mellitus (GDM) and Adverse Pregnancy Outcome in South Asia: A Systematic Review. *Endocrinol. Diabetes Metab.* **2021**, *4*, e00285. [CrossRef]
24. Nunes, J.S.; Ladeiras, R.; Machado, L.; Coelho, D.; Duarte, C.; Furtado, J.M. The Influence of Preeclampsia, Advanced Maternal Age and Maternal Obesity in Neonatal Outcomes among Women with Gestational Diabetes. *Rev. Bras. Ginecol. Obstet.* **2020**, *42*, 607–613. [CrossRef] [PubMed]
25. Dmitrenko, O.P.; Karpova, N.S.; Nurbekov, M.K.; Papysheva, O.V. I/D Polymorphism Gene ACE and Risk of Preeclampsia in Women with Gestational Diabetes Mellitus. *Dis. Markers* **2020**, *2020*, 8875230. [CrossRef]
26. Lin, Y.-W.; Lin, M.-H.; Pai, L.-W.; Fang, J.-W.; Mou, C.-H.; Sung, F.-C.; Tzeng, Y.-L. Population-Based Study on Birth Outcomes among Women with Hypertensive Disorders of Pregnancy and Gestational Diabetes Mellitus. *Sci. Rep.* **2021**, *11*, 17391. [CrossRef]
27. European Society of Gynecology (ESG); Association for European Paediatric Cardiology (AEPC); German Society for Gender Medicine (DGesGM); Regitz-Zagrosek, V.; Lundqvist, C.B.; Borghi, C.; Cifkova, R.; Ferreira, R.; Foidart, J.-M.; Gibbs, J.S.R.; et al. ESC Guidelines on the Management of Cardiovascular Diseases during Pregnancy: The Task Force on the Management of Cardiovascular Diseases during Pregnancy of the European Society of Cardiology (ESC). *Eur. Heart J.* **2011**, *32*, 3147–3197. [CrossRef]
28. Whiting, D.R.; Guariguata, L.; Weil, C.; Shaw, J. IDF Diabetes Atlas: Global Estimates of the Prevalence of Diabetes for 2011 and 2030. *Diabetes Res. Clin. Pract.* **2011**, *94*, 311–321. [CrossRef]
29. World Medical Association. World Medical Association Declaration of Helsinki: Ethical Principles for Medical Research Involving Human Subjects. *JAMA* **2013**, *310*, 2191–2194. [CrossRef]
30. Persson, M.; Norman, M.; Hanson, U. Obstetric and Perinatal Outcomes in Type 1 Diabetic Pregnancies: A Large, Population-Based Study. *Diabetes Care* **2009**, *32*, 2005–2009. [CrossRef]
31. Knight, K.M.; Thornburg, L.L.; Pressman, E.K. Pregnancy Outcomes in Type 2 Diabetic Patients as Compared with Type 1 Diabetic Patients and Nondiabetic Controls. *J. Reprod. Med.* **2012**, *57*, 397–404. [PubMed]

32. Nerenberg, K.A.; Johnson, J.A.; Leung, B.; Savu, A.; Ryan, E.A.; Chik, C.L.; Kaul, P. Risks of Gestational Diabetes and Preeclampsia over the Last Decade in a Cohort of Alberta Women. *J. Obstet. Gynaecol. Can.* **2013**, *35*, 986–994. [CrossRef]
33. de Guimarães, M.F.B.R.; Brandão, A.H.F.; de Rezende, C.A.L.; Cabral, A.C.V.; Brum, A.P.; Leite, H.V.; Capuruço, C.A.B. Assessment of Endothelial Function in Pregnant Women with Preeclampsia and Gestational Diabetes Mellitus by Flow-Mediated Dilation of Brachial Artery. *Arch. Gynecol. Obstet.* **2014**, *290*, 441–447. [CrossRef] [PubMed]
34. Karacay, O.; Sepici-Dincel, A.; Karcaaltincaba, D.; Sahin, D.; Yalvaç, S.; Akyol, M.; Kandemir, O.; Altan, N. A Quantitative Evaluation of Total Antioxidant Status and Oxidative Stress Markers in Preeclampsia and Gestational Diabetic Patients in 24–36 Weeks of Gestation. *Diabetes Res. Clin. Pract.* **2010**, *89*, 231–238. [CrossRef]
35. Kapustin, R.V.; Drobintseva, A.O.; Alekseenkova, E.N.; Onopriychuk, A.R.; Arzhanova, O.N.; Polyakova, V.O.; Kvetnoy, I.M. Placental Protein Expression of Kisspeptin-1 (KISS1) and the Kisspeptin-1 Receptor (KISS1R) in Pregnancy Complicated by Diabetes Mellitus or Preeclampsia. *Arch. Gynecol. Obstet.* **2020**, *301*, 437–445. [CrossRef]
36. Abo-Elmatty, D.M.; Mehanna, E.T. MIR146A Rs2910164 (G/C) Polymorphism Is Associated with Incidence of Preeclampsia in Gestational Diabetes Patients. *Biochem. Genet.* **2019**, *57*, 222–233. [CrossRef]
37. Li, Y.; Wang, W.; Zhang, D. Maternal Diabetes Mellitus and Risk of Neonatal Respiratory Distress Syndrome: A Meta-Analysis. *Acta Diabetol.* **2019**, *56*, 729–740. [CrossRef]
38. Bourbon, J.R.; Farrell, P.M. Fetal Lung Development in the Diabetic Pregnancy. *Pediatr. Res.* **1985**, *19*, 253–267. [CrossRef]
39. Gorgal, R.; Gonçalves, E.; Barros, M.; Namora, G.; Magalhães, A.; Rodrigues, T.; Montenegro, N. Gestational Diabetes Mellitus: A Risk Factor for Non-Elective Cesarean Section. *J. Obstet. Gynaecol. Res.* **2012**, *38*, 154–159. [CrossRef]
40. Kc, K.; Shakya, S.; Zhang, H. Gestational Diabetes Mellitus and Macrosomia: A Literature Review. *Ann. Nutr. Metab.* **2015**, *66* (Suppl. 2), 14–20. [CrossRef]
41. Nuzzo, A.M.; Giuffrida, D.; Moretti, L.; Re, P.; Grassi, G.; Menato, G.; Rolfo, A. Placental and Maternal SFlt1/PlGF Expression in Gestational Diabetes Mellitus. *Sci. Rep.* **2021**, *11*, 2312. [CrossRef] [PubMed]
42. Cohen, A.; Lim, K.-H.; Lee, Y.; Rana, S.; Karumanchi, S.A.; Brown, F. Circulating Levels of the Antiangiogenic Marker Soluble FMS-like Tyrosine Kinase 1 Are Elevated in Women with Pregestational Diabetes and Preeclampsia: Angiogenic Markers in Preeclampsia and Preexisting Diabetes. *Diabetes Care* **2007**, *30*, 375–377. [CrossRef] [PubMed]
43. Kapustin, R.V.; Kopteeva, E.V.; Alekseenkova, E.N.; Tral, T.G.; Tolibova, G.K.; Arzhanova, O.N. Placental Expression of Endoglin, Placental Growth Factor, Leptin, and Hypoxia-Inducible Factor-1 in Diabetic Pregnancy and Pre-Eclampsia. *Gynecol. Endocrinol.* **2021**, *37*, 35–39. [CrossRef] [PubMed]
44. Vieira, M.C.; Begum, S.; Seed, P.T.; Badran, D.; Briley, A.L.; Gill, C.; Godfrey, K.M.; Lawlor, D.A.; Nelson, S.M.; Patel, N.; et al. Gestational Diabetes Modifies the Association between PlGF in Early Pregnancy and Preeclampsia in Women with Obesity. *Pregnancy Hypertens.* **2018**, *13*, 267–272. [CrossRef] [PubMed]
45. Troncoso, F.; Acurio, J.; Herlitz, K.; Aguayo, C.; Bertoglia, P.; Guzman-Gutierrez, E.; Loyola, M.; Gonzalez, M.; Rezgaoui, M.; Desoye, G.; et al. Gestational Diabetes Mellitus Is Associated with Increased Pro-Migratory Activation of Vascular Endothelial Growth Factor Receptor 2 and Reduced Expression of Vascular Endothelial Growth Factor Receptor 1. *PLoS ONE* **2017**, *12*, e0182509. [CrossRef]
46. Wolf, M.; Sauk, J.; Shah, A.; Smirnakis, K.V.; Jimenez-Kimble, R.; Ecker, J.L.; Thadhani, R. Inflammation and Glucose Intolerance: A Prospective Study of Gestational Diabetes Mellitus. *Diabetes Care* **2004**, *27*, 21–27. [CrossRef]
47. Harmon, A.C.; Cornelius, D.C.; Amaral, L.M.; Faulkner, J.L.; Cunningham, M.W.; Wallace, K.; LaMarca, B. The Role of Inflammation in the Pathology of Preeclampsia. *Clin. Sci.* **2016**, *130*, 409–419. [CrossRef]
48. Pietro, L.; Daher, S.; Rudge, M.V.C.; Calderon, I.M.P.; Damasceno, D.C.; Sinzato, Y.K.; Bandeira, C.; Bevilacqua, E. Vascular Endothelial Growth Factor (VEGF) and VEGF-Receptor Expression in Placenta of Hyperglycemic Pregnant Women. *Placenta* **2010**, *31*, 770–780. [CrossRef]
49. Rochlani, Y.; Pothineni, N.V.; Kovelamudi, S.; Mehta, J.L. Metabolic Syndrome: Pathophysiology, Management, and Modulation by Natural Compounds. *Ther. Adv. Cardiovasc. Dis.* **2017**, *11*, 215–225. [CrossRef]
50. Vernini, J.M.; Nicolosi, B.F.; Arantes, M.A.; Costa, R.A.; Magalhães, C.G.; Corrente, J.E.; Lima, S.A.M.; Rudge, M.V.; Calderon, I.M. Metabolic Syndrome Markers and Risk of Hyperglycemia in Pregnancy: A Cross-Sectional Cohort Study. *Sci. Rep.* **2020**, *10*, 21042. [CrossRef]
51. Grieger, J.A.; Bianco-Miotto, T.; Grzeskowiak, L.E.; Leemaqz, S.Y.; Poston, L.; McCowan, L.M.; Kenny, L.C.; Myers, J.E.; Walker, J.J.; Dekker, G.A.; et al. Metabolic Syndrome in Pregnancy and Risk for Adverse Pregnancy Outcomes: A Prospective Cohort of Nulliparous Women. *PLoS Med.* **2018**, *15*, e1002710. [CrossRef] [PubMed]
52. Hooijschuur, M.C.E.; Ghossein-Doha, C.; Kroon, A.A.; De Leeuw, P.W.; Zandbergen, A.A.M.; Van Kuijk, S.M.J.; Spaanderman, M.E.A. Metabolic Syndrome and Pre-Eclampsia. *Ultrasound Obstet. Gynecol.* **2019**, *54*, 64–71. [CrossRef] [PubMed]
53. Melchiorre, K.; Sharma, R.; Thilaganathan, B. Cardiovascular Implications in Preeclampsia: An Overview. *Circulation* **2014**, *130*, 703–714. [CrossRef] [PubMed]
54. Rana, S.; Schnettler, W.T.; Powe, C.; Wenger, J.; Salahuddin, S.; Cerdeira, A.S.; Verlohren, S.; Perschel, F.H.; Arany, Z.; Lim, K.-H.; et al. Clinical Characterization and Outcomes of Preeclampsia with Normal Angiogenic Profile. *Hypertens. Pregnancy* **2013**, *32*, 189–201. [CrossRef] [PubMed]

55. Oe, Y.; Ko, M.; Fushima, T.; Sato, E.; Karumanchi, S.A.; Sato, H.; Sugawara, J.; Ito, S.; Takahashi, N. Hepatic Dysfunction and Thrombocytopenia Induced by Excess SFlt1 in Mice Lacking Endothelial Nitric Oxide Synthase. *Sci. Rep.* **2018**, *8*, 102. [CrossRef] [PubMed]
56. Levine, R.J.; Lam, C.; Qian, C.; Yu, K.F.; Maynard, S.E.; Sachs, B.P.; Sibai, B.M.; Epstein, F.H.; Romero, R.; Thadhani, R.; et al. Soluble Endoglin and Other Circulating Antiangiogenic Factors in Preeclampsia. *N. Engl. J. Med.* **2006**, *355*, 992–1005. [CrossRef]
57. Pankiewicz, K.; Szczerba, E.; Fijalkowska, A.; Szamotulska, K.; Szewczyk, G.; Issat, T.; Maciejewski, T.M. The Association between Serum Galectin-3 Level and Its Placental Production in Patients with Preeclampsia. *J. Physiol. Pharmacol.* **2020**, *71*, 1–12. [CrossRef]

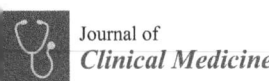

Journal of
Clinical Medicine

Article

Corin—The Early Marker of Preeclampsia in Pregestational Diabetes Mellitus

Daniel Boroń [1,2,*], Jakub Kornacki [1], Paweł Gutaj [1], Urszula Mantaj [1], Przemysław Wirstlein [1] and Ewa Wender-Ozegowska [1]

1 Department of Reproduction, Poznań University of Medical Sciences, 61-701 Poznan, Poland
2 PUMS Doctoral School, 61-701 Poznan, Poland
* Correspondence: boron.daniel92@gmail.com

Abstract: Preeclampsia (PE) is one of the leading causes of mortality and morbidity in pregnant women. Pregestational diabetes (PGDM) patients are prone to vascular complications and preeclampsia, whereas vascular exposure to hyperglycemia induces inflammation, vascular remodeling, and arterial stiffness. Corin is a serine protease, converting inactive pro-atrial natriuretic peptide (pro-ANP) into an active form. It also promotes salt and water excretion by activating atrial natriuretic peptide (ANP), and significantly increases trophoblast invasion. The study aimed to determine whether corin may be a predictor of PE in a high-risk group—women with long-term PGDM. The nested case-control prospective study involved 63 patients with long-term pregestational type 1 diabetes (PGDM). In total, 17 patients developed preeclampsia (the study group), whereas 43 patients without PE constituted the control group. To assess corin concentration, blood samples were collected at two time points: between 18th–22nd week of gestation and 28th–32nd week of gestation. PE patients presented significantly higher mid-gestation corin levels, urine protein loss in each trimester, serum creatinine in the third trimester, and lower creatinine clearance in the third trimester. The results of our study indicate that serum corin assessment may play a role in predicting preeclampsia. Thus, it may be included in the PE risk calculator, initially in high-risk groups, such as patients with PGDM.

Keywords: corin; preeclampsia; pregestational diabetes

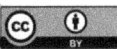

1. Introduction

Preeclampsia constitutes one of the leading causes of mortality and morbidity in pregnant women. Moreover, it remains a challenge for the public health, particularly in high-income countries. In fact, approximately 10–15% of pregnancy-associated maternal deaths are due to complications related to preeclampsia (PE) [1–3]. Nevertheless, effective diagnostic tools to predict the development of preeclampsia remain scarce, as well as the methods of treating it, other than the symptomatic treatment (anti-hypertensive drugs) or timing the delivery, which is the only effective PE treatment.

It is suggested that PE results from impaired cytotrophoblast invasion [4]. This, in turn, leads to early subclinical malfunction of the placenta and is transferred to the maternal uterine arteries, resulting in an increased pulsatility index (PI) [5]. In order to assess PE risk, uterine artery PI is determined in the first trimester scan [3]. The association between the maternal arterial stiffness and PE development has been shown both before and during pregnancy [6,7]. Nevertheless, patients with only minor vascular changes, which may lead to an increased arterial stiffness, frequently experience no symptoms prior to the pregnancy and are usually unaware of their condition. In contrast, patients with pregestational diabetes (PGDM), particularly long-term PGDM, are a group particularly susceptible to vascular complications and preeclampsia. It is worth bearing in mind that vascular exposure to hyperglycemia induces inflammation, vascular remodeling, and arterial stiffness [8,9], whereas local inflammation affects the intima-media complex, increasing its thickness and pulsatility index [10,11]. Hence, it is essential to identify a group of patients at risk of developing PE, not only because of pregnancy complications and different follow up in the course of pregnancy, but also due to the increased risk of cardiovascular disease (CVD) and death associated with an acute cardiovascular event [12–14].

Natriuretic peptides, involved in the prevention of hypertension, increase urine production; thus, reducing intravascular volume. In view of the reduced a intravascular volume, the initial thesis assumed that women with preeclampsia would present lower serum levels of natriuretic peptides [15]. However, the published studies indicate that patients with preeclampsia show significantly higher levels of natriuretic peptides due to the increased peripheral vascular resistance [16]. Nonetheless, the prediction value based on natriuretic peptide levels is limited. Most publications show increased levels of natriuretic peptides in patients with PE, although the concentration is unremarkable in patients prior to PE development [17].

Corin is a serine protease found in the heart, converting inactive pro-atrial natriuretic peptide (pro-ANP) into an active form [18]. It promotes salt and water excretion by atrial natriuretic peptide (ANP) activation. Animal models show that a lack of corin leads to salt-sensitive hypertension, gestational cardiomyopathy, and preeclampsia in mice [19,20]. Interestingly, decreased corin plasma levels in humans were reported in patients with heart failure and corin was suggested as a biochemical marker of cardiovascular disease [21–23]. Similarly, reduced corin renal expression was observed among patients with glomerular diseases associated with salt retention [24].

During pregnancy, particularly in late pregnancy, corin serum concentration increases compared to the pre-pregnancy level and then, returns to the basal level following delivery. It is of note that gestational corin elevation is more significant among women with preeclampsia and gestational hypertension [25]. This, in turn, corresponds with how the increased afterload impacts maternal circulation during normotensive pregnancy and pregnancy complicated by the increased peripheral/placental resistance, causing hypertensive disorders of pregnancy. Moreover, corin expression was found in the uteri of pregnant women, and its expression was significantly lower among patients with PE [26]. Animal models and human observations support the hypothesis that corin significantly promotes trophoblast invasion and spiral artery remodeling [27]. In fact, an elevated corin serum level was found in pregnancies complicated by preeclampsia and fetal growth restriction (FGR). However, corin mRNA expression was not increased in either of these complications. Therefore, the upregulation of corin may not only be associated with hypertension, but may also play a role in the common pathway of PE and FGR pathogenesis [28].

The presented study aimed to determine whether corin may be effective in predicting preeclampsia, fetal growth restriction, and gestational hypertension in a high-risk group—women with long-term pregestational diabetes. The other goal was to identify the determinants of elevated corin levels in PGDM patients.

2. Materials and Methods

2.1. Patients

This prospective study involved 63 patients in a singleton pregnancy with long-term pregestational type 1 diabetes (PGDM). Recruitment of patients was conducted at the Department of Reproduction at Poznań University of Medical Sciences, a tertiary-care center specializing in PGDM treatment, between April 2019 and July 2022. Patients were all Caucasian and received a standard pregnancy care for diabetes, as recommended by the Polish Diabetes Association and Polish Gynecological Society, targeting a fasting glucose level of 3.8–5.0 mmol/L, 1-h postprandial glucose below 7.0 mmol/L, and glycated hemoglobin (HbA$_{1c}$) below 6.0% (42 mmol/mol) [29]. All the women were treated with intensive insulin therapy, either with multiple daily insulin (MDI) injections or continuous subcutaneous insulin infusion (CSII). According to the Polish recommendations, all the patients received 150 mg of aspirin daily from the 12th–the 36th week of gestation as a form of preventing preeclampsia [29].

In all, 63 women met the inclusion criteria: singleton pregnancy, long-term type 1 diabetes (class C, D, F, R, according to the White classification [30]), no history of preeclampsia or gestational hypertension. In total, 3 patients were excluded from the study due to the withdrawal of consent (n = 2) and spontaneous abortion (n = 1). No major fetal anatomical abnormality or aneuploidy was diagnosed in these pregnancies.

In order to diagnose preeclampsia, the ISSHP (International Society for the Study of Hypertension in Pregnancy) criteria [31] were used, with adjustments for patients with diabetes according to Kornacki et al. [32]: in patients who had not been previously diagnosed with chronic hypertension (n = 48) [31]—systolic blood pressure (BP) $\geq$ 140 mmHg or diastolic BP $\geq$ 90 mmHg on two specific instants which occurred for the first time after 20 weeks of gestation, and one of the following complications with the onset in the second half of pregnancy: (1) proteinuria ($\geq$300 mg/24 h or >100% increase in proteinuria in proteinuric patients); (2) serum creatinine > 1 mg/dL (>90 µmol/L) or >50% increase in serum creatinine within 7 days; (3) elevation of transaminase levels > 40 IU/L; (4) neurological complications (eclampsia, altered mental status, blindness, stroke, clonus, severe headache, persistent visual scotomata); (5) hematological complications (thrombocytopenia < 150 G/L, disseminated intravascular coagulation, hemolysis); and (6) uteroplacental dysfunction (fetal growth restriction, Doppler indices of placental insufficiency [33]). Moreover, in patients with chronic hypertension (n = 12), PE was diagnosed following the onset of severe hypertension (systolic BP > 160 mmHg or diastolic BP > 110 mmHg) after 20 weeks of gestation or the need to increase treatment to maintain BP < 160/110 mmHg in the second half of pregnancy. These had to be accompanied by at least one of the abovementioned criteria for patients without previous chronic hypertension, except uteroplacental dysfunction, according to ISSHP [31]. Fetal growth restriction (FGR) was diagnosed according to the Delphi consensus criteria [33].

2.2. Monitoring of Laboratory and Clinical Measurements

The following laboratory tests were performed in each trimester in all the patients: (1) glycated hemoglobin (HbA1c), (2) daily urine protein loss, (3) serum creatinine, (4) creatinine clearance, and (5) concentration of serum triglycerides (TG). In terms of the clinical characteristics, they comprised maternal height, pregestational weight, body weight just before the delivery, weight gain, Doppler ultrasound examination, insulin intake, and the data concerning the delivery (method, timing, complications, neonatal results) presented in Table 1.

Table 1. Maternal characteristics in PE patients and the control group.

Parameter	Controls (n = 43)	Preeclampsia (n = 17)	p
Maternal age	30.47 ± 5.67	32 ± 6.24	0.36
Maternal height (m)	1.65 ± 0.077	1.63 ± 0.055	0.44
Maternal bmi at admission (kg/m^2)	24.28 ± 6.25	24.85 ± 3.88	0.72
Maternal bmi at delivery (kg/m^2)	27.53 (25.21–31.06)	28.42 (25.8–30.86)	0.74
Weight gain (kg)	10.6 (7.3–15)	9 (6–14)	0.72
Nulliparous	26 (60.47%)	13 (76.47%)	0.38
Vascular complications at admission	14 (32.56%)	10 (58.82%)	0.11
Age at diabetes diagnosis (years)	9 (7–12.5)	11 (9–14)	0.18
Diabetes duration (years)	20 (16–23)	22 (18–23)	0.56
Treatment with the insulin pump	37 (86.05%)	13 (76.47%)	0.37
Chronic hypertension	4 (9.3%)	8 (47.06%)	0.001
Fetal FGR	1 (2.38%)	4 (23.53%)	0.008
Gestational age at delivery (weeks)	38 (37–38)	35 (33–37)	0.00003
Newborns' weight	3348.3 ± 524.9	2591.7 ± 907.3	0.0002
Cesarean section	34 (85%)	17 (100%)	0.09
Emergency cesarian section	8 (23.53%)	6 (35.29%)	0.37

Blood samples for all the routine analyses were collected following overnight fasting and immediately transported to the accredited university hospital laboratory, with the ISO 9000 quality management certification. HbA1c in whole blood was determined using the turbidimetric inhibition immunoassay (TINIA), Tina-quant Hemoglobin A1c II test in a Cobas c311 analyzer (Roche Diagnostics). The normal range for a non-pregnant population amounts to 29–42 mmol/mol (4.8–6.0%). In the presented study, three HbA1c values were used: the first was measured in the first trimester or at first admission, the second was measured in the second trimester between 18 + 0 and 22 + 0 gestational weeks, and the third was measured prior to the delivery (up to six days before). The mean value was used if two HbA1c values were measured in the second trimester.

Blood samples for corin concentration assessment were collected at two time points: between the 18th–22nd and the 28th–32nd week of gestation. In total, 119 blood samples were collected and maternal-corin serum levels were measured in all cases. A nested case-control study was performed, and all women were divided into the PE group ($n = 13$) and controls ($n = 47$) based on pregnancy outcome.

In order to determine corin concentration, 7.5 mL of venous blood was collected from patients with PE and from the control group. After centrifugation ($2000 \times g$) of the blood samples, the obtained serum was frozen at $-20\,^{\circ}\mathrm{C}$ for further assessment. Corin concentrations were determined by immuno-enzymatic tests (enzyme-linked immunosorbent assay [ELISA] kit) procured from Develop (DLR-CRN-Hu; Wuxi Donglin Sci & Tech Development Co., Ltd. Jangsu, China). The assays were performed according to the manufacturer's instructions. Plate reading was conducted using an MRX reader (Dynex Technologies, Chantilly, VA, USA) at $\lambda = 450$ nm, with corrections at 570 nm.

Written informed consent was obtained from each patient prior to enrolment and blood sampling. The study was approved by the Bioethics Committee at Poznań University of Medical Sciences and conducted in accordance with the Declaration of Helsinki (No. 291/21). The Bioethics Committee at Poznan University of Medical Sciences reviewed the study protocol and confirmed that the conducted research was not a clinical trial.

2.3. Statistical Analysis

The analysis was conducted in the PQStat 1.8.4 program (PQStat software, Poznan, Poland). The Lilliefors test was applied for the verification of normality and compared the groups using the *t*-student test for data that followed a normal distribution. To compare the data that did not follow a normal distribution, the Mann–Whitney test was used; and for categorical variables, the chi-square test with Yates modification was applied. Multivariate multiple regression analysis was performed to determine factors affecting corin serum concentration.

3. Results

In the studied population, 17 patients developed preeclampsia, whereas 43 women without PE constituted the control group. There were no significant differences between the preeclampsia and the control group in terms of the maternal age, height, BMI (neither pregestational, nor at term), weight gain during pregnancy, parity, diabetes duration, and presence of vascular complications on admission. Vascular complications in PGDM included nephropathy, retinopathy, peripheral neuropathy, and major vascular events described in the patients' history. The number of patients with chronic hypertension and fetal growth restriction was higher in the PE group (Table 1).

Patients with preeclampsia presented significantly higher mid-gestation corin levels, urine protein loss in each trimester, as well as serum creatinine in the third trimester, and lower creatinine clearance in the third trimester (Table 2) (Figure 1). Gestational age at delivery and neonate weight were lower in the preeclampsia group. However, the ratio of cesarean and emergency cesarean sections were unremarkable in the two groups.

Table 2. Differences in biochemical parameters between PE patients and the control group.

Parameter	Controls (n = 43)	Preeclampsia (n = 17)	p
Corin—18th–22nd week of gestation (ng/mL)	2.64 (2.382–3.142)	3.286 (2.684–4.31)	0.002
Corin—28th–32nd week of gestation (ng/mL)	2.93 (2.652–4.174)	2.754 (2.668–3.537)	0.55
Hba1c—I trimester (%)	6.50 (6.09–7.31)	6.61 (6.29–7.27)	0.46
Hba1c—II trimester (%)	5.66 ± 0.65	5.99 ± 0.95	0.13
Hba1c—III trimester (%)	5.88 ± 0.61	6.09 ± 0.77	0.27
Triglycerides—I trimester (mg/dL)	64.6 (52.75–85.35)	65.7 (46.6–82.6)	0.84
Triglycerides—II trimester (mg/dL)	132.6 (107.2–158.1)	117.2 (102.5–178.1)	0.94
Triglycerides—III trimester (mg/dL)	280.61 ± 86.41	241.71 ± 51.43	0.09
Proteinuria—I trimester (g/24 h)	0.18 (0.14–0.21)	0.3 (0.2–0.73)	0.003
Proteinuria—II trimester (g/24 h)	0.16 (0.14–0.22)	0.34 (0.15-0.91)	0.02
Proteinuria—III trimester (g/24 h))	0.22 (0.16–0.31)	0.78 (0.38–1.82)	0.000001
Creatinine clearance—I trimester (mL/min)	126.79 ± 41.24	130.59 ± 53.64	0.77
Creatinine clearance—II trimester (mL/min)	138.74 ± 43.15	112.01 ± 53.7	0.054
Creatinine clearance—III trimester (mL/min)	127.87 ± 37.64	99.26 ± 41.8	0.01
Serum creatinine—I trimester (mg/dL)	0.57 (0.52–0.62)	0.62 (0.52–0.79)	0.34
Serum creatinine—II trimester (mg/dL)	0.595 (0.49–0.62)	0.62 (0.49–0.72)	0.13
Serum creatinine—III trimester (mg/dL)	0.6 (0.52–0.69)	0.7 (0.64–0.81)	0.007

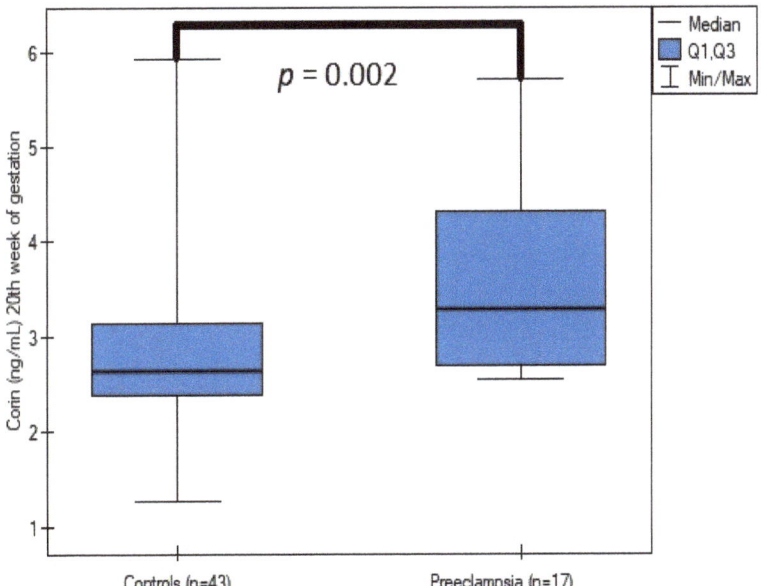

Figure 1. The comparison of corin serum concentrations at the 20th week of gestation between the patients with and without preeclampsia.

The duration of diabetes ($p = 0.81$), vascular complications ($p = 0.22$), in each trimester additionally: HbA1c ($p = 0.47$; $p = 0.97$; $p = 0.81$, respectively), triglycerides ($p = 0.49$; $p = 0.46$; $p = 0.21$, respectively), protein loss within 24 h of urine collection ($p = 0.74$; $p = 0.85$; $p = 0.67$, respectively), creatinine clearance ($p = 0.19$; $p = 0.59$; $p = 0.5$, respectively), and serum creatinine concentration ($p = 0.73$; $p = 0.94$; $p = 0.82$ respectively) were considered as the potential determinants of corin concentration, although none of the above affected protease concentration. Maternal parameters, such as height ($p = 0.13$), weight ($p = 0.99$), pregestational BMI ($p = 0.51$), weight gain ($p = 0.99$), insulin intake ($p = 0.21$), and parity ($p = 0.69$) also did not significantly impact corin concentration.

4. Discussion

Our results demonstrate the role of corin in the early stages of the pathogenesis of preeclampsia, and indicate the potential use of corin as a biomarker of impaired placental function and trophoblast invasion in patients with pregestational diabetes. The increased corin serum concentration was associated with a higher PE incidence ($p = 0.002$). Moreover, our study indicated a potential role of corin in preeclampsia screening in patients with PGDM. Corin sensitivity and specificity at a cut-off value of 2.676 ng/mL were 88.24% and 58.14%, with an AUC = 0.760 (95% CI, 0.637–0.883) (Figure 2). Additionally, all the parameters considered as the potential determinants of corin concentration did not show statistical significance. The aforementioned results reduce the potential bias created by maternal obesity or preexisting proteinuria, which frequently challenges preeclampsia diagnosis in the day-to-day clinical practice.

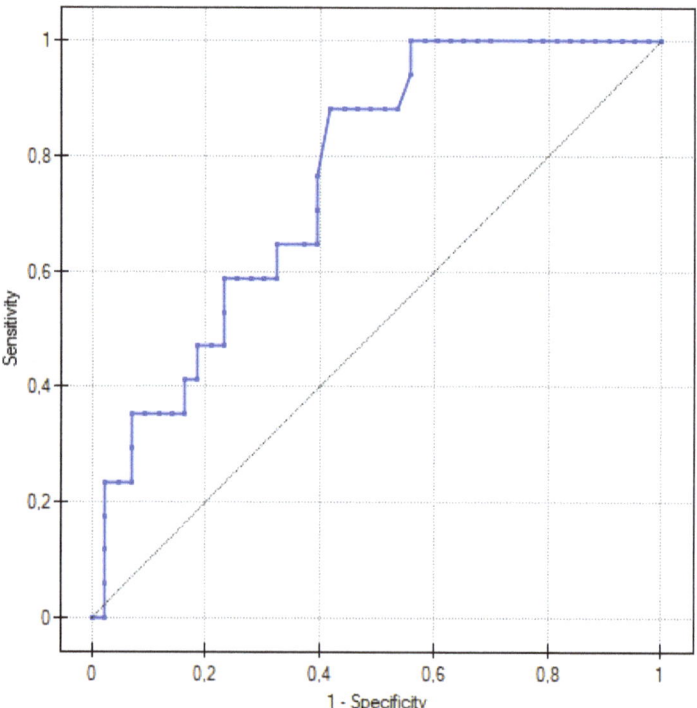

Figure 2. ROC curve for predicting preeclampsia according to corin serum levels in 20th week of gestation. At a corin cut-off value of 2.676 ng/mL, the sensitivity was 88.24% and the specificity was 58.14%, with an AUC = 0.760 (95% CI, 0.637–0.883).

Recent studies have showed a correlation between corin serum levels and preeclampsia [19,27,28,34]. Furthermore, the data indicate that serum corin measurements may be applicable not only in terms of detecting preeclampsia itself, but also in predicting it [35]. Corin serum levels may be affected by cardiac expression, which activates natriuretic peptides reducing blood pressure (BP) by means of increasing salt excretion and urine production. Corin expression was observed in the uterus during pregnancy, which, in turn, was related to the fact that uterine expression affected corin serum levels due to the direct contact of syncytiotrophoblast with maternal circulation [36]. Therefore, potentially, the changes in uterine corin expression may participate in the pathomechanism of preeclampsia, whereas cardiac expression of soluble corin may be interpreted as a response to the increased peripheral vascular resistance. Additionally, corin is a transmembrane serine protease, and it was demonstrated that the soluble form found in serum showed the same activity as the membrane-bound form [37].

In our study, the patients and control groups were relatively homogenous. Nevertheless, certain differences in fetal weight, chronic hypertension, and gestational age at delivery in patients with preeclampsia were expected. In fact, placental dysfunction leading to PE development impairs fetal growth and may result in earlier induction of labor or planned caesarian section, as recommended by international and Polish guidelines [38,39].

The role of corin in the pathogenesis of PE remains unclear. Corin expression was detected in the uteri of pregnant women, and by means of activating ANP, trophoblast invasion and spiral arteries remodeling were promoted [26]. Moreover, knocking out corin and ANP genes in the murine model led to salt-sensitive hypertension, preeclampsia, and cardiac hypertrophy [40–42]. Hyperinsulinemia in patients with type 2 diabetes is a different risk factor for lower corin expression and immunoreactivity in the placenta, which may also participate in the impaired trophoblast invasion [43]. Mutations in the corin gene were found in humans, more frequently in black individuals; and when present, they significantly increase the risk of hypertension, due to the impaired natriuretic peptide BP regulation [44,45].

Zaki et al. showed that patients with increased blood pressure presented higher corin and natriuretic peptide serum levels [46]. The assumption in our study was that the increased soluble corin levels in patients who subsequently developed preeclampsia may be used as a marker of subclinical increase of peripheral resistance due to the impaired spiral artery remodeling. This hypothesis is supported by the study assessing mid-pregnancy levels of soluble corin and its elevation in patients developing hypertensive disorders in pregnancy [47]. However, Khalil et al., in their longitudinal observation of corin levels throughout pregnancy, presented decreased corin levels until the 20th week of gestation in PE patients, as compared to the controls, as well as increased corin levels in the late second and in the third trimester [34]. Our results demonstrate that in patients with pregestational diabetes, vascular changes are present before conception, and may accelerate placental insufficiency and its impact on the peripheral resistance, leading to earlier corin overexpression aimed to maintain normal blood pressure.

Interestingly, adding plasma-soluble corin to the preeclampsia prediction model improved its effectiveness [35,48]. A combination of corin with the currently used sFlt-1/PLGF ratio may be an ideal marker with respect to predicting preeclampsia, presented by Liu et al., as a marker with the highest AUC in ROC curves analysis comparing different methods [48]. Moreover, our results advocate the inclusion of corin to the standard preeclampsia screening [3]. Patients with pregestational diabetes frequently present with subclinical vascular complications and are particularly at risk of developing hypertensive disorders in pregnancy. Therefore, in view of our research, the incorporation of corin in PGDM patients for PE screening as the most beneficial, providing a greater risk stratification and a better follow-up model, simultaneously reducing the number of complications.

The strengths of this research include the number of pregnant women with pregestational diabetes enrolled for the purpose of the nested case-control study, as well as the homogeneity of the studied groups. In contrast, the study's limitations comprise the still undetermined pathomechanisms of PE development, as well as the failure to differentiate the serum corin fractions based on the origin of its expression. An additionally increased number of participants would provide stronger evidence for corin assessment in PE prediction. Hopefully, further studies will provide data sufficient to implement corin assessment in clinical practice.

5. Conclusions

As the obtained results demonstrate, the assessment of corin serum concentration may play a role in the prediction of preeclampsia. Possibly, it may be included in the PE risk calculator, although initially only in high-risk patient groups, such as patients with PGDM. Further studies on larger populations are essential to establish the most effective protocol for determining the PE risk by means of comparing its efficiency using new biomarkers, such as corin, with the currently used ones; e.g., sFLT-1/PlGF.

Author Contributions: Conceptualization, D.B., J.K. and E.W.-O.; methodology, J.K., P.W.; software, D.B. and P.W.; data curation, D.B. and U.M.; writing—original draft preparation, D.B. and E.W.-O.; writing—review and editing, D.B., J.K., P.G. and E.W.-O.; visualization, D.B.; supervision, J.K. and E.W.-O. All authors have read and agreed to the published version of the manuscript.

Funding: This research received no external funding.

Institutional Review Board Statement: The study was approved by the Bioethics Committee at Poznań University of Medical Sciences and conducted in accordance with the Declaration of Helsinki (No. 291/21). The Bioethics Committee at Poznan University of Medical Sciences reviewed the study protocol and confirmed that the conducted research was not a clinical trial.

Informed Consent Statement: Informed consent was obtained from all the subjects involved in the study.

Data Availability Statement: All the raw data are on the clinical server, available upon request.

Conflicts of Interest: The authors declare no conflict of interest.

References

1. Duley, L. The Global Impact of Pre-eclampsia and Eclampsia. *Semin. Perinatol.* **2009**, *33*, 130–137. [CrossRef] [PubMed]
2. Redman, C.W.G. Pre-eclampsia and the placenta. *Placenta* **1991**, *12*, 301–308. [CrossRef] [PubMed]
3. Poon, L.C.; Shennan, A.; Hyett, J.A.; Kapur, A.; Hadar, E.; Divakar, H.; McAuliffe, F.; da Silva Costa, F.; von Dadelszen, P.; McIntyre, H.D.; et al. The International Federation of Gynecology and Obstetrics (FIGO) initiative on pre-eclampsia: A pragmatic guide for first-trimester screening and prevention. *Int. J. Gynaecol. Obstet. Off. Organ Int. Fed. Gynaecol. Obstet.* **2019**, *145*, 1–33. [CrossRef] [PubMed]
4. Granger, J.P.; Alexander, B.T.; Llinas, M.T.; Bennett, W.A.; Khalil, R.A. Pathophysiology of hypertension during preeclampsia linking placental ischemia with endothelial dysfunction. *Hypertension* **2001**, *38*, 718–722. [CrossRef]
5. Ridder, A.; Giorgione, V.; Khalil, A.; Thilaganathan, B. Preeclampsia: The Relationship between Uterine Artery Blood Flow and Trophoblast Function. *Int. J. Mol. Sci.* **2019**, *20*, 3263. [CrossRef] [PubMed]
6. Hausvater, A.; Giannone, T.; Sandoval, Y.H.G.; Doonan, R.J.; Antonopoulos, C.N.; Matsoukis, I.L.; Ioannis, L.; Petridou, E.T.; Daskalopoulou, S.S. The association between preeclampsia and arterial stiffness. *J. Hypertens.* **2012**, *30*, 17–33. [CrossRef]
7. Hale, S.A.; Badger, G.J.; McBride, C.; Magness, R.; Bernstein, I.M. Prepregnancy Vascular Dysfunction in Women who Subsequently Develop Hypertension During Pregnancy. *Pregnancy Hypertens.* **2013**, *3*, 140–145. [CrossRef] [PubMed]
8. Vajnerova, O.; Kafka, P.; Kratzerova, T.; Chalupsky, K.; Hampl, V. Pregestational diabetes increases fetoplacental vascular resistance in rats. *Placenta* **2018**, *63*, 32–38. [CrossRef]
9. Hausvater, A.; Giannone, T.; Sandoval, Y.-H.G.; Doonan, R.J.; Antonopoulos, C.N.; Matsoukis, I.L.; Petridou, E.T.; Daskalopoulou, S.S. Pregnancy Outcomes in Women with Long-Duration Type 1 Diabetes-25 Years of Experience. *J. Clin. Med.* **2020**, *9*, E3223.
10. Boroń, D.; Kornacki, J.; Wender-Ozegowska, E. The Assessment of Maternal and Fetal Intima-Media Thickness in Perinatology. *J. Clin. Med.* **2022**, *11*, 1168. [CrossRef]
11. Cosmi, E.; Visentin, S.; Fanelli, T.; Mautone, A.J.; Zanardo, V. Aortic intima media thickness in fetuses and children with intrauterine growth restriction. *Obstet. Gynecol.* **2009**, *114*, 1109–1114. [CrossRef] [PubMed]
12. Smith, G.C.; Pell, J.P.; Walsh, D. Pregnancy complications and maternal risk of ischaemic heart disease: A retrospective cohort study of 129,290 births. *Lancet* **2001**, *357*, 2002–2006. [CrossRef] [PubMed]
13. Bellamy, L.; Casas, J.-P.; Hingorani, A.D.; Williams, D.J. Pre-eclampsia and risk of cardiovascular disease and cancer in later life: Systematic review and meta-analysis. *BMJ* **2007**, *335*, 974. [CrossRef]
14. Irgens, H.U.; Reisæter, L.; Irgens, L.M.; Lie, R.T.; Roberts, J.M. Long term mortality of mothers and fathers after pre-eclampsia: Population based cohort study. *BMJ* **2001**, *323*, 1213–1217. [CrossRef] [PubMed]
15. Hatjis, C.G.; Greelish, J.P.; Kofinas, A.D.; Stroud, A.; Hashimoto, K.; Rose, J.C. Atrial natriuretic factor maternal and fetal concentrations in severe preeclampsia. *Am. J. Obstet. Gynecol.* **1989**, *161*, 1015–1019. [CrossRef]

16. Tihtonen, K.M.; Kööbi, T.; Vuolteenaho, O.; Huhtala, H.S.; Uotila, J.T. Natriuretic peptides and hemodynamics in preeclampsia. *Am. J. Obstet. Gynecol.* **2007**, *196*, 328.e1–328.e7. [CrossRef]
17. Borghi, C.; Esposti, D.D.; Immordino, V.; Cassani, A.; Boschi, S.; Bovicelli, L. Relationship of systemic hemodynamics, left ventricular structure and function, and plasma natriuretic peptide concentrations during pregnancy complicated by preeclampsia. *Am. J. Obstet. Gynecol.* **2000**, *183*, 140–147. [CrossRef]
18. Yan, W.; Wu, F.; Morser, J.; Wu, Q. Corin, a transmembrane cardiac serine protease, acts as a pro-atrial natriuretic peptide-converting enzyme. *Proc. Natl. Acad. Sci. USA* **2000**, *97*, 8525–8529. Available online: https://pubmed.ncbi.nlm.nih.gov/10880574/ (accessed on 15 September 2022). [.150149097CrossRef]
19. Zhou, Y.; Wu, Q. Corin in natriuretic peptide processing and hypertension. *Curr. Hypertens. Rep.* **2014**, *16*, 415. [CrossRef]
20. Wu, Q.; Xu-cai, Y.O.; Chen, S.; Wang, W. Corin: New insights into the natriuretic peptide system. *Kidney Int.* **2009**, *75*, 142–146. Available online: https://pubmed.ncbi.nlm.nih.gov/18716601/ (accessed on 15 September 2022). [CrossRef]
21. Dong, N.; Chen, S.; Yang, J.; He, L.; Liu, P.; Zheng, D.; Li, L.; Zhou, Y.; Ruan, C.; Plow, E.; et al. Plasma soluble corin in patients with heart failure. *Circ. Heart Fail.* **2010**, *3*, 207–211. Available online: https://pubmed.ncbi.nlm.nih.gov/20061521/ (accessed on 15 September 2022). [CrossRef] [PubMed]
22. Ibebuogu, U.N.; Gladysheva, I.P.; Huong, A.K.; Reed, G.L. Decompensated heart failure is associated with reduced corin levels and decreased cleavage of pro-atrial natriuretic peptide. *Circ. Heart Fail.* **2011**, *4*, 114–120. Available online: https://pubmed.ncbi.nlm.nih.gov/21216831/ (accessed on 15 September 2022). [CrossRef] [PubMed]
23. Yu, R.; Han, X.; Zhang, X.; Wang, Y.; Wang, T. Circulating soluble corin as a potential biomarker for cardiovascular diseases: A translational review. *Clin. Chim. Acta* **2018**, *485*, 106–112. [CrossRef] [PubMed]
24. Polzin, D.; Kaminski, H.J.; Kastner, C.; Wang, W.; Krämer, S.; Gambaryan, S.; Russwurm, M.; Peters, H.; Wu, Q.; Vandewalle, A.; et al. Decreased renal corin expression contributes to sodium retention in proteinuric kidney diseases. *Kidney Int.* **2010**, *78*, 650–659. Available online: https://pubmed.ncbi.nlm.nih.gov/20613715/ (accessed on 15 September 2022). [CrossRef] [PubMed]
25. Badrov, M.B.; Park, S.Y.; Yoo, J.-K.; Hieda, M.; Okada, Y.; Jarvis, S.S.; Stickford, A.S.; Best, S.A.; Nelson, D.B.; Fu, Q. Role of Corin in Blood Pressure Regulation in Normotensive and Hypertensive Pregnancy. *Hypertension* **2019**, *73*, 432–439. [CrossRef]
26. Cui, Y.; Wang, W.; Dong, N.; Lou, J.; Srinivasan, D.K.; Cheng, W.; Huang, X.; Liu, M.; Fang, C.; Peng, J.; et al. Role of corin in trophoblast invasion and uterine spiral artery remodelling in pregnancy. *Nature* **2012**, *484*, 246–250. [CrossRef]
27. Zhou, Y.; Wu, Q. Role of corin and atrial natriuretic peptide in preeclampsia. *Placenta* **2013**, *34*, 89–94. [CrossRef]
28. Miyazaki, J.; Nishizawa, H.; Kambayashi, A.; Ito, M.; Noda, Y.; Terasawa, S.; Kato, T.; Miyamura, H.; Shiogama, K.; Sekiya, T.; et al. Increased levels of soluble corin in pre-eclampsia and fetal growth restriction. *Placenta* **2016**, *48*, 20–25. [CrossRef]
29. Wender-Ożegowska, E.; Bomba-Opoń, D.; Brązert, J.; Celewicz, Z.; Czajkowski, K.; Gutaj, P.; Malinowska-Polubiec, A.; Zawiejska, A.; Wielgoś, M. Standards of Polish Society of Gynecologists and Obstetricians in management of women with diabetes. *Ginekol. Polska* **2018**, *89*, 341–350. [CrossRef]
30. Hare, J.W.; White, P. Gestational Diabetes and the White Classification. *Diabetes Care* **1980**, *3*, 394. [CrossRef]
31. Brown, M.A.; Magee, L.A.; Kenny, L.C.; Karumanchi, S.A.; McCarthy, F.P.; Saito, S.; Hall, D.R.; Warren, C.E.; Adoyi, G.; Ishaku, S. The hypertensive disorders of pregnancy: ISSHP classification, diagnosis & management recommendations for international practice. *Pregnancy Hypertens.* **2018**, *13*, 291–310. [PubMed]
32. Kornacki, J.; Boroń, D.; Gutaj, P.; Mantaj, U.; Wirstlein, P.; Wender-Ozegowska, E. Diagnosis of preeclampsia in women with diabetic kidney disease. *Hypertens. Pregnancy* **2021**, *40*, 322–329. [CrossRef] [PubMed]
33. Gordijn, S.J.; Beune, I.M.; Thilaganathan, B.; Papageorghiou, A.; Baschat, A.A.; Baker, P.N.; Silver, R.M.; Wynia, K.; Ganzevoort, W. Consensus definition of fetal growth restriction: A Delphi procedure. *Ultrasound Obstet. Gynecol.* **2016**, *48*, 333–339. [CrossRef] [PubMed]
34. Khalil, A.; Maiz, N.; Garcia-Mandujano, R.; Elkhouli, M.; Nicolaides, K.H. Longitudinal changes in maternal corin and mid-regional proatrial natriuretic peptide in women at risk of pre-eclampsia. *Ultrasound Obstet. Gynecol.* **2015**, *45*, 190–198. [CrossRef] [PubMed]
35. Zhang, W.; Zhou, Y.; Dong, Y.; Liu, W.; Li, H.; Song, W. Correlation between N-terminal pro-atrial natriuretic peptide, corin, and target organ damage in hypertensive disorders of pregnancy. *J. Clin. Hypertens.* **2022**, *24*, 644–651. [CrossRef] [PubMed]
36. Degrelle, S.A.; Chissey, A.; Stepanian, A.; Fournier, T.; Guibourdenche, J.; Mandelbrot, L.; Tsatsaris, V. Placental Overexpression of Soluble CORIN in Preeclampsia. *Am. J. Pathol.* **2020**, *190*, 970–976. [CrossRef]
37. Knappe, S.; Wu, F.; Masikat, M.R.; Morser, J.; Wu, Q. Functional analysis of the transmembrane domain and activation cleavage of human corin: Design and characterization of a soluble corin. *J. Biol. Chem.* **2003**, *278*, 52363–52370. [CrossRef]
38. Figueras, F.; Gratacós, E. Update on the diagnosis and classification of fetal growth restriction and proposal of a stage-based management protocol. *Fetal Diagn. Ther.* **2014**, *36*, 86–98. [CrossRef]
39. Kwiatkowski, S.; Torbe, A.; Borowski, D.; Breborowicz, G.; Czajkowski, K.; Huras, H.; Kajdy, A.; Kalinka, J.; Kosinska-Kaczynska, K.; Leszczynska-Gorzelak, B.; et al. Polish Society of Gynecologists and Obstetricians Recommendations on diagnosis and management of fetal growth restriction. *Ginekol. Polska* **2020**, *91*, 634–643. [CrossRef]
40. Wang, W.; Cui, Y.; Shen, J.; Jiang, J.; Chen, S.; Peng, J.; Wu, Q. Salt-sensitive hypertension and cardiac hypertrophy in transgenic mice expressing a corin variant identified in blacks. *Hypertension* **2012**, *60*, 1352–1358. [CrossRef]

41. Melo, L.G.; Veress, A.T.; Chong, C.K.; Pang, S.C.; Flynn, T.G.; Sonnenberg, H. Salt-sensitive hypertension in ANP knockout mice: Potential role of abnormal plasma renin activity. *Am. J. Physiol. Integr. Comp. Physiol.* **1998**, *274*, R255–R261. [CrossRef] [PubMed]
42. Chan, J.C.Y.; Knudson, O.; Wu, F.; Morser, J.; Dole, W.P.; Wu, Q. Hypertension in mice lacking the proatrial natriuretic peptide convertase corin. *Proc. Natl. Acad. Sci. USA* **2005**, *102*, 785–790. [CrossRef] [PubMed]
43. Abassi, Z.; Kinaneh, S.; Skarzinski, G.; Cinnamon, E.; Smith, Y.; Bursztyn, M.; Ariel, I. Aberrant corin and PCSK6 in placentas of the maternal hyperinsulinemia IUGR rat model. *Pregnancy Hypertens.* **2020**, *21*, 70–76. [CrossRef] [PubMed]
44. Dries, D.L.; Victor, R.G.; Rame, J.E.; Cooper, R.S.; Wu, X.; Zhu, X.; Leonard, D.; Ho, S.-I.; Wu, Q.; Post, W.; et al. Corin gene minor allele defined by 2 missense mutations is common in blacks and associated with high blood pressure and hypertension. *Circulation* **2005**, *112*, 2403–2410. [CrossRef]
45. Wang, W.; Liao, X.; Fukuda, K.; Knappe, S.; Wu, F.; Dries, D.L.; Qin, J.; Wu, Q. Corin variant associated with hypertension and cardiac hypertrophy exhibits impaired zymogen activation and natriuretic peptide processing activity. *Circ. Res.* **2008**, *103*, 502–508. [CrossRef]
46. Zaki, M.A.; El-Banawy, S.E.-D.S.; El-Gammal, H.H. Plasma soluble corin and N-terminal pro-atrial natriuretic peptide levels in pregnancy induced hypertension. *Pregnancy Hypertens.* **2012**, *2*, 48–52. [CrossRef]
47. Liu, Y.; Hu, J.; Yu, Q.; Zhang, P.; Han, X.; Peng, H. Increased Serum Soluble Corin in Mid Pregnancy Is Associated with Hypertensive Disorders of Pregnancy. *J. Women's Health* **2015**, *24*, 572–577. [CrossRef]
48. Liu, M.; Wang, R.B.; Xing, J.H.; Tang, Y.X. Nested Case–Control Study of Corin Combined with sFlt-1/PLGF in Predicting the Risk of Preeclampsia. *Int. J. Gen. Med.* **2021**, *14*, 2313–2320. [CrossRef]

Disclaimer/Publisher's Note: The statements, opinions and data contained in all publications are solely those of the individual author(s) and contributor(s) and not of MDPI and/or the editor(s). MDPI and/or the editor(s) disclaim responsibility for any injury to people or property resulting from any ideas, methods, instructions or products referred to in the content.

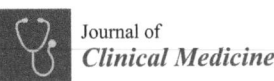

Article

Predictive Model for Preeclampsia Combining sFlt-1, PlGF, NT-proBNP, and Uric Acid as Biomarkers

Carmen Garrido-Giménez [1,2,3,†], Mónica Cruz-Lemini [1,2,3,†], Francisco V. Álvarez [4], Madalina Nicoleta Nan [5], Francisco Carretero [4,6], Antonio Fernández-Oliva [1,2], Josefina Mora [5], Olga Sánchez-García [2,3], Álvaro García-Osuna [5], Jaume Alijotas-Reig [7,8,*], Elisa Llurba [1,2,3] and on behalf of the EuroPE Working Group[‡]

1. Department of Obstetrics and Gynecology, Maternal-Fetal Medicine Unit (Hospital de la Santa Creu i Sant Pau, Sant Antoni Maria Claret, 167), Universitat Autònoma de Barcelona, 08025 Barcelona, Spain
2. Women and Perinatal Health Research Group, Institut d'Investigació Biomèdica Sant Pau (IIB SANT PAU), Sant Quintí 77–79, 08041 Barcelona, Spain
3. Primary Care Interventions to Prevent Maternal and Child Chronic Diseases of Perinatal and Developmental Network (SAMID-RICORS, RD21/0012) and Maternal and Child Health Development Network (SAMID, RD16/0022), Instituto de Salud Carlos III, 28040 Madrid, Spain
4. Clinical Biochemistry, Laboratory Medicine, Hospital Universitario Central de Asturias and Department of Biochemistry and Molecular Biology, Universidad de Oviedo, 33011 Oviedo, Spain
5. Clinical Biochemistry, Hospital de la Santa Creu i Sant Pau, Universitat Autònoma de Barcelona, 08025 Barcelona, Spain
6. Cátedra de Inteligencia Analítica, Universidad de Oviedo, 33011 Oviedo, Spain
7. Systemic Autoimmune Disease Unit, Internal Medicine Department, Vall d'Hebron University Hospital, Departament de Medicina de la Universitat Autònoma de Barcelona, 08025 Barcelona, Spain
8. Systemic Autoimmune Diseases Research Group, Vall d'Hebron Research Institute/Vall d'Hebron Hospital, 08025 Barcelona, Spain
* Correspondence: jaume.alijotas@vallhebron.cat
† These authors contributed equally to this work.
‡ EuroPE Working Group are listed in acknowledgments.

Abstract: N-terminal pro-brain natriuretic peptide (NT-proBNP) and uric acid are elevated in pregnancies with preeclampsia (PE). Short-term prediction of PE using angiogenic factors has many false-positive results. Our objective was to validate a machine-learning model (MLM) to predict PE in patients with clinical suspicion, and evaluate if the model performed better than the sFlt-1/PlGF ratio alone. A multicentric cohort study of pregnancies with suspected PE between 24^{+0} and 36^{+6} weeks was used. The MLM included six predictors: gestational age, chronic hypertension, sFlt-1, PlGF, NT-proBNP, and uric acid. A total of 936 serum samples from 597 women were included. The PPV of the MLM for PE following 6 weeks was 83.1% (95% CI 78.5–88.2) compared to 72.8% (95% CI 67.4–78.4) for the sFlt-1/PlGF ratio. The specificity of the model was better; 94.9% vs. 91%, respectively. The AUC was significantly improved compared to the ratio alone [0.941 (95% CI 0.926–0.956) vs. 0.901 (95% CI 0.880–0.921), $p < 0.05$]. For prediction of preterm PE within 1 week, the AUC of the MLM was 0.954 (95% CI 0.937–0.968); significantly greater than the ratio alone [0.914 (95% CI 0.890–0.934), $p < 0.01$]. To conclude, an MLM combining the sFlt-1/PlGF ratio, NT-proBNP, and uric acid performs better to predict preterm PE compared to the sFlt-1/PlGF ratio alone, potentially increasing clinical precision.

Keywords: angiogenic factors; machine-learning; N-terminal pro-brain natriuretic peptide (NT-proBNP); placental growth factor (PlGF); prediction; preeclampsia; soluble fms-like tyrosine kinase 1 (sFlt-1); uric acid

1. Introduction

Preeclampsia (PE) is a pregnancy-related hypertensive and multisystemic disorder that affects 2–5% of pregnancies worldwide [1]. Although obstetrical care has significantly improved and reduced its mortality, it remains a leading cause of maternal morbidity and pregnancy complications such as preterm delivery, intrauterine growth restriction (IUGR), placental abruption, stillbirth, and perinatal morbidity/mortality due to prematurity [2]. Although the pathophysiology of PE is not fully understood, it is well known that it is a placental disorder with impaired trophoblast invasion and differentiation [3] that leads to an unbalance of angiogenic and antiangiogenic factors [4]. Soluble fms-like tyrosine kinase-1 (sFlt-1, an inhibitor of vascular endothelial growth factor) is responsible for maternal dysfunction, causing peripheral vasoconstriction in an attempt to raise maternal blood pressure [5]. Elevated levels of sFlt-1, reduced levels of placental growth factor (PlGF), and an increased sFlt-1/PlGF ratio have been reported both in women with established PE, and before clinical development of the disease [6,7]. A high sFlt-1/PlGF ratio seems to be a better predictor of disease severity than either marker alone [8–10], and these findings have led to incorporation of the sFlt-1/PlGF ratio into clinical practice to improve diagnosis and prognosis of PE [11]. It is widely accepted that the cut-off value of <38 for the sFlt-1/PlGF ratio between 24^{+0} and 36^{+6} weeks of gestation rules out PE in patients with clinical suspicion for up to four weeks [12], and the use of this ratio is cost effective [13]. However, evidence is more limited regarding management and prognosis of women that present an abnormally high sFlt-1/PlGF ratio during pregnancy.

Pregnancy promotes several changes that are stressful to the cardiovascular system in order to maintain utero–placental circulation: maternal cardiac output and heart rate increase, while blood pressure and vascular resistances decrease [14]. Cardiovascular adaptation in pregnancy is abnormal in patients with PE due to cardiac diastolic dysfunction [15]. As cardiovascular changes represent a stressful scenario for the heart, cardiac myocytes respond, producing cardiac damage markers. In particular, N-terminal pro-brain natriuretic peptide (NT-proBNP), which is used as a biomarker for heart failure in non-obstetric populations [16], has been described with higher concentrations in preeclamptic pregnancies in response to abnormal cardiovascular adaptation. Furthermore, there is a correlation between NT-proBNP levels and severity of PE [17], and higher levels are described in early vs. late-onset PE [18]. Thus, NT-proBNP could be a useful tool for the evaluation of PE and prediction of maternal cardiovascular complications reflecting cardiac changes. Serum urid acid is consistently elevated in PE secondary to reduced glomerular filtration, increased resorption, and decreased secretion in the proximal tubule, although the reasons for such an elevation are incompletely understood [19]. Thus, hyperuricemia has been classically considered a good biomarker for PE, since high concentrations have been associated with more severe disease and adverse outcomes at time of delivery [20].

Neither NT-proBNP nor uric acid individually have been shown to be good predictors for PE [21], but models combining these biomarkers show promise. Lafuente-Ganuza et al. [22], published in 2020 a predictive machine-learning algorithm for early-onset PE using a combination of the sFlt-1/PlGF ratio, NT-proBNP and uric acid as biomarkers, with apparent better positive predictive values (PPV) than the sFlt-1/PlGF ratio alone. External validation is necessary to determine reproducibility for a prediction model and applicability to different populations. For this study, our primary objectives were, first, to perform external validation of this machine-learning model (MLM) to predict preterm PE in patients with clinical suspicion and, second, to study if the model performed better than the sFlt-1/PlGF ratio alone.

2. Materials and Methods

2.1. Study Design

Our real-world dataset included pregnant women with suspected PE between 24^{+0} and 36^{+6} weeks admitted to the Obstetrics Department of seven Spanish University Hospitals between March 2018 and December 2020. Patients were part of the EuroPE study cohort, a randomized open-label controlled trial to evaluate if the incorporation of sFlt1/PlGF ratio in diagnosis and classification of PE improved maternal and perinatal outcomes in women with suspicion of the disease (NCT03231657). Blood samples were obtained at inclusion (upon suspicion of PE), and multiple samples per patient were allowed but restricted to one sample per gestational week. The study protocol was approved by the institutional Ethics Committee (IIBSP-EUR-2017-20) and all patients provided written informed consent. Exclusion criteria were pregnant women outside 24^{+0} and 36^{+6} weeks, multiple pregnancies, fetal chromosomal or congenital anomalies, those lost to follow-up and conditions that required immediate delivery (eclampsia, pulmonary edema, uncontrolled hypertension, severe visual disturbances, severe headache, fetal demise, and non-reassuring fetal status).

2.2. Diagnostic Criteria

Criteria for diagnosis of PE were those of the International Society for the Study of Hypertension in Pregnancy [23]. PE was defined as a previously normotensive woman who presented with systolic or diastolic blood pressure > 140/90 mmHg, measured twice (at least 4 h apart), and proteinuria > 300 mg in a 24-h urine specimen or 2+ protein on dipsticks in urine after 20 weeks' gestation. A diagnosis of PE before 33^{+6} weeks of gestation was considered early-preterm PE, and between 34^{+0} and 36^{+6} weeks, late-preterm PE.

Suspected PE was considered upon high blood pressure or aggravation of pre-existing hypertension, new onset of proteinuria or aggravation of pre-existing proteinuria, or one or more preeclampsia-related symptoms such as epigastric pain, severe edema (face, hands, feet), persistent headache, visual disturbances, sudden weight gain (>1 kg/week in the third trimester). It was also suspected when low platelets (<100.000) or elevated liver enzymes were detected in blood analysis, as well as when abnormal uterine perfusion was detected by Doppler sonography with mean pulsatility index > 95th percentile in the second trimester and/or bilateral uterine artery notching. PE was also suspected when IUGR was detected, and was defined as an estimated fetal weight below the 3rd centile for gestational age (GA) according to local reference curves [24], or an estimated fetal weight below the 10th centile together with umbilical artery or mean uterine arteries pulsatility index above the 95th centile [25].

Adverse maternal outcome was defined as admission to the intensive care unit (ICU), eclampsia, placental abruption, disseminated intravascular coagulation, pulmonary edema, and HELLP syndrome. HELLP syndrome is a severe form of PE diagnosed when hemolysis, elevated liver enzymes (>100 U/L) and low platelet counts $< 100 \times 10^9$ /L were detected, with or without proteinuria or severe hypertension [26]. Adverse perinatal outcomes were defined as preterm delivery before 34^{+0} weeks, IUGR, stillbirth, and placental abruption. Adverse neonatal outcomes included neonatal ICU admission for >48 h, proven and/or suspected sepsis, respiratory distress syndrome, intraventricular hemorrhage (grades II–VI), necrotizing enterocolitis, retinopathy, and bronchopulmonary dysplasia.

2.3. Laboratory Methods

Blood samples were collected in serum separator tubes and centrifuged at $3000 \times g$ for 15 min. Serum concentrations of PlGF, sFlt-1, and NT-proBNP were measured using automated electrochemiluminescence immunoassays on the Roche Cobas® e601 platform (Roche Diagnostics GmbH, Mannheim, Germany) with a turnaround time of 18 min for PlGF and sFlt-1, and a turnaround time of 9 min for NT-proBNP. Serum concentration of uric acid was measured using an automated colorimetric uricase method on the Abbott Alinity® c platform (Abbott Laboratories, Chicago, IL, USA) with a turnaround time of 10 min. Product codes of reagents are 08P5620 for uric acid, 09315284190 for NT-proBNP, 07027818190 for sFlt-1, and 07027648190 for PlGF. The measuring ranges were 3–10,000 pg/mL for PlGF, 10–85,000 pg/mL for sFlt-1, 10–35,000 ng/L for NT-proBNP, and 60–1950 µmol/L for uric acid. The limits of quantification were 10 pg/mL for PlGF, 15 pg/mL for sFlt-1, 50 ng/L for NT-proBNP, and 10 µmol/L for uric acid. No high-dose hook effect has been described for concentrations up to 100,000 pg/mL for PlGF, 200,000 pg/mL for sFlt-1, 300,000 ng/L for NT-proBNP. Intra- and interassay coefficients of variation, evaluated with PreciControl Multimarkers 1 and 2 (Roche Diagnostics) for PlGF and sFlt-1, with PreciControl Cardiac 1 and 2 (Roche Diagnostics) for NT-proBNP, and with Multichem S Plus 1, 2 and 3 (Technopath) for uric acid, were found to be <5% in all assays.

2.4. Statistical Analysis

Demographic data were analyzed using the IBM SPSS Statistics 26 statistical package. Variables studied were tested for normal distribution using the Kolmogorov–Smirnov test. Comparisons between study groups were performed with analysis of variance (ANOVA) or Chi-squared test when appropriate, and are presented as mean (standard deviation) or percentage (*n*) *p*-values below 0.05 were considered statistically significant for all tests performed.

The MLM to predict PE included six predictors, as previously published [22]. Briefly, GA at admission, chronic hypertension, and biomarker serum levels (sFlt-1, PlGF, NT-proBNP, uric acid), corrected for GA at sampling, were included. Pregnancy data and outcomes were blinded to the professional who applied the random forest-based supervised MLM to predict the risk or probability of PE (low, moderately low, moderately high, or high) of a patient with clinical suspicion. We defined a patient as negative (no PE) if none of the patient's repeated measurements presented a moderately high risk or above. Otherwise, the patient was considered positive, and with high probability of developing PE. True positive and true negative patients are those coincident with the final decision of the clinician. The predictive model and the decision thresholds for being positive (high or very high) or being negative (low or very low) are found in the Supplementary Methods and Table S1. Scikit-learn (version 0.23.2), an open-source python library, was used to support the best machine-learning practices for setting up the predictive model of the software. The *p*-values and 95% confidence intervals were calculated by using the bootstrap method. Statistical significance of sensitivity, specificity, predictive values, and area under curve (AUC) were calculated using the 95% percentile bootstrap confidence intervals with 10,000 bootstrap samples.

3. Results

3.1. Characteristics of the Study Population

A total of 792 women with suspected PE were initially recruited. A total of 4 twin pregnancies, 9 pregnancies lost to follow-up, and 182 pregnancies included at term were excluded, so the final analysis included 597 participants and 936 serum samples, obtained between 24^{+0} and 36^{+6} weeks. The global incidence of PE was 34.7% (207/597): 90 women (15.1%) developed early-preterm PE ($<34^{+0}$), 67 (11.2%) had late-preterm PE (34–36^{+6}), 50 (6.3%) had term PE ($\geq 37^{+0}$), and 390 women (65.3%) did not develop PE.

Table 1 shows the demographic, clinical, and perinatal characteristics of the study population, divided into those women that developed early-preterm PE, late-preterm PE, and those without PE. There were no differences in baseline characteristics between these groups. Women with PE had significantly higher levels of sFlt-1, sFlt-1/PlGF ratio, NT-proBNP, and uric acid compared to those without PE ($p < 0.001$ for all variables mentioned), and patients with early-preterm PE had higher levels than those with late-preterm PE. GA at delivery was significantly earlier in the early-preterm PE group. The mode of delivery showed a significantly higher prevalence of caesarean section and maternal admission to the obstetric ICU in the early-preterm PE group. Regarding neonatal outcomes, birth weight was significantly lower in the early-preterm PE group, with higher rate of IUGR, as well as lower Apgar test, and higher rate of admission to the neonatal ICU and of adverse neonatal outcomes.

Table 1. Demographic, clinical, and perinatal characteristics of the study population.

	No Preeclampsia ($n = 390$)	Early-Preterm Preeclampsia ($n = 90$)	Late-Preterm Preeclampsia ($n = 67$)	p-Value
	Maternal characteristics			
Age (years)	34.02 ± 6	35.5 ± 5.9	34.8 ± 7.6	0.422
Ethnicity Caucasian Black Asian	88.1 (258) 7.2 (21) 4.8 (14)	76.5 (26) 11.8 (4) 11.8 (4)	94.2 (49) 1.9 (1) 3.8 (2)	0.143
Smoking	7.6 (22)	8.8 (3)	0 (0)	0.112
Nulliparity	39.8 (117)	55.9 (19)	44.2 (23)	0.184
	Maternal morbidity			
Diabetes mellitus type 1	1.4 (4)	2.9 (1)	3.8 (2)	0.415
Diabetes mellitus type 2	1.7 (5)	0 (0)	5.8 (5)	0.114
Hypertension	17 (50)	17.6 (6)	13.5 (7)	0.806
Cardiovascular disease	0.7 (2)	0 (0)	0 (0)	0.745
Renal disease	2.4 (7)	2.9 (1)	1.9 (1)	0.955
	Biomarker data			
GA at sampling (weeks)	33.6 ± 3.3	30.8 ± 2.1 *	34.9 ± 1.2 ¥	<0.001
sFlt-1 (pg/mL)	3252 ± 2815.2	15043.1 ± 9289 *	12044.8 ± 9167.7 *,¥	<0.001
PlGF (pg/mL)	361.2 ± 394.7	66.9 ± 84.4	83.4 ± 72.9	0.227
sFlt-1/PlGF ratio	28.9 ± 56.8	443.7 ± 329.1 *	220.8 ± 229.9 *,¥	<0.001
NT-proBNP (ng/L)	44.3 ± 46.3	883.5 ± 2391.5 *	261.6 ± 247.2 *,¥	<0.001
Uric acid (mg/dL)	3.9 ± 1	5.9 ± 1.4 *	5.8 ± 1.5 *,¥	<0.001
	Pregnancy outcomes			
GA at delivery (weeks)	38.3 ± 2.3	31.4 ± 2.1 *	35.3 ± 1 *,¥	<0.001
Mode of delivery Vaginal Operative vaginal Cesarean section	53.3 (154) 6.6 (19) 39.9 (115)	11.8 (4) * 0 (0) 88.2 (30) *	32.7 (17) * 0 (0) 67.3 (35) *	<0.001
Maternal admission to OICU	0.7 (2)	70.6 (24) *	63.5 (33) *	<0.001
	Neonatal outcomes			
Birth weight (grams)	2755.4 ± 654.5	1315.5 ± 372 *	2249.1 ± 458.1 *,¥	<0.001
IUGR	23.7 (72)	82.9 (29) *	43.6 (24) *,¥	<0.001
1′ Apgar score	8 ± 1	6 ± 2 *	8 ± 0 ¥	<0.001
5′ Apgar score	9 ± 0	8 ± 1 *	9 ± 1 ¥	<0.001
Umbilical artery pH	7.2 ± 0.6	7.3 ± 0.1	7.2 ± 0.1	0.943
Umbilical vein pH	7.3 ± 0.1	7.3 ± 0.1	7.3 ± 0.1	0.05
Admission to NICU	13 (37)	97 (32) *	52.9 (27) *,¥	<0.001
Adverse neonatal outcome	11.3 (32)	87.9 (29) *	28.8 (15) *,¥	<0.001

Data shown as mean ± SD or %(n). GA, gestational age; IUGR, intrauterine growth restriction; NT-proBNP, N-terminal pro-brain natriuretic peptide; NICU, neonatal intensive care unit; OICU, obstetric intensive care unit; PlGF, placental growth factor; sFlt-1, soluble fms-like tyrosine kinase 1. p-values obtained by ANOVA or Chi-squared test, where appropriate, and comparisons were performed between groups. * p-value < 0.05 compared to no preeclampsia; ¥ p-value < 0.05 compared to early-preterm PE.

3.2. Predictive Model Results

Table 2 and Figure 1 show validation of the MLM compared to the sFlt-1/PlGF ratio alone in predicting preterm PE. A decreased false-positive rate was observed with this model compared to the sFlt-1/PlGF ratio alone (23% vs. 41%, respectively). There was also decreased false-negative rate with the model compared to the sFlt-1/PlGF ratio alone (29% vs. 32%, respectively), and to those patients with a clinical diagnosis of PE, but with normal values of biomarkers. Table 3 shows the validation models for predicting early-preterm and late-preterm PE individually. The complete ROC curve analysis comparing the model to the sFlt-1/PlGF ratio is shown in Figure S1 in the Supplementary Materials.

Table 2. Validation of models for predicting preterm PE.

	sFlt-1/PlGF Ratio	sFlt-1/PlGF Ratio + NT-proBNP + Uric Acid	*p*-Value
Sensitivity (%)	77.5 (71.9–83.0)	79.6 (74.4–84.5)	0.210
Specificity (%)	91.0 (89.0–93.0)	94.9 (93.4–96.5)	<0.05
PPV (%)	72.8 (67.4–78.4)	83.1 (78.5–88.2)	<0.05
NPV (%)	92.8 (91.0–94.7)	93.7 (92.0–95.3)	0.140

sFlt-1, soluble fms-like tyrosine kinase 1; PlGF, placental growth factor; NT-proBNP, N-terminal pro-brain natriuretic peptide; PPV, positive predictive value; NPV, negative predictive value. Preterm PE was defined as PE below 37^{+0} weeks. Sensitivity to rule in was calculated as the proportion of positives that were correctly classified as patients in whom preeclampsia developed at any time between 24 and 36^{+6} weeks of gestation. Specificity to rule in was calculated as 1-proportion of positives that were incorrectly classified as patients in whom preeclampsia developed any time between 24 and 36^{+6} weeks of gestation.

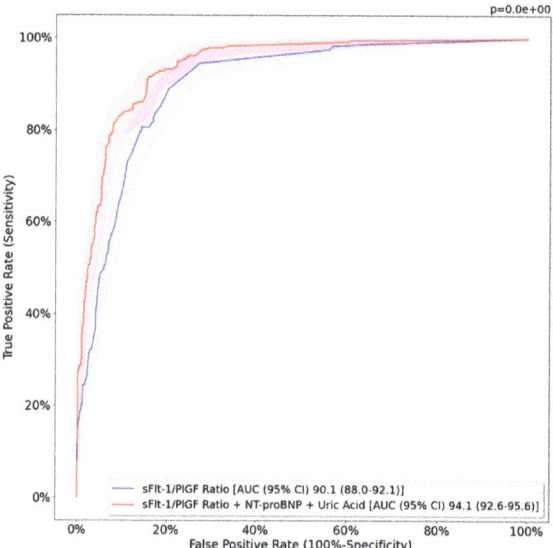

Figure 1. Performance of studied models for predicting preterm PE. sFlt-1, soluble fms-like tyrosine kinase 1; PlGF, placental growth factor; NT-proBNP, N-terminal pro-brain natriuretic peptide; AUC, area under the curve; CI, confidence interval. Preterm PE was defined as PE below 37^{+0} weeks.

Table 3. Validation of models for predicting early-preterm and late-preterm PE.

Biomarkers	sFlt-1/PlGF Ratio	sFlt-1/PlGF Ratio + NT-proBNP + Uric Acid
Early-preterm PE		
Sensitivity (%)	82.2 (76.3–88.5)	86.7 (81.8–92.6)
Specificity (%)	90.8 (88.4–93.5)	93.8 (91.7–95.9) *
PPV (%)	72.5 (66.1–79.4)	80.4 (74.2–86.4) *
NPV (%)	94.5 (92.6–96.6)	96.0 (94.3–97.8)
Late-preterm PE		
Sensitivity (%)	63.5 (53.1–75.0)	63.5 (53.1–75.0)
Specificity (%)	90.2 (87.6–92.8)	96.0 (94.2–97.8) *
PPV (%)	55.0 (45.7–64.9)	75.0 (65.2–86.2) *
NPV (%)	92.9 (90.7–95.5)	93.3 (91.1–95.7)

sFlt-1, soluble fms-like tyrosine kinase 1; PlGF, placental growth factor; NT-proBNP, N-terminal pro-brain natriuretic peptide; PPV, positive predictive value; NPV, negative predictive value. Early-preterm PE was defined as PE below 34^{+0} weeks, late-preterm PE was defined as PE between 34^{+0} and 36^{+6} weeks. Sensitivity to rule in was calculated as the proportion of positives that were correctly classified as patients in whom preeclampsia developed at any time between 24 and 36^{+6} weeks of gestation. Specificity to rule in was calculated as 1-proportion of positives that were incorrectly classified as patients in whom preeclampsia developed any time between 24 and 36^{+6} weeks of gestation. * p-value < 0.05.

The ROC curves of the combined model and the sFlt-1/PlGF ratio for predicting preterm PE within 1 and 3 weeks of clinical suspicion are observed in Figure 2. Results of specificity, sensitivity, and predictive values comparing both tests for predicting early-preterm PE and late-preterm PE within 1 and 2 or 3 weeks of clinical suspicion are shown in Table 4. ROC curves show that the algorithm performed better as the delivery date grew closer, within one and three weeks, and are shown as Figures S2 and S3 in the Supplementary Materials.

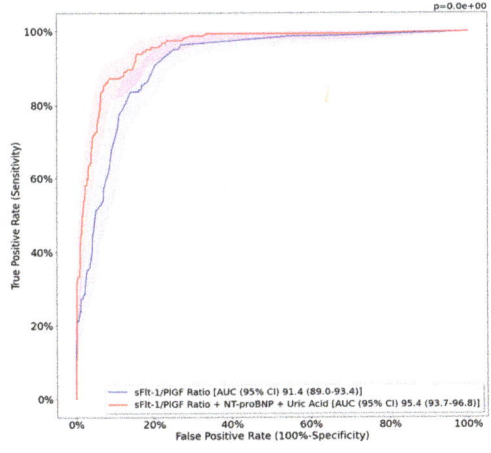
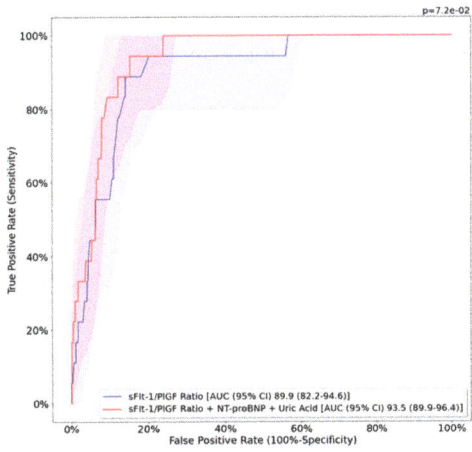

(a) (b)

Figure 2. Performance of studied models for predicting preterm PE within 1 and 3 weeks to delivery. (a) Prediction of preterm PE within 1 week to delivery, (b) prediction of preterm PE within 3 weeks to delivery. sFlt-1, soluble fms-like tyrosine kinase 1; PlGF, placental growth factor; NT-proBNP, N-terminal pro-brain natriuretic peptide; AUC, area under the curve; CI, confidence interval. Preterm PE was defined as PE below 37^{+0} weeks.

Table 4. Prediction of early and late-preterm PE using the combined model vs. sFlt-1/PlGF ratio alone.

Early-Preterm PE	sFlt-1/PlGF Ratio	sFlt-1/PlGF Ratio + NT-proBNP + Uric Acid	Late-Preterm PE	sFlt-1/PlGF Ratio	sFlt-1/PlGF Ratio + NT-proBNP + Uric Acid
	Within 1 week			Within 1 week	
Sensitivity (%)	87.0 (81.4–92.7)	90.9 (86.0–95.9)	Sensitivity (%)	65.3 (54.8–75.9)	65.3 (54.8–75.9)
PPV (%)	70.5 (63.8–77.6)	78.7 (72.3–84.9) *	PPV (%)	54.2 (44.7–63.6)	74.4 (64.3–84.0) *
Specificity (%)	90.8 (88.1–93.2)	93.8 (91.8–95.8) *	Specificity (%)	90.2 (87.6–92.9)	96.0 (94.3–97.8) *
NPV (%)	96.5 (94.9–98.2)	97.6 (96.2–98.9)	NPV (%)	93.6 (91.5–95.9)	94.0 (92.0–96.1)
	Within 3 weeks			Within 2 weeks	
Sensitivity (%)	71.4 (50.0–100.0)	50 (25.0–71.4)	Sensitivity (%)	40.0 (18.2–60.0)	40.0 (18.2–60.0)
PPV (%)	26.3 (13.6–36.4)	26.9 (11.8–40.0)	PPV (%)	18.2 (5.9–27.8)	35.3 (15.4–55.6)
Specificity (%)	90.8 (88.4–93.3)	93.8 (91.7–95.9) *	Specificity (%)	90.2 (87.6–92.9) *	96.0 (94.3–97.8) *
NPV (%)	98.6 (97.7–100.0)	97.6 (96.3–99.0)	NPV (%)	96.5 (94.8–98.2)	96.7 (95.1–98.3)

sFlt-1, soluble fms-like tyrosine kinase 1; PlGF, placental growth factor; NT-proBNP, N-terminal pro-brain natriuretic peptide; PPV, positive predictive value; NPV, negative predictive value. * p-value < 0.05.

4. Discussion

4.1. Principal Findings

Our study demonstrates the high performance of a predictive model combining the sFlt-1/PlGF ratio, NT-proBNP, and uric acid to rule in and rule out preterm PE in women with clinical suspicion. The PPV (to develop PE in the subsequent 6 weeks) and specificity (false positives) of the model were significantly better than the sFlt-1/PlGF ratio alone. Although differences were not significant, sensitivity and NPV of the model to rule out PE were slightly better than the sFlt-1/PlGF ratio alone. These differences were observed mainly in early-preterm PE, but also in late-preterm PE, and the model performed better as the delivery date approached. The short-term prediction of early-onset and late-preterm PE within 1 week was also better with the combined model.

4.2. Interpretation of Results and Comparison with Existing Literature

The sFlt-1/PlGF ratio is a good predictor of PE and serious pregnancy complications, since it increases before the first clinical symptoms appear [4]. Other biomarkers used individually have not shown to improve the predictive results of the sFlt-1/PlGF ratio [9]. We and others have previously demonstrated that the sFlt-1/PlGF ratio is increased in early and severe cases of placental insufficiency (i.e., IUGR with or without PE) because of increased levels of sFlt-1 [4,10]. It is known that high values of the sFlt-1/PlGF ratio are associated with shorter intervals to delivery [8], but hospitalization and intense monitoring in test-positive patients are often required because of high false positives. The reason why an antiangiogenic state does not always result in development of PE is still unclear, but maternal predisposition is probably necessary, added to a severe and prolonged endothelial insult.

NT-proBNP has shown higher concentrations in women with hypertensive disorders of pregnancy [18,27], especially those complicated with severe and preterm PE [27,28]. A recent study reported mean NT-proBNP levels of 349.1 ± 93.5 pg/mL in PE without severe clinical signs and 725.3 ± 290.5 pg/mL in severe PE [29]. In our data, NT-proBNP levels were also higher in preterm PE, with early-preterm showing the highest values, and higher levels were observed in the most severe cases. NT-proBNP levels are higher in pregnant women with chronic hypertension [30,31]; therefore, this was taken into account in the MLM of our study and the necessary adjustments were performed.

The prospective, multicenter, and observational PROGNOSIS study [9] reported that an sFlt-1/PlGF ratio of 38 was the optimal cut off in pregnancies between 24^{+0} and 36^{+6} weeks to rule out PE in women with clinical suspicion. This cut off performed with an NPV of 99.3% (95% CI, 97.9 to 99.9) within 1 week, and remained high at 2 (97.9%), 3 (95.7%), and 4 weeks (94.3%) after testing [12]; that is, a woman with results in this range was extremely unlikely to progress to PE or HELLP within the next month. In our study, the combined model rules out preterm PE in the next 6 weeks with 93.7% probability, slightly better than the sFlt-1/PlGF ratio alone, and performs better for early-preterm PE, ruling out with a 96% probability. Although the NPV of the sFlt-1/PlGF ratio to rule out early-preterm PE within 1 week was slightly lower than that reported in the PROGNOSIS study, this improved with the MLM (96.5% to 97.6%).

On the other hand, an sFlt-1/PlGF ratio > 38 was characterized by poor PPV: within 1 week 16.7% (95% CI, 12.3–21.9), and in the next 4 weeks 36.7% (95% CI, 28.4 to 45.7%), with 66.2% sensitivity (95% CI, 54.0–77.0) and 83.1% specificity (95% CI, 79.4–86.3) [9]. In addition, the reported ability of NT-proBNP to predict PE alone is modest, with an AUC of 0.55 [32] and 0.69 [31] in the first and third trimesters, respectively. The strategy of adding NT-proBNP to the sFlt/PlGF ratio to try to improve short-term prediction of PE has previously been reported. Lafuente-Ganuza et al. [22] identified that when maternal serum NT-proBNP value > 174 pg/mL was combined with an sFlt-1/PlGF ratio > 45, the PPV for diagnosis of early-onset PE (24^{+0} to 33^{+6} weeks) was 86% (95% CI: 79.2–92.6) at any point in time, with a sensitivity of 72.5% (95% CI 70.5–81.8) and specificity of 97.7% (95% CI 96.7–98.5). Similar results have been obtained in our study. In our cohort the PPV of the model is somewhat lower to predict preterm PE in the subsequent 6 weeks, but is statistically superior to those obtained with the sFlt1/PlGF ratio alone [72.5% (95% CI 66.1–79.4) vs. 80.4% (95% CI 74.2–86.4)], with statistically better specificity. This is the first time this model was applied to pregnancies between 34^{+0} and 36^{+6} weeks but it performed better for early-preterm PE, and also surpassed the PPV and specificity of the sFlt-1/PlGF ratio alone. Our data did not allow us to perform analysis for a 4-week period, but the model's precision for PE was also better than the sFlt1/PlGF ratio alone from 1 to 3 weeks, improving clinical decisions regarding monitoring intervals. Sabrià et al. [33] described a prediction model where the addition of NT-proBNP assessment to an sFlt/PlGF ratio $\geq$ 38 yielded a superior ability for detecting delivery in the subsequent week in women with suspected PE. The AUC was 0.845 (95% CI 0.7870.896), which was significantly greater than the AUC of the sFlt-1/PlGF ratio alone 0.786 (95% CI: 0.722–0.844). This means that when adding NT-proBNP to the sFlt1/PlGF ratio, a false-positive rate reduction of 18.2% could be achieved. Finally, in line with previous studies, serum levels of uric acid were higher in pregnancies complicated with PE [34,35]. Hyperuricemia precedes the onset of proteinuria and hypertension in PE, but its prognostic value is debated [36]. It seems that among women with diagnosed PE, higher levels may help to identify those who will develop a more severe disease, but a cut-off value has not been stablished.

Multiple sFlt-1/PlGF ratio cut offs have been studied to enhance the diagnostic accuracy of this maternal syndrome. The MLM produced a cut-off value of 45 for the sFlt/PlGF ratio, 174 pg/mL for NT-proBNP, and 5.6 mg/dL for uric acid for PE prediction of early-preterm PE. A retrospective cohort study [22] described that the PPV to rule in early-onset PE of the sFlt-1/PlGF ratio > 45 was 49.5% (95% CI 41.9–51.8), with a specificity of 79.8% (95% CI 78.5–83.6). A multicenter case–control study including a total of 1149 patients concluded that the sFlt-1/PlGF ratio $\geq$ 85 for early-onset PE and $\geq$110 for late-onset PE resulted in a sensitivity/specificity of 88%/99.5% and 58.2%/95.5%, respectively [37]. A recent study has reported that uric acid has similar specificity to the sFlt-1/PlGF ratio for the diagnosis of PE, although the sensitivity appears to be much lower [38]. The NT-proBNP cut-off point to associate pregnancy complications is not known. Serum NT-proBNP < 125 pg/mL excludes heart failure in non-obstetric populations [39], and it seems that maternal serum NT-proBNP levels < 40.6 pg/mL could rule out PE with a high NPV of 92% [40]. Alvarez et al. [18] described that a cut-off point of NT-proBNP 219 ng/L predicted development of an adverse outcome in pregnant women < 34 weeks, with a sensitivity of 76% and specificity of 94%. Another study of this group demonstrated similar performance in the prediction of adverse outcomes with cut-off points of 178 and 219 for the sFlt-1/PlGF ratio and NT-proBNP, with a sensitivity/specificity of

95/84% and 94/76%, respectively [18]. Therefore, it seems that maternal serum NT-proBNP levels > 129.5 g/mL would warrant close follow-up during pregnancy [27,41,42].

Pregnancies with placental-related disorders, such as isolated IUGR or placental abruption, also show increased sFlt-1/PlGF ratio levels, exceeding the cut-off points for PE diagnosis explained above, but it is unknown how these entities affect NT-proBNP levels [43]. Elevated NT-proBNP levels may reflect ventricular stress and subclinical cardiac dysfunction, worsening if IUGR is present. When PE is associated with IUGR, patients present higher peripheral vascular resistance and lower cardiac output compared to isolated IUGR [44]. Few studies have evaluated NT-proBNP levels in pregnant women with IUGR, and higher maternal serum NT-proBNP levels have been detected in pregnancies with early-onset PE, with or without IUGR, than in pregnancies with isolated IUGR [22,41]. Therefore, when a high sFlt/PlGF ratio is detected, lower levels of NT-proBNP could discriminate between those pregnant women that are not going to develop PE.

4.3. Clinical Implications and Future Research Directions

Clinical presentation of PE is heterogeneous, and a daily challenge to the practicing obstetrician. This diagnostic model using a combination of cardiac, renal, and placental biomarkers has been validated to predict preterm PE in patients with clinical suspicion, with better PPV, sensitivity, and specificity than the sFlt-1/PlGF ratio alone. This information could help clinicians decide which women may be followed up on safely on an outpatient basis, and which women need careful and close surveillance, and hospitalization. If expectant management is considered, this MLM could also provide more accurate and valuable information for the frequency of patient assessment and follow-up. Furthermore, a specific software could be developed and studied to calculate the risk of maternal and fetal-adverse outcomes, and indicate imminent delivery, evaluating also the cost effectiveness of the routinely incorporation of uric acid and NT-proBNP in women with suspected PE.

4.4. Strengths and Limitations

This study externally validates an MLM previously published to predict PE. This is the first study that improves the sFlt-1/PlGF ratio's prognosis of PE using other related maternal serum PE biomarkers. It is a nested study, with a very strict selection process for patients, prospectively included in the database but not managed based on these results; therefore, it has no bias with regard to our findings. However, more data from randomized trials is needed to establish whether the use of this algorithm in clinical practice could really reduce unnecessary hospitalization and costs. Another limitation of this study is that the different cut-off values proposed for the sFlt-1/PlGF ratio can only be applied when using Elecsys immunoassays, since differences have been reported with other brands or platforms.

5. Conclusions

An MLM combining the sFlt-1/PlGF ratio, NT-proBNP, and uric acid performs better to predict preterm PE compared to the sFlt-1/PlGF ratio alone, potentially increasing clinical precision, decreasing false-positive rates, and increasing PPV and specificity. This model also performed better than the sFlt-1/PlGF ratio for prediction of PE within 1 and 3 weeks. These results could avoid unnecessary interventions in women with suspected PE. Our work highlights the need of further studies combining different biomarkers and supports the use of NT-proBNP and uric acid added to maternal serum angiogenic factors to increase PE prediction.

Supplementary Materials: The following supporting information can be downloaded at: https://www.mdpi.com/article/10.3390/jcm12020431/s1, Figure S1: Performance of studied models for predicting preterm PE; Figure S2: Performance of studied models for predicting early-preterm PE within 1 and 3 weeks to delivery; Figure S3: Performance of studied models for predicting late-preterm PE within 1 and 2 weeks to delivery. Table S1: Decision thresholds.

Author Contributions: Conceptualization, E.L.; methodology, F.V.Á., J.A.-R. and E.L.; software, F.V.Á. and F.C.; Validation, C.G.-G. and M.C.-L.; formal analysis, M.C.-L., F.V.Á. and F.C.; investigation, C.G.-G., M.N.N., A.F.-O., J.M., O.S.-G. and Á.G.-O.; resources, E.L.; data curation, C.G.-G., M.N.N. and F.C.; writing—original draft, C.G.-G.; writing—review and editing, M.C.-L., J.A.-R. and E.L.; visualization, C.G.-G.; supervision, J.A.-R.; project administration, E.L.; funding acquisition, E.L. The EuroPE Working Group contributed on investigation (inclusion of patients). All authors have read and agreed to the published version of the manuscript.

Funding: This work was supported by public funds obtained in competitive calls with peer review (grant PI19/00702), Insituto de Salud Carlos III, Spanish Ministry of Health, by the Maternal and Child Health and Development Network (SAMID, RD16/0022/0015), Instituto de Salud Carlos III, Madrid, Spain, the Spanish Clinical Research and Clinical Trials Platform, SCReN (Spanish Clinical Research Network), funded by the ISCIII-General Subdirectorate for Evaluation and Promotion of Research, through project PT13/0002/0028, integrated in the 2013–2016 R + D + I State Plan and co-financed by and the European Regional Development Fund (FEDER); and by the Primary Care Interventions to Prevent Maternal and Child Chronic Diseases of Perinatal and Developmental Origin Network (RICORS, RD21/0012/0001), Instituto de Salud Carlos III, Madrid, Spain, funded by the Recovery, Transformation and Resilience Plan 2017–2020, ISCIII, and by the European Union-Next Generation EU. Dr Cruz-Lemini is supported by Juan Rodés contract JR19/00047, Instituto de Salud Carlos III-Spanish Ministry of Health. Funding sources were not involved in study design, collection, analysis, and interpretation of data.

Institutional Review Board Statement: All subjects gave their informed consent for inclusion before they participated in this study. This study was conducted in accordance with the Declaration of Helsinki and approved by the Ethics Committee of Institut de Recerca de l'Hospital de la Santa Creu i Sant Pau–IIB Sant Pau (IIBSP-EUR-2017-20, 02/03/2017).

Informed Consent Statement: Written informed consent has been obtained from the patients to publish this paper.

Data Availability Statement: The data presented in this study are available upon request from the corresponding author. The data are not publicly available due to privacy policies.

Acknowledgments: The authors greatly appreciate collaboration from the different hospitals and participants who agreed to take part in the EuroPE study. Collaborators of the EuroPE working group: M Vila-Cortés, (Department of Obstetrics and Gynecology, Hospital Universitari Son Espases, Palma, Spain); MJ Pelegay, (Department of Obstetrics and Gynecology, Hospital Universitari Arnau de Vilanova, Lleida, Spain); M Ricart, (Department of Obstetrics and Gynecology, Hospital Universitari Germans Trias i Pujol, Universitat Autònoma de Barcelona, Barcelona, Spain); B Muñoz-Abellana, (Department of Obstetrics and Gynecology, Hospital Universitari Sant Joan de Reus, Tarragona, Spain); X Gabaldó Barrios, (Clinical Laboratory Department, Hospital Universitari Sant Joan de Reus, Reus and Universitat Rovira I Virgili, Tarragona, Spain).

Conflicts of Interest: Llurba reports receiving fees for lectures from Cook, Roche, and serving on advisory boards for Roche Diagnostics. The remaining authors report no conflict of interest.

References

1. Abalos, E.; Cuesta, C.; Grosso, A.L.; Chou, D.; Say, L. Global and regional estimates of preeclampsia and eclampsia: A systematic review. *Eur. J. Obstet. Gynecol. Reprod. Biol.* **2013**, *170*, 1–7. [CrossRef] [PubMed]
2. Ronsmans, C.; Graham, W.J. Maternal mortality: Who, when, where, and why. *Lancet* **2006**, *368*, 1189–1200. [CrossRef] [PubMed]
3. Fantone, S.; Mazzucchelli, R.; Giannubilo, S.R.; Ciavattini, A.; Marzioni, D.; Tossetta, G. AT-rich interactive domain 1A protein expression in normal and pathological pregnancies complicated by preeclampsia. *Histochem. Cell Biol.* **2020**, *154*, 339–346. [CrossRef]
4. Levine, R.J.; Maynard, S.E.; Qian, C.; Lim, K.-H.; England, L.J.; Yu, K.F.; Schisterman, E.F.; Thadhani, R.; Sachs, B.P.; Epstein, F.H.; et al. Circulating angiogenic factors and the risk of preeclampsia. *N. Engl. J. Med.* **2004**, *350*, 672–683. [CrossRef]
5. Staff, A.C.; Braekke, K.; Harsem, N.K.; Lyberg, T.; Holthe, M.R. Circulating concentrations of sFlt1 (soluble fms-like tyrosine kinase 1) in fetal and maternal serum during pre-eclampsia. *Eur. J. Obstet. Gynecol. Reprod. Biol.* **2005**, *122*, 33–39. [CrossRef] [PubMed]
6. Maynard, S.E.; Min, J.Y.; Merchan, J.; Lim, K.H.; Li, J.; Mondal, S.; Libermann, T.A.; Morgan, J.P.; Sellke, F.W.; Stillman, I.E.; et al. Excess placental soluble fms-like tyrosine kinase 1 (sFlt1) may contribute to endothelial dysfunction hypertension, and proteinuria in preeclampsia. *J. Clin. Investig.* **2003**, *111*, 649–658. [CrossRef]

7. Staff, A.C.; Benton, S.J.; von Dadelszen, P.; Roberts, J.M.; Taylor, R.N.; Powers, R.W.; Charnock-Jones, D.S.; Redman, C.W.G. Redefining preeclampsia using placenta-derived biomarkers. *Hypertension* **2013**, *61*, 932–942. [CrossRef]
8. Zeisler, H.; Llurba, E.; Chantraine, F.; Vatish, M.; Staff, A.C.; Sennström, M.; Olovsson, M.; Brennecke, S.P.; Stepan, H.; Allegranza, D.; et al. Soluble fms-Like Tyrosine Kinase-1-to-Placental Growth Factor Ratio and Time to Delivery in Women with Suspected Preeclampsia. *Obstet. Gynecol.* **2016**, *128*, 261–269. [CrossRef]
9. Zeisler, H.; Llurba, E.; Chantraine, F.; Vatish, M.; Staff, A.C.; Sennström, M.; Olovsson, M.; Brennecke, S.P.; Stepan, H.; Allegranza, D.; et al. Predictive Value of the sFlt-1: PlGF Ratio in Women with Suspected Preeclampsia. *N. Engl. J. Med.* **2016**, *374*, 13–22. [CrossRef]
10. Verlohren, S.; Herraiz, I.; Lapaire, O.; Schlembach, D.; Moertl, M.; Zeisler, H.; Calda, P.; Holzgreve, W.; Galindo, A.; Engels, T.; et al. The sFlt-1/PlGF ratio in different types of hypertensive pregnancy disorders and its prognostic potential in preeclamptic patients. *Am. J. Obstet. Gynecol.* **2012**, *206*, 58.e1-8. [CrossRef]
11. Herraiz, I.; Llurba, E.; Verlohren, S.; Galindo, A.; Bartha, J.L.; De La Calle, M.; Delgado, J.L.; De Paco, C.; Escudero, A.I.; Moreno, F.; et al. Update on the Diagnosis and Prognosis of Preeclampsia with the Aid of the sFlt-1/PlGF Ratio in Singleton Pregnancies. *Fetal Diagn. Ther.* **2018**, *43*, 81–89. [CrossRef] [PubMed]
12. Zeisler, H.; Llurba, E.; Chantraine, F.J.; Vatish, M.; Staff, A.C.; Sennström, M.; Olovsson, M.; Brennecke, S.P.; Stepan, H.; Allegranza, D.; et al. Soluble fms-like tyrosine kinase-1 to placental growth factor ratio: Ruling out pre-eclampsia for up to 4 weeks and value of retesting. *Ultrasound Obstet. Gynecol.* **2019**, *53*, 367–375. [CrossRef] [PubMed]
13. Vatish, M.; Strunz-McKendry, T.; Hund, M.; Allegranza, D.; Wolf, C.; Smare, C. sFlt-1/PlGF ratio test for pre-eclampsia: An economic assessment for the UK. *Ultrasound Obstet. Gynecol.* **2016**, *48*, 765–771. [CrossRef] [PubMed]
14. Sanghavi, M.; Rutherford, J.D. Cardiovascular physiology of pregnancy. *Circulation* **2014**, *130*, 1003–1008. [CrossRef]
15. Melchiorre, K.; Sutherland, G.R.; Baltabaeva, A.; Liberati, M.; Thilaganathan, B. Maternal cardiac dysfunction and remodeling in women with preeclampsia at term. *Hypertension* **2011**, *57*, 85–93. [CrossRef]
16. Chow, S.L.; Maisel, A.S.; Anand, I.; Bozkurt, B.; De Boer, R.A.; Felker, G.M.; Fonarow, G.C.; Greenberg, B.; Januzzi, J.L.; Kiernan, M.S.; et al. Role of biomarkers for the prevention, assessment, and management of heart failure: A scientific statement from the American Heart Association. *Circulation* **2017**, *135*, e1054–e1091. [CrossRef]
17. Seong, W.J.; Kim, S.C.; Hong, D.G.; Koo, T.B.; Park, S. Amino-terminal pro-brain natriuretic peptide levels in hypertensive disorders complicating pregnancy. *Hypertens. Pregnancy* **2011**, *30*, 287–294. [CrossRef]
18. Álvarez-Fernández, I.; Prieto, B.; Rodríguez, V.; Ruano, Y.; Escudero, A.I.; Álvarez, F.V. N-terminal pro B-type natriuretic peptide and angiogenic biomarkers in the prognosis of adverse outcomes in women with suspected preeclampsia. *Clin. Chim. Acta* **2016**, *463*, 150–157. [CrossRef]
19. Lam, C.; Lim, K.H.; Kang, D.H.; Karumanchi, S.A. Uric acid and preeclampsia. *Semin. Nephrol.* **2005**, *25*, 56–60. [CrossRef]
20. Germany Paula, L.; Ercília Pinheiro Da Costa, B.; Eduardo Poli-De-Figueiredo, C.; Carlos Ferreira Antonello, I. Does uric acid provide information about maternal condition and fetal outcome in pregnant women with hypertension? *Hypertens. Pregnancy* **2008**, *27*, 413–420. [CrossRef]
21. Townsend, R.; Khalil, A.; Premakumar, Y.; Allotey, J.; Snell, K.I.E.; Chan, C.; Chappell, L.C.; Hooper, R.; Green, M.; Mol, B.W.; et al. Prediction of pre-eclampsia: Review of reviews. *Ultrasound Obstet. Gynecol.* **2019**, *54*, 16–27. [CrossRef] [PubMed]
22. Lafuente-Ganuza, P.; Lequerica-Fernandez, P.; Carretero, F.; Escudero, A.I.; Martinez-Morillo, E.; Sabria, E.; Herraiz, I.; Galindo, A.; Lopez, A.; Martinez-Triguero, M.L.; et al. A more accurate prediction to rule in and rule out pre-eclampsia using the sFlt-1/PlGF ratio and NT-proBNP as biomarkers. *Clin. Chem. Lab. Med.* **2020**, *58*, 399–407. [CrossRef] [PubMed]
23. Tranquilli, A.L.; Brown, M.A.; Zeeman, G.G.; Dekker, G.; Sibai, B.M. The definition of severe and early-onset preeclampsia. Statements from the International Society for the Study of Hypertension in Pregnancy (ISSHP). *Pregnancy Hypertens. Int. J. Women's Cardiovasc. Health* **2013**, *3*, 44–47. [CrossRef] [PubMed]
24. Figueras, F.; Meler, E.; Iraola, A.; Eixarch, E.; Coll, O.; Figueras, J.; Francis, A.; Gratacos, E.; Gardosi, J. Customized birthweight standards for a Spanish population. *Eur. J. Obstet. Gynecol. Reprod. Biol.* **2008**, *136*, 20–24. [CrossRef]
25. Arduini, D.; Rizzo, G. Normal values of Pulsatility Index from fetal vessels: A cross-sectional study on 1556 healthy fetuses. *J. Perinat. Med.* **1990**, *18*, 165–172. [CrossRef]
26. American College of Obstetricians; Task Force on Hypertension in Pregnancy Hypertension in Pregnancy. Report of the American College of Obstetricians and Gynecologists' Task Force on Hypertension in Pregnancy. *Obstet. Gynecol.* **2013**, *122*, 1122–1131. [CrossRef]
27. Borghi, C.; Esposti, D.D.; Immordino, V.; Cassani, A.; Boschi, S.; Bovicelli, L.; Ambrosioni, E. Relationship of systemic hemodynamics, left ventricular structure and function, and plasma natriuretic peptide concentrations during pregnancy complicated by preeclampsia. *Am. J. Obstet. Gynecol.* **2000**, *183*, 140–147. [CrossRef]
28. Zhang, Y.; Tan, X.; Yu, F. The diagnostic and predictive values of N-terminal pro-B-type natriuretic peptides in pregnancy complications and neonatal outcomes. *Am. J. Transl. Res.* **2021**, *13*, 10372–10379.
29. Nguyen, T.X.; Nguyen, V.T.; Nguyen-Phan, H.N.; Hoang Bui, B. Serum Levels of NT-Pro BNP in Patients with Preeclampsia. *Integr. Blood Press. Control* **2022**, *15*, 43–51. [CrossRef]
30. Fleming, S.M.; O'Byrne, L.; Grimes, H.; Daly, K.M.; Morrison, J.J.; Morrison, J.J. Amino-terminal pro-brain natriuretic peptide in normal and hypertensive pregnancy. *Hypertens. Pregnancy* **2001**, *20*, 169–175. [CrossRef]

31. Verlohren, S.; Perschel, F.H.; Thilaganathan, B.; Dröge, L.A.; Henrich, W.; Busjahn, A.; Khalil, A. Angiogenic Markers and Cardiovascular Indices in the Prediction of Hypertensive Disorders of Pregnancy. *Hypertension* **2017**, *69*, 1192–1197. [CrossRef] [PubMed]
32. Pihl, K.; Sørensen, S.; Stener Jørgensen, F. Prediction of Preeclampsia in Nulliparous Women according to First Trimester Maternal Factors and Serum Markers. *Fetal Diagn. Ther.* **2020**, *47*, 277–283. [CrossRef] [PubMed]
33. Sabriá, E.; Lequerica-Fernández, P.; Lafuente-Ganuza, P.; Eguia-Ángeles, E.; Escudero, A.I.; Martínez-Morillo, E.; Barceló, C.; Álvarez, F.V. Addition of N-terminal pro-B natriuretic peptide to soluble fms-like tyrosine kinase-1/placental growth factor ratio > 38 improves prediction of pre-eclampsia requiring delivery within 1 week: A longitudinal cohort study. *Ultrasound Obstet. Gynecol.* **2018**, *51*, 758–767. [CrossRef] [PubMed]
34. Kumar, N.; Singh, A.K. Maternal Serum Uric Acid as a Predictor of Severity of Hypertensive Disorders of Pregnancy: A Prospective Cohort Study. *Curr. Hypertens. Rev.* **2018**, *15*, 154–160. [CrossRef]
35. Hawkins, T.L.A.; Roberts, J.M.; Mangos, G.J.; Davis, G.K.; Roberts, L.M.; Brown, M.A. Plasma uric acid remains a marker of poor outcome in hypertensive pregnancy: A retrospective cohort study. *BJOG Int. J. Obstet. Gynaecol.* **2012**, *119*, 484–492. [CrossRef]
36. Bellomo, G.; Venanzi, S.; Saronio, P.; Verdura, C.; Narducci, P.L. Prognostic significance of serum uric acid in women with gestational hypertension. *Hypertension* **2011**, *58*, 704–708. [CrossRef]
37. Verlohren, S.; Herraiz, I.; Lapaire, O.; Schlembach, D.; Zeisler, H.; Calda, P.; Sabria, J.; Markfeld-Erol, F.; Galindo, A.; Schoofs, K.; et al. New gestational phase-specific cutoff values for the use of the soluble fms-like tyrosine kinase-1/placental growth factor ratio as a diagnostic test for preeclampsia. *Hypertension* **2014**, *63*, 346–352. [CrossRef]
38. Álvarez-Fernández, I.; Prieto, B.; Rodríguez, V.; Ruano, Y.; Escudero, A.I.; Álvarez, F.V. New biomarkers in diagnosis of early onset preeclampsia and imminent delivery prognosis. *Clin. Chem. Lab. Med.* **2014**, *52*, 1159–1168. [CrossRef]
39. Ponikowski, P.; Voors, A.A.; Anker, S.D.; Bueno, H.; Cleland, J.G.F.; Coats, A.J.S.; Falk, V.; González-Juanatey, J.R.; Harjola, V.P.; Jankowska, E.A.; et al. 2016 ESC Guidelines for the diagnosis and treatment of acute and chronic heart failure: The Task Force for the diagnosis and treatment of acute and chronic heart failure of the European Society of Cardiology (ESC). Developed with the special contribution of the Heart Failure Association (HFA) of the ESC. *Eur. J. Heart Fail.* **2016**, *18*, 891–975. [CrossRef]
40. Resnik, J.L.; Hong, C.; Resnik, R.; Kazanegra, R.; Beede, J.; Bhalla, V.; Maisel, A. Evaluation of B-type natriuretic peptide (BNP) levels in normal and preeclamptic women. *Am. J. Obstet. Gynecol.* **2005**, *193*, 450–454. [CrossRef]
41. Lafuente-Ganuza, P.; Carretero, F.; Lequerica-FernÃindez, P.; Fernandez-Bernardo, A.; Escudero, A.I.; De La Hera-Galarza, J.M.; Garcia-Iglesias, D.; Alvarez-Velasco, R.; Alvarez, F.V. NT-proBNP levels in preeclampsia, intrauterine growth restriction as well as in the prediction on an imminent delivery. *Clin. Chem. Lab. Med.* **2021**, *59*, 1077–1085. [CrossRef]
42. Zheng, Z.; Lin, X.; Cheng, X. Serum Levels of N-Terminal Pro-Brain Natriuretic Peptide in Gestational Hypertension, Mild Preeclampsia, and Severe Preeclampsia: A Study from a Center in Zhejiang Province, China. *Med. Sci. Monit.* **2021**, *28*, e934285-1. [CrossRef] [PubMed]
43. Herraiz, I.; Dröge, L.A.; Gómez-Montes, E.; Henrich, W.; Galindo, A.; Verlohren, S. Characterization of the soluble fms-like tyrosine kinase-1 to placental growth factor ratio in pregnancies complicated by fetal growth restriction. *Obstet. Gynecol.* **2014**, *124*, 265–273. [CrossRef] [PubMed]
44. Tay, J.; Foo, L.; Masini, G.; Bennett, P.R.; McEniery, C.M.; Wilkinson, I.B.; Lees, C.C. Early and late preeclampsia are characterized by high cardiac output, but in the presence of fetal growth restriction, cardiac output is low: Insights from a prospective study. *Am. J. Obstet. Gynecol.* **2018**, *218*, 517.e1–517.e12. [CrossRef] [PubMed]

Disclaimer/Publisher's Note: The statements, opinions and data contained in all publications are solely those of the individual author(s) and contributor(s) and not of MDPI and/or the editor(s). MDPI and/or the editor(s) disclaim responsibility for any injury to people or property resulting from any ideas, methods, instructions or products referred to in the content.

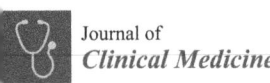

Article

Combination of Maternal Serum ESM-1 and PLGF with Uterine Artery Doppler PI for Predicting Preeclampsia

Xianjing Xie [1,2,†], Dan Chen [1,2,3,†], Xingyu Yang [1,2,4], Yunyun Cao [1], Yuna Guo [1,*] and Weiwei Cheng [1,2,*]

1. International Peace Maternity and Child Health Hospital, School of Medicine, Shanghai Jiao Tong University, Shanghai 200030, China
2. Shanghai Key Laboratory of Embryo Original Diseases, Shanghai 200030, China
3. Department of Obstetrics and Gynecology, Renji Hospital, School of Medicine, Shanghai Jiao Tong University, Shanghai 200127, China
4. Institute of Birth Defects and Rare Diseases, School of Medicine, Shanghai Jiao Tong University, Shanghai 200030, China
* Correspondence: gyna@live.com (Y.G.); wwcheng29@shsmu.edu.cn (W.C.); Tel./Fax: +86-21-64070434 (Y.G. & W.C.)
† These authors contributed equally to this work.

Abstract: Objective: This study aimed to determine whether the combination of pregnancy-associated endothelial cell-specific molecule 1 (ESM-1), the placental growth factor (PLGF) in the first- and second-trimester maternal serum, and the uterine artery Doppler pulsatility index (PI) in the second trimester can predict preeclampsia (PE). Methods: The serum levels of ESM-1 and PLGF in 33 severe preeclampsia (SPE) patients, 18 mild preeclampsia patients (MPE), and 60 age-matched normal controls (CON) were measured. The Doppler ultrasonography was performed, and the artery pulsatility index (PI) was calculated for the same subjects. Results: The 2nd PLGF level was significantly lower and the 2nd PI was higher than those in the MPE group. Combining the 2nd PLGF with the 2nd PI yielded an AUC of 0.819 (83.33% sensitivity and 70.00% specificity). In the SPE group, the 1st ESM-1 level and the 2nd PLGF level were significantly lower, and the 2nd ESM-1 level and the 2nd PI were significantly higher in the SPE group. The combination of the 1st ESM-1, the 2nd PLGF, and the 2nd PI yielded an AUC of 0.912 (72.73% sensitivity and 95.00% specificity). Conclusions: The 1st ESM-1 and the 2nd PLGF levels and the 2nd PI were associated with PE. The combination of serum biomarkers and the PI improved the screening efficiency of the PE prediction, especially for SPE.

Keywords: preeclampsia; ESM-1; PLGF; uterine artery Doppler; PI; prediction

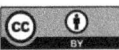

1. Introduction

Preeclampsia (PE) is a major cause of morbidity and mortality among pregnant women and infants, resulting in an estimated 76,000 maternal deaths and 500,000 fetal and newborn deaths every year [1]. The etiology of PE is still an enigma; currently, the most widely accepted theory for the development of PE is the "two-stage" theory. The first stage is reduced placental perfusion, and the second stage is generalized maternal endothelial dysfunction. Abnormal vascular growth and impaired endothelial function are considered to be the main components of the pathogenesis [2]. The imbalance between the antiangiogenic and proangiogenic factors is considered to be the link between the two stages. The expression of the antiangiogenic and angiogenic factors is altered in PE [3].

Endocan, an antiangiogenic factor which is also called endothelial cell-specific molecule-1 (ESM-1), was originally identified in cultured endothelial cells [4]. Several studies have shown that ESM-1 could be a novel biomarker of various diseases with endothelial dysfunction and inflammation, such as newly diagnosed hypertension [5]. A recent meta-analysis suggested that women with PE had a higher level of circulating ESM-1 than women with normal pregnancies [6].

Placental growth factor (PLGF), produced by villous syncytiotrophoblasts, is thought to induce nonbranching angiogenesis, leading to a low-resistance placental vascular network [7,8]. Limited angiogenesis in early PE pregnancies, with a shallow vascular invasion of the maternal spiral arteries, results in the subsequent placental hypoperfusion [9]. Many studies have revealed that angiogenic factors such as PLGF are decreased in the serum of PE patients [10,11]. PLGF has been proven to be a useful screening tool for PE prediction [12].

Spiral artery transformation failure in PE could lead to an increase in uterine artery blood flow resistance [13], which could be captured as an abnormality, such as by the presence of an impedance on the uterine artery Doppler. These changes support the uterine artery Doppler velocimetry-based screening of patients who are at risk of developing PE [14]. Furthermore, some studies have shown that uterine artery PI is a promising marker for predicting PE [15,16].

The objective of our study was to evaluate the maternal serum ESM-1 and the PLGF levels in the first and second trimesters and the uterine artery Doppler PI in the second trimester and to determine whether the integration of these biomarkers with the 2nd PI would be helpful in the prediction of PE.

2. Patients and Methods

2.1. Patients

This was a prospective study. Women with singleton pregnancies who presented at the International Peace Maternity and Child Health Hospital, Shanghai, China, from 2020 to 2021 for prenatal examination were eligible for inclusion. The exclusion criteria were multiple pregnancies, chronic hypertension, chronic renal disease or pre-existing proteinuria, diabetes, malignancy, autoimmune disorders, acute systemic inflammation, fever, premature rupture of membranes, preterm labor, or major congenital fetal anomaly. The study was conducted according to the Declaration of Helsinki guidelines and the approval of the National Ethics Committee for Science and Technology (number: GKLW2020-03). All the participants were followed from the first trimester to delivery, with pregnancy outcomes recorded and written informed consent provided.

The definition of the severe preeclampsia (SPE) group was as follows:

(1) Blood pressure $\geq 160/110$ mm Hg on two occasions at least 4 h apart (unless antihypertensive therapy was initiated before this time);
(2) Thrombocytopenia: platelet count $<100 \times 10^9$/L;
(3) Renal insufficiency: serum creatinine concentrations >1.1 mg/dL or a doubling of the serum creatinine concentration in the absence of other renal diseases;
(4) Impaired liver function: elevated blood concentrations of liver transaminases to twice the normal concentration;
(5) Pulmonary edema;
(6) New-onset headache unresponsive to medication and not accounted for by alternative diagnoses or visual symptoms.

The mild preeclampsia (MPE) group was described as follows:

(1) Blood pressure $\geq 140/90$ mmHg on two occasions at least 4 h apart after 20 weeks of gestation in a woman with previously normal blood pressure;
(2) Three hundred milligrams or more per 24 h of urine collection (or this amount extrapolated from a timed collection) or a protein/creatinine ratio ≥ 0.3 mg/dL or a dipstick reading of 2+.

2.2. Maternal Serum Analytes

Peripheral venous blood samples were collected from all the participants during two different periods: the first trimester, at 9–13^{+6} weeks of gestation, and the second trimester, at 24–28 weeks of gestation. All the blood samples were centrifuged at 3000 rpm for 10 min, and the serum samples were stored at -80 °C until use.

All the samples from the subsequently diagnosed PE patients based on the ACOG guidelines [17] and gestational age and storage time-matched control (CON) pregnancies were retrieved. The ESM-1 and PLGF levels were measured using the enzyme-linked immunosorbent assay (ELISA) (R&D Systems, Minneapolis, MN, USA) by technicians who were blinded to the identity of the samples. The accuracy and stability of the ELISA method were validated in the pilot experiments. Each sample was measured three times and the average level was used as the final value for the sample. The ESM-1 kit detection range was 10.3–2500 pg/mL. The kit performance characteristics were a sensitivity of 1.08 pg/mL and a coefficient of variation (CV%) of <10. The PLGF kit detection range was 2.88–700 pg/mL. The kit performance characteristics were a sensitivity of 1.9 pg/mL and a coefficient of variation (CV%) of <10.

2.3. Uterine Artery PI

The patients without fetal defects on routine ultrasound performed at 22–28 weeks of gestation also underwent a bilateral uterine artery Doppler assessment. The uterine artery PI was determined as the average PI from three continuous similar waveforms. All the examinations were evaluated by ultrasound by simultaneous B-mode scanning (GE Healthcare, Milwaukee, WI, USA). The carrier frequency was from 1 to 5 MHz for the transabdominal probers.

2.4. Statistical Analysis

The data analysis was performed using SPSS 25.0 (SPSS Inc., Chicago, IL, USA) and MedCalc (version 11.4.2.0). The data are presented as the mean ± SD or median (min-max). Logistic regression analysis was used to evaluate the combination of these indicators. Receiver operating characteristic (ROC) curve analysis was performed to assess the predictive value. Statistically significant differences were estimated utilizing the Student's t-tests or chi-square tests. A p value < 0.05 was considered statistically significant.

3. Results

In total, 2086 pregnant women were recruited for the study. Among them, 1927 pregnant women completed the study, and 159 (7.6%) did not give birth in our hospital and were lost to the follow-up. Fifty-one women developed PE (severe preeclampsia (SPE) 33 cases and mild preeclampsia (MPE) 18 cases), with an incidence rate of 2.6%, which was consistent with that in the literature [18]. The CON group comprised 60 women with normal pregnancies who were randomly chosen and matched for gestational age to the women with PE. The flowchart of our prospective cohort study was shown in Figure 1.

The clinical and demographic characteristics of the participants are presented in Table 1. Compared with those in the CON group, the blood pressures of all those in the PE groups were higher ($p < 0.001$). The gestational age at delivery and the fetal weights were significantly lower in the PE group, especially in the SPE group ($p < 0.001$). The placental weights were lower in the SPE group ($p < 0.05$). However, there was no significant difference in maternal age, pre-pregnancy BMI, or the 5′ Apgar scores among the groups.

The results of the serum analytes from the PE group and the CON group samples collected in the first and second trimesters are shown in Table 2 and Figures 2–4. In the first trimester, compared with those in the gestational age-matched controls, the ESM-1 level (285.82 ± 89.53 vs. 357.61 ± 80.40, $p < 0.001$) in the SPE group was significantly lower. There was no significant difference in the ESM-1 level between the control and the MPE groups (Figure 2A). Additionally, there was also no significant difference in the PLGF level between the control group and any PE group (Figure 2B). In the second trimester, compared with those in the gestational age-matched controls, the ESM-1 level (206.24 ± 132.53 vs. 152.35 ± 29.00, $p = 0.0032$) in the SPE group was significantly higher and the PLGF level (14.03 ± 6.21 vs. 29.52 ± 17.26, $p < 0.001$) in the SPE group was significantly lower (Figure 3A,B). Moreover, compared to those in the control group, the PLGF level was significantly lower (16.82 ± 6.25 vs. 29.52 ± 17.26, $p < 0.001$) in the MPE group (Figure 3B). There was no significant difference in the ESM-1 level between the control and the MPE groups (Figure 3A). Compared with those in the gestational age-matched controls, the 2nd

PI (1.35 ± 0.39 vs. 0.89 ± 0.22, $p < 0.001$) in the SPE group and the 2nd PI (1.15 ± 0.34 vs. 0.89 ± 0.22, $p < 0.001$) in the MPE group were also significantly higher (Figure 4).

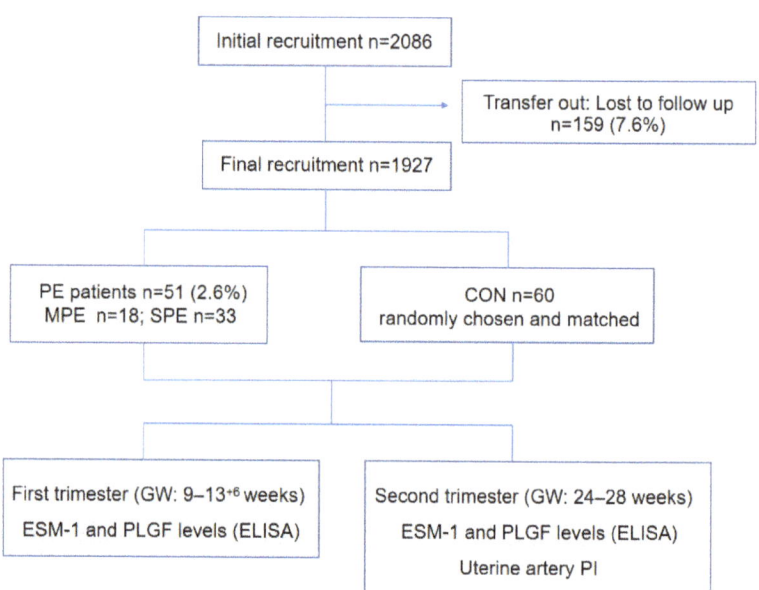

Figure 1. The flowchart of the prospective cohort study. CON, control group; MPE, mild preeclampsia group; SPE, severe preeclampsia group; GW, gestational week.

Table 1. Demographic characteristics of the participants.

Characteristic	SPE (n = 33)	MPE (n = 18)	CON (n = 60)
Maternal age, y	31.06 ± 4.34	31.89 ± 4.38	30.03 ± 3.61
Pre-BMI, kg/m^2	21.02 ± 2.55	21.51 ± 2.02	20.60 ± 1.82
SBP (mmHg)	166.18 ± 9.74 **	144.39 ± 5.38 **	117.00 ± 9.39
DBP (mmHg)	97.91 ± 8.91 **	92.33 ± 5.24 **	74.78 ± 9.11
Nulliparous, n (%)	29 (87.88%)	16 (88.89%)	52 (86.67%)
GA at delivery, weeks	37.09 ± 3.01 **	38.73 ± 1.20 *	39.45 ± 0.81
Fetal weight, g	2660.45 ± 754.43 **	3161.39 ± 266.34 *	3375.50 ± 297.29
Placental weight, g	537.27 ± 165.52 *	622.50 ± 84.53	614.08 ± 67.01
5′ Apgar score	9.33 ± 1.83	9.61 ± 0.61	9.81 ± 0.62

SPE, severe preeclampsia; MPE, mild preeclampsia; CON, control; pre-BMI: pre-pregnancy body mass index; SBP, systolic blood pressure; DBP, diastolic blood pressure; GA, gestational age. * $p < 0.05$; ** $p < 0.001$ compared to the CON.

Furthermore, the details of the AUCs are shown in Table 3, and the ROC curves for the biomarkers in the SPE prediction are presented in Figure 5. The ROC analysis for the SPE and control subjects yielded AUCs for the 1st ESM-1, the 2nd PLGF, and the 2nd PI of 0.714 (95% CI: 0.611–0.803, $p = 0.0002$), 0.802 (95% CI: 0.706–0.877, $p < 0.0001$), and 0.843 (95% CI: 0.753–0.911, $p < 0.0001$), respectively. Logistic regression analysis was used to evaluate the combination of these indicators. In the SPE group, the AUCs for the combinations of the 1st ESM-1 and 2nd PLGF, the 1st ESM-1 and 2nd PI, and the 2nd PLGF and 2nd PI were 0.856 (93.90% sensitivity and 66.70% specificity), 0.876 (84.85% sensitivity and 80.00% specificity), and 0.890 (69.70% sensitivity and 95.00% specificity), respectively. The combination of the 1st ESM-1, the 2nd PLGF, and the 2nd PI yielded an AUC of 0.912 (72.73% sensitivity and 95.00% specificity) ($p < 0.0001$ for all).

Table 2. Comparison of biomarker levels among study groups.

	SPE (n = 33)	MPE (n = 18)	CON (n = 60)	p Value SPE	p Value MPE
1st ESM-1 (pg/mL)	285.82 ± 89.53	304.00 ± 121.59	357.61 ± 80.40	<0.001 **	0.093
2nd ESM-1 (pg/mL)	206.24 ± 132.53	142.58 ± 60.68	152.35 ± 29.00	0.0032 *	0.347
1st PLGF (pg/mL)	2.67 ± 1.07	2.87 ± 1.27	3.13 ± 1.10	0.0524	0.400
2nd PLGF (pg/mL)	14.03 ± 6.21	16.82 ± 6.25	29.52 ± 17.26	<0.001 **	<0.001 **
2nd PI	1.35 ± 0.39	1.15 ± 0.34	0.89 ± 0.22	<0.001 **	<0.001 **

SPE, severe preeclampsia; MPE, mild preeclampsia; CON, control; ESM-1, endothelial cell-specific molecule 1; PLGF, placental growth factor; PI, pulsatility index. 1st/2nd ESM-1, ESM-1 level measured in the first/second trimester; 1st/2nd PLGF, PLGF level measured in the first/second trimester; 2nd PI, PI measured in the second trimester. * $p < 0.05$; ** $p < 0.001$ compared to the CON.

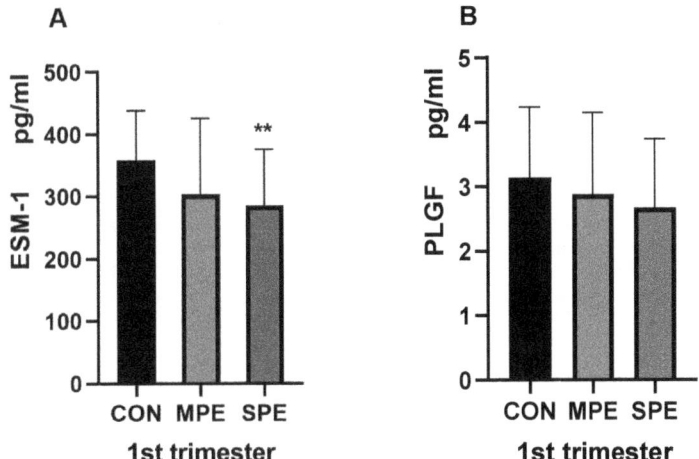

Figure 2. ESM-1 and PLGF in first-trimester maternal serum (**A**,**B**). CON, n = 60; MPE, n = 18; SPE, n = 33, ** $p < 0.001$.

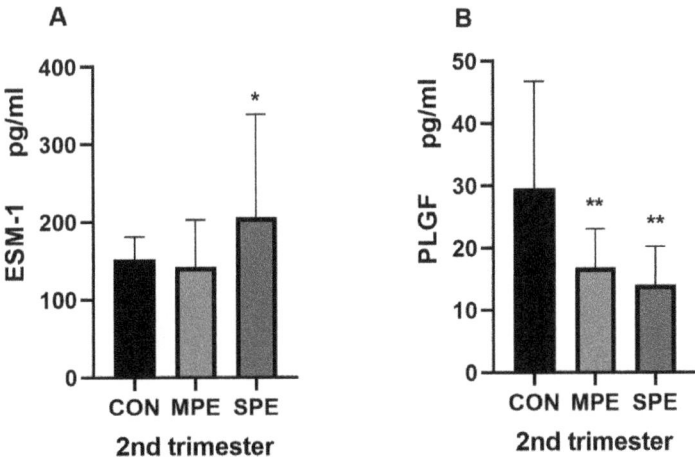

Figure 3. ESM-1 and PLGF in second-trimester maternal serum (**A**,**B**). CON, n = 60; MPE, n = 18; SPE, n = 33, * $p < 0.05$, ** $p < 0.001$.

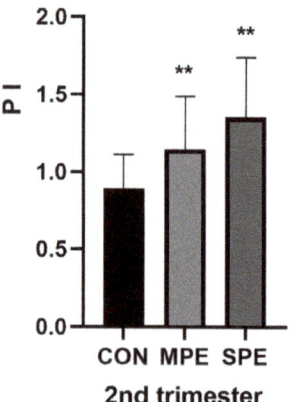

Figure 4. Uterine artery Doppler PI in the second trimester. CON, $n = 60$; MPE, $n = 18$; SPE, $n = 33$, ** $p < 0.001$.

Table 3. Predictive efficiency of biomarker levels and PI for severe preeclampsia.

Variable	AUC	p Value	95%CI	Cutoff	Specificity (%)	Sensitivity (%)
1st ESM-1	0.714	0.0002	0.611–0.803	262.33	91.67	45.50
2nd PLGF	0.802	<0.0001	0.706–0.877	19.12	70.00	84.85
2nd PI	0.843	<0.0001	0.753–0.911	1.12	86.67	75.76
1st ESM-1 + 2nd PLGF	0.856	<0.0001	0.767–0.920	-	66.70	93.90
1st ESM-1 + 2nd PI	0.876	<0.0001	0.792–0.935	-	80.00	84.85
2nd PLGF + 2nd PI	0.890	<0.0001	0.808–0.945	-	95.00	69.70
1st ESM-1 + 2nd PLGF + 2nd PI	0.912	<0.0001	0.835–0.961	-	95.00	72.73

CI: confidence interval; ESM-1, endothelial cell-specific molecule 1; PLGF, placental growth factor; PI, pulsatility index; 1st/2nd ESM-1, ESM-1 level measured in the first/second trimester; 1st/2nd PLGF, PLGF level measured in the first/second trimester.

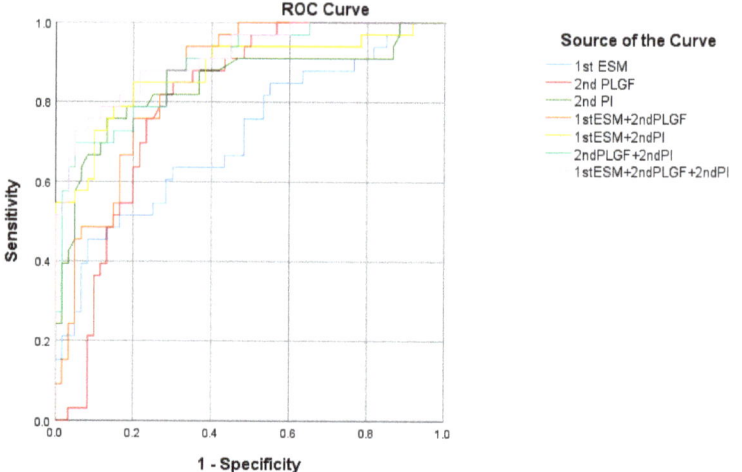

Figure 5. Receiver operating characteristic curve showing the clinical discrimination of different markers alone or in combination in the detection of severe preeclampsia.

The ROC curves for the biomarkers in the MPE prediction are presented in Figure 6. The ROC analysis for the MPE and control subjects yielded areas under the curve (AUCs) for the 2nd PLGF and the 2nd PI of 0.738 (95% CI: 0.626–0.831, $p < 0.0001$) and (95% CI: 0.636–0.839, $p = 0.0007$), respectively. In the MPE group, combining the 2nd PLGF with the 2nd PI yielded an AUC of 0.819 (83.33% sensitivity and 70.00% specificity).

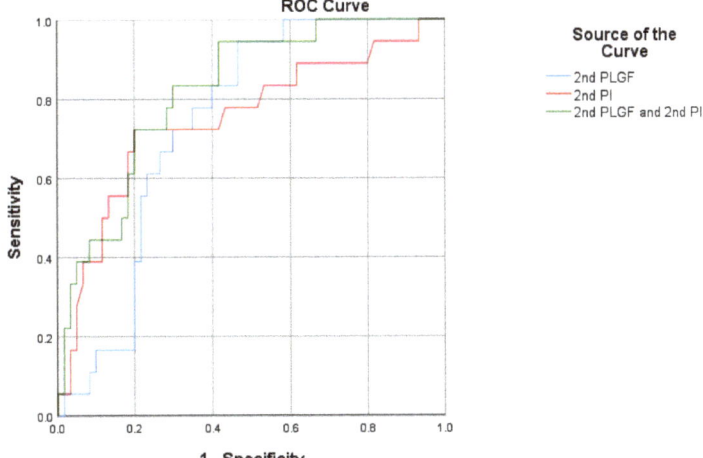

Figure 6. Receiver operating characteristic curve showing the clinical discrimination of different markers alone or in combination in the detection of mild preeclampsia.

4. Discussion

Accumulative evidence has revealed that inflammation and endothelial dysfunction are vitally important to the pathophysiology of PE [19]. ESM-1 might be involved in endothelial-related processes, including cell adhesion, angiogenesis, inflammation, and endothelial dysfunction [20]. Thus, ESM-1 could be regarded as a biomarker for hypertension [5,21], sepsis [22], malignancy [23], and PE [6].

The results showed that the ESM-1 level in the maternal plasma was lower during the first trimester (12–16 weeks of gestation) but increased in the second and third trimesters (≥24 weeks of gestation) in the SPE group [24]. Some studies in 2015 and 2016 reported higher ESM-1 concentrations in PE maternal plasma and a negative correlation with the clinical data, indicating its crucial role in the pathogenesis of PE progression [25,26]. Moreover, the stratified results from a meta-analysis conducted to determine the potential role of ESM-1 in PE suggested the upregulation of ESM-1 levels in PE [6]. The results obtained in our study were consistent with these studies, except that ESM-1 was detected earlier in the first trimester in our study.

As an explanation for the lower 1st ESM-1 level in PE, some researchers have suggested that ESM-1 functions as a protective cytokine by inhibiting leukocyte aggregation to protect tissues and organs from inflammatory damage and is consumed in early pregnancy [25]. It was also indicated that a positive feedback loop exists between the vascular endothelial growth factor (VEGF) and ESM-1 [27]; therefore, as the results revealed, the 2nd ESM-1 level was reduced with the advancement of the placental vasculature in the CON group and PE groups. In addition, ESM-1 can be upregulated by proinflammatory factors and growth factors, such as TNF-α, IL-6, and VEGF [28]. With the development of PE, the inflammatory response and endothelial dysfunction were aggravated, and the ESM-1 level was elevated in the second and third trimesters. Regarding the lack of a significant difference in the ESM-1 level between the MPE group and the normal pregnancy group in the first and second trimesters, it was speculated that inflammation and endothelial dysfunction were too minor to distinguish.

PLGF, which is expressed in the human placenta, heart, and lungs, is a member of the VEGF family [29]. It can directly activate its angiogenic pathway through PLGF/VEGFR1 (known as FLT1) and compete with VEGF-A for VEGFR1, further stimulating angiogenesis via the VEGFA/VEGFR2 (known as FLK1) interaction. During normal pregnancy, the PLGF level is relatively low in the first trimester. It gradually increases with the advancement of the utero-placental circulation and remodeling of the myometrial spiral arteries and finally reaches its peak at approximately 30 weeks of gestation, after which it drops [8]. Given the vital role of the placenta in PE, the usefulness of PLGF in PE prediction was investigated. A previous study revealed that at 9–12^{+6} weeks of gestation, the PLGF expression was significantly lower in PE pregnancies than in the CON pregnancies [30]. Another study examined the concentrations of PLGF in women with PE during two periods (8–14 weeks of gestation and 20–34 weeks of gestation). The results suggested that the PLGF level in the PE group was significantly lower in the first period, but no difference was found in the second period between the PE group and the CON group [31]. The study investigated the remarkably lower PLGF level in PE pregnancies at 24–28 weeks of gestation [32], and another study found that the PLGF concentration was also significantly lower before 35 weeks in the PE pregnancy compared to the normal pregnancy [33]. Moreover, the PLGF change was relevant to disease severity [34]. Our study had similar results. Specifically, a lack of a significant difference in the 1st PLGF level was found between the PE group and the CON group. Additionally, the 2nd PLGF concentrations were elevated compared to the 1st PLGF concentrations, but they were significantly lower than the 2nd PLGF concentration in the CON group, especially for SPE. With pregnancy progression in PE, the PLGF might compete with the VEGF for binding to sFlt-1, resulting in a significant drop emerging in the second trimester before the onset of PE symptoms [8].

Some studies have shown that uterine artery PI is a significant marker for predicting PE. The Doppler ultrasound of the maternal uterine artery PI might be the most effective method for screening women with PE in the second trimester [35]. In our study, 75.76% sensitivity and 86.67% specificity were achieved with the uterine artery PI. The uterine artery PI was increased in the second-trimester pregnancies in the PE patients, especially the SPE patients, which was consistent with the reported literature.

Many recent studies have suggested that the combination of biochemical indicators and the uterine artery Doppler could improve the screening efficiency for the prediction of PE [36,37]. Notably, our study similarly indicated that the overall predictive efficiency for SPE achieved by combining serum biomarkers and the uterine artery Doppler PI was improved compared with the single use of any marker alone.

5. Conclusions

The 1st ESM-1, 2nd PLGF levels and the 2nd uterine artery Doppler PI were associated with PE. The combination of serum biomarkers and the uterine artery Doppler PI strengthened the screening efficiency for the prediction of PE, especially for SPE. Our study is the first to assess the predictive combination of the 1st ESM-1, the 2nd PLGF, and the 2nd uterine artery Doppler PI for PE. Unfortunately, due to the COVID-19 outbreak, the blood samples of the participants in the third trimester were lost, resulting in a lack of data on the serum concentrations of ESM-1 and PLGF. Further studies are needed in a larger population to determine the potential for use of the aforementioned indicators.

Author Contributions: Conception and design, X.X. and D.C.; acquisition of data, X.X., D.C., and Y.C.; analysis and interpretation of data, X.X. and X.Y.; drafting of the manuscript, X.X. and D.C.; critical revision of the manuscript, X.X., D.C., Y.G. and W.C. All authors have read and agreed to the published version of the manuscript.

Funding: This study was supported by the Shanghai Municipal Health Commission (20194Y0050), the project of International Peace Maternal and Child Health Hospital Affiliated to Shanghai Jiaotong University (CR2018WX04), the National Natural Science Foundation of China (81370727), the Interdisciplinary Program of Shanghai Jiao Tong University (ZH2018ZDA31), and the establishment of preeclampsia–eclampsia cohort database (Clinical Research Plan of SHDC, SHDC2020CR6021).

Institutional Review Board Statement: The study was conducted according to the Declaration of Helsinki guidelines and the approval of the National Ethics Committee for Science and Technology (number: GKLW2020-03).

Informed Consent Statement: Written informed consent was obtained from all the participants.

Data Availability Statement: All the study data will be made available upon request to the corresponding author.

Acknowledgments: We thank all our participants for their cooperation and help during this study.

Conflicts of Interest: The authors report no conflict of interest in this work.

References

1. Kassebaum, N.J.; Barber, R.M.; Bhutta, Z.A.; Dandona, L.; Gething, P.W.; Hay, S.I.; Kinfu, Y.; Larson, H.J.; Liang, X.; Lim, S.S.; et al. Global, regional, and national levels of maternal mortality, 1990–2015: A systematic analysis for the Global Burden of Disease Study 2015. *Lancet* **2016**, *388*, 1775–1812. [CrossRef] [PubMed]
2. Roberts, J.M.; Lain, K.Y. Recent Insights into the pathogenesis of pre-eclampsia. *Placenta* **2002**, *23*, 359–372. [CrossRef] [PubMed]
3. Kornacki, J.; Wender-Ożegowska, E. Utility of biochemical tests in prediction, diagnostics and clinical management of preeclampsia: A review. *Arch. Med. Sci.* **2020**, *16*, 1370–1375. [CrossRef] [PubMed]
4. Lassalle, P.; Molet, S.; Janin, A.; Van der Heyden, J.; Tavernier, J.; Fiers, W.; Devos, R.; Tonnel, A.-B. ESM-1 is a novel human endothelial cell-specific molecule expressed in lung and regulated by cytokines. *J. Biol. Chem.* **1996**, *271*, 20458–20464. [CrossRef] [PubMed]
5. Balta, S.; Mikhailidis, D.P.; Demirkol, S.; Ozturk, C.; Kurtoglu, E.; Demir, M.; Celik, T.; Turker, T.; Iyisoy, A. Endocan—A novel inflammatory indicator in newly diagnosed patients with hypertension: A pilot study. *Angiology* **2014**, *65*, 773–777. [CrossRef]
6. Lan, X.; Liu, Z. Circulating endocan and preeclampsia: A meta-analysis. *Biosci. Rep.* **2020**, *40*, 1–9. [CrossRef]
7. Kingdom, J.; Huppertz, B.; Seaward, G.; Kaufmann, P. Development of the placental villous tree and its consequences for fetal growth. *Eur. J. Obstet. Gynecol. Reprod. Biol.* **2000**, *92*, 35–43. [CrossRef]
8. Chau, K.; Hennessy, A.; Makris, A. Placental growth factor and pre-eclampsia. *J. Hum. Hypertens.* **2017**, *31*, 782–786. [CrossRef]
9. Agrawal, S.; Shinar, S.; Cerdeira, A.S.; Redman, C.; Vatish, M. Predictive Performance of PlGF (Placental Growth Factor) for Screening Preeclampsia in Asymptomatic Women: A Systematic Review and Meta-Analysis. *Hypertension* **2019**, *74*, 1124–1135. [CrossRef]
10. Levine, R.J.; Maynard, S.E.; Qian, C.; Lim, K.-H.; England, L.J.; Yu, K.F.; Schisterman, E.F.; Thadhani, R.; Sachs, B.P.; Epstein, F.H.; et al. Circulating Angiogenic Factors and the Risk of Preeclampsia. *N. Engl. J. Med.* **2004**, *350*, 672–683. [CrossRef]
11. Polliotti, B.M.; Fry, A.G.; Saller, D.N.; Mooney, R.A.; Cox, C.; Miller, R.K. Second-trimester maternal serum placental growth factor and vascular endothelial growth factor for predicting severe, early-onset preeclampsia. *Obstet. Gynecol.* **2003**, *101*, 1266–1274. [CrossRef] [PubMed]
12. Perry, H.; Binder, J.; Kalafat, E.; Jones, S.; Thilaganathan, B.; Khalil, A. Angiogenic Marker Prognostic Models in Pregnant Women with Hypertension. *Hypertension* **2020**, *75*, 755–761. [CrossRef] [PubMed]
13. Carbillon, L.; Challier, J.; Alouini, S.; Uzan, M.; Uzan, S. Uteroplacental Circulation Development: Doppler Assessment and Clinical Importance. *Placenta* **2001**, *22*, 795–799. [CrossRef] [PubMed]
14. Lloyd-Davies, C.; Collins, S.L.; Burton, G.J. Understanding the uterine artery Doppler waveform and its relationship to spiral artery remodelling. *Placenta* **2021**, *105*, 78–84. [CrossRef]
15. Cui, S.; Gao, Y.; Zhang, L.; Wang, Y.; Zhang, L.; Liu, P.; Liu, L.; Chen, J. Combined use of serum MCP-1/IL-10 ratio and uterine artery Doppler index significantly improves the prediction of preeclampsia. *Clin. Chim. Acta* **2017**, *473*, 228–236. [CrossRef]
16. Papageorghiou, A.T.; Yu, C.K.H.; Bindra, R.; Pandis, G.; Nicolaides, K. Multicenter screening for pre-eclampsia and fetal growth restriction by transvaginal uterine artery Doppler at 23 weeks of gestation. *Ultrasound Obstet. Gynecol.* **2001**, *18*, 441–449. [CrossRef]
17. American College of Obstetricians and Gynecologists. Gestational Hypertension and Preeclampsia: ACOG Practice Bulletin Summary, Number 222. *Obstet. Gynecol.* **2020**, *135*, 1492–1495. [CrossRef] [PubMed]
18. Ives, C.W.; Sinkey, R.; Rajapreyar, I.; Tita, A.T.; Oparil, S. Preeclampsia—Pathophysiology and Clinical Presentations: JACC State-of-the-Art Review. *J. Am. Coll. Cardiol.* **2020**, *76*, 1690–1702. [CrossRef]
19. Chappell, L.C.; Cluver, C.A.; Kingdom, J.; Tong, S. Pre-eclampsia. *Lancet* **2021**, *398*, 341–354. [CrossRef]
20. Balta, S.; Mikhailidis, D.P.; Demirkol, S.; Ozturk, C.; Celik, T.; Iyisoy, A. Endocan: A novel inflammatory indicator in cardiovascular disease? *Atherosclerosis* **2015**, *243*, 339–343. [CrossRef]
21. Oktar, S.F.; Guney, I.; Eren, S.A.; Oktar, L.; Kosar, K.; Buyukterzi, Z.; Alkan, E.; Biyik, Z.; Erdem, S.S. Serum endocan levels, carotid intima-media thickness and microalbuminuria in patients with newly diagnosed hypertension. *Clin. Exp. Hypertens.* **2019**, *41*, 787–794. [CrossRef] [PubMed]
22. Mihajlovic, D.M.; Lendak, D.F.; Draskovic, B.G.; Brkic, S.V.; Mitic, G.P.; Mikic, A.S.N.; Cebovic, T.N. Corrigendum to "Endocan is useful biomarker of survival and severity in sepsis" [Microvasc. Res. 93 (2014) 92–97]. *Microvasc. Res.* **2020**, *129*, 103992. [CrossRef] [PubMed]

23. Scherpereel, A.; Gentina, T.; Grigoriu, B.; Sénéchal, S.; Janin, A.; Tsicopoulos, A.; Plénat, F.; Béchard, D.; Tonnel, A.-B.; Lassalle, P. Overexpression of endocan induces tumor formation. *Cancer Res.* **2003**, *63*, 6084–6089. [PubMed]
24. Schuitemaker, J.; Woudenberg, J.; Wijbenga, G.; Scherjon, S.; van Pampus, M.; Faas, M. PPNew prognostic marker for the risk to develop early-onset preeclampsia. *Pregnancy Hypertens.* **2013**, *3*, 95–96. [CrossRef]
25. Hentschke, M.R.; Lucas, L.S.; Mistry, H.D.; Pinheiro da Costa, B.E.; Poli-de-Figueiredo, C.E. Endocan-1 concentrations in maternal and fetal plasma and placentae in pre-eclampsia in the third trimester of pregnancy. *Cytokine* **2015**, *74*, 152–156. [CrossRef]
26. Cakmak, M.; Yılmaz, H.; Bağlar, E.; Darçın, T.; Inan, O.; Aktas, A.; Celik, H.T.; Özdemir, O.; Atalay, C.R.; Akcay, A. Serum levels of endocan correlate with the presence and severity of pre-eclampsia. *Clin. Exp. Hypertens.* **2015**, *38*, 137–142. [CrossRef]
27. Roudnicky, F.; Poyet, C.; Wild, P.; Krampitz, S.; Negrini, F.; Huggenberger, R.; Rogler, A.; Stöhr, R.; Hartmann, A.; Provenzano, M.; et al. Endocan Is Upregulated on Tumor Vessels in Invasive Bladder Cancer Where It Mediates VEGF-A–Induced Angiogenesis. *Cancer Res.* **2013**, *73*, 1097–1106. [CrossRef]
28. Zhang, H.; Shen, Y.-W.; Zhang, L.-J.; Chen, J.-J.; Bian, H.-T.; Gu, W.-J.; Zhang, H.; Chen, H.-Z.; Zhang, W.-D.; Luan, X. Targeting Endothelial Cell-Specific Molecule 1 Protein in Cancer: A Promising Therapeutic Approach. *Front. Oncol.* **2021**, *11*, 687120. [CrossRef]
29. Lohela, M.; Bry, M.; Tammela, T.; Alitalo, K. VEGFs and receptors involved in angiogenesis versus lymphangiogenesis. *Curr. Opin. Cell Biol.* **2009**, *21*, 154–165. [CrossRef]
30. Myatt, L.; Clifton, R.G.; Roberts, J.M.; Spong, C.Y.; Hauth, J.C.; Varner, M.W.; Thorp, J.M.; Mercer, B.M.; Peaceman, A.M.; Ramin, S.M.; et al. First-Trimester Prediction of Preeclampsia in Nulliparous Women at Low Risk. *Obstet. Gynecol.* **2012**, *119*, 1234–1242. [CrossRef]
31. Andersen, L.B.; Dechend, R.; Jørgensen, J.S.; Luef, B.M.; Nielsen, J.; Barington, T.; Christesen, H.T. Prediction of preeclampsia with angiogenic biomarkers. Results from the prospective Odense Child Cohort. *Hypertens. Pregnancy* **2016**, *35*, 405–419. [CrossRef] [PubMed]
32. De Vivo, A.; Baviera, G.; Giordano, D.; Todarello, G.; Corrado, F.; D'Anna, R. Endoglin, PlGF and sFlt-1 as markers for predicting pre-eclampsia. *Acta Obstet. Gynecol. Scand.* **2008**, *87*, 837–842. [CrossRef] [PubMed]
33. Chappell, L.C.; Duckworth, S.; Seed, P.T.; Griffin, M.; Myers, J.; Mackillop, L.; Simpson, N.; Waugh, J.; Anumba, D.; Kenny, L.; et al. Diagnostic Accuracy of Placental Growth Factor in Women with Suspected Preeclampsia: A prospective multicenter study. *Circulation* **2013**, *128*, 2121–2131. [CrossRef] [PubMed]
34. Robinson, C.J.; Johnson, D.D.; Chang, E.Y.; Armstrong, D.M.; Wang, W. Evaluation of placenta growth factor and soluble Fms-like tyrosine kinase 1 receptor levels in mild and severe preeclampsia. *Am. J. Obstet. Gynecol.* **2006**, *195*, 255–259. [CrossRef]
35. Cnossen, J.S.; Morris, R.K.; ter Riet, G.; Mol, B.W.; van der Post, J.A.; Coomarasamy, A.; Zwinderman, A.H.; Robson, S.C.; Bindels, P.J.; Kleijnen, J.; et al. Use of uterine artery Doppler ultrasonography to predict pre-eclampsia and intrauterine growth restriction: A systematic review and bivariable meta-analysis. *Can. Med. Assoc. J.* **2008**, *178*, 701–711. [CrossRef]
36. Poon, L.C.; Nicolaides, K.H. Early Prediction of Preeclampsia. *Obstet. Gynecol. Int.* **2014**, *2014*, 1–11. [CrossRef]
37. Yu, N.; Cui, H.; Chen, X.; Chang, Y. First trimester maternal serum analytes and second trimester uterine artery Doppler in the prediction of preeclampsia and fetal growth restriction. *Taiwan J. Obstet. Gynecol.* **2017**, *56*, 358–361. [CrossRef]

Disclaimer/Publisher's Note: The statements, opinions and data contained in all publications are solely those of the individual author(s) and contributor(s) and not of MDPI and/or the editor(s). MDPI and/or the editor(s) disclaim responsibility for any injury to people or property resulting from any ideas, methods, instructions or products referred to in the content.

Article

Sonographic Flow-Mediated Dilation Imaging versus Electronic EndoCheck Flow-Mediated Slowing by VICORDER in Pregnant Women—A Comparison of Two Methods to Evaluate Vascular Function in Pregnancy

Charlotte Lößner [1], Anna Multhaup [1], Thomas Lehmann [2], Ekkehard Schleußner [1] and Tanja Groten [1,*]

1 Department of Obstetrics, University Hospital Jena, 07747 Jena, Germany
2 Institute of Medical Statistics, Information Sciences and Documentation, University Hospital Jena, 07747 Jena, Germany
* Correspondence: tanja.groten@med.uni-jena.de

Abstract: The evaluation of endothelial function is gaining interest and importance during pregnancy, since the impaired adaptation in early pregnancy has been associated with an increased risk in preeclampsia and fetal growth restriction. To standardize the risk assessment and to implement the evaluation of vascular function in routine pregnancy care, a suitable, accurate and easy to use method is needed. Flow-mediated dilatation (FMD) of the brachial artery assessed by ultrasound is considered to be the gold standard for measuring the vascular endothelial function. The challenges of the FMD measurement have so far prevented its introduction into clinical routine. The VICORDER® device allows an automated determination of the flow-mediated slowing (FMS). The equivalence of FMD and FMS has not yet been proven in pregnant women. We collected data of 20 pregnant women randomly and consecutively while they presented for a vascular function assessment in our hospital. The gestational age at investigation was between 22 and 32 weeks of gestation, three had preexisting hypertensive pregnancy disease and three were twin pregnancies. The results for FMD or FMS below 11.3% were considered to be abnormal. Comparing FMD to FMS results in our cohort revealed a convergence in 9/9 cases, indicating normal endothelial function (specificity of 100%) and a sensitivity of 72.7%. In conclusion, we verify that the FMS measurement is a convenient, automated and operator-independent test method of endothelial function in pregnant women.

Keywords: pregnancy; hypertension; flow-mediated dilatation; flow-mediated slowing; vascular function

1. Introduction

Endothelial dysfunction is thought to be an important factor in the development of a placenta-associated disease such as preeclampsia, which is further associated with fetal growth restriction, chronic immune activation and multi-organ endothelial disease. In preeclampsia, the placenta secretes excess anti-angiogenic factors into the maternal circulation, leading to widespread endothelial damage and inflammation. Growing evidence links vascular dysfunction and the prediction of preeclampsia and fetal growth restriction in pregnancy. Diverse studies in high-risk women who developed preeclampsia have demonstrated that the endothelial dysfunction precedes the onset of clinical disease [1–4]. A recent systematic review of the vascular structure and function in preeclampsia demonstrates that an impaired endothelial function was consistently reported prior to, during and immediately after pregnancy, as evidenced by differences in the FMD of 1.7–12.2% [5]. Other publications verified that the FMD is decreased during a preeclamptic pregnancy [6,7]. Thus, measuring the cardiovascular function in obstetric routine care is increasingly discussed [8].

The endothelial function can be measured in coronary arteries and the periphery by measuring the vasomotor function after an intra-arterial infusion of pharmacologic substances, which enhance the release of endothelial nitric oxide. The disadvantage of these methods is their invasive nature, making them unsuitable for diverse studies. Celermajer et al. [9] developed the technique of flow-mediated dilatation (FMD) as a noninvasive method to measure the vascular endothelial function, and Coretti et al. [10] published the initial guidelines for the ultrasonic assessment of the FMD of the brachial artery. The method has been documented to correlate with the mentioned invasively assessed endothelial function in coronary arteries [11] and is considered today as the gold standard for measuring endothelial function [12]. However, there are various challenges in using the FMD measurement in daily clinical practice. The precision of measurement is highly dependent on the investigators' experience and expertise, and the procedure is time and material-consuming. The VICORDER® SMT medical device [13] mimics the FMD test procedure by analyzing flow-mediated slowing (FMS). The test allows for an automated and operator-independent testing of the endothelial function. The interchangeability of both test procedures has been shown [12–14], but an explicit investigation of pregnant women has not yet been done.

In order to promote the introduction of the evaluation of the maternal hemodynamics into the routine care of pregnant women, we aimed to prove the equivalency of the FMD and FMS measurement in a cohort of pregnant women. We compared the FMD measuring by ultrasound to the FMS measuring by VICORDER® in pregnant women for the first time.

2. Materials and Methods

During the assessment period between July 2020 and March 2021, pregnant women, scheduled for a routine assessment of cardiovascular function by FMD, received an additional measurement of FMS using VICORDER®. The women were consecutively included in our study. There were no exclusion criteria defined. In order to reduce the inter-observer variability the same examiner carried out all measurements. The clinical outcome data were collected from obstetric records following delivery. Ethical approval to include patient data for the analysis was obtained by the ethical committee of the Friedrich–Schiller University in Jena (2022-2683-Daten). The anonymous use of clinical data for research and educational purposes is covered by the governmental rules of Thuringia.

For the FMD measurement, we used the ultrasound system Canon Aplio 500 (Canon Medical Systems GmbH, Neuss, Germany), which was equipped with a vascular software (Precision + APure +) for 2D-imaging (Preset Carotid), color and spectral Doppler, an internal electrocardiogram (ECG) monitor and a high-frequency vascular transducer. Our test subjects were in supine position with their arms in comfortable position for imaging the brachial artery. The artery was imaged above the antecubital fossa in a longitudinal plane. A segment with clear anterior and posterior intimal interfaces was chosen. To induce a flow stimulus, a conventional blood pressure cuff was placed on the patients' forearm. The arterial occlusion was then created by a cuff inflation to the suprasystolic pressure (50 mmHg above systolic pressure) and held for 5 min. The occlusion caused ischemia and the consequent dilation of downstream resistance vessels via autoregulatory mechanisms. The cuff deflation then induced reactive hyperemia to accommodate the dilated resistance vessels. The resulting increase in shear stress caused the brachial artery to dilate. The brachial artery was measured at the same time in the cardiac circle by using ECG-gating during the image acquisition. We referred to the peak of the R-wave as the peak of systole, where the artery's diameter is known to be at its largest state. Determined from the ultrasound image, the diameter of the brachial artery was compared before and after occlusion, and the percentage of change was determined. Measurements were performed in triplicates for each participant. We then referred to the respective mean value of the three measurements before and after vascular congestion.

To determine FMS, we used the VICORDER® EndoCheck FMS Model. The test procedure was according to the device manual. The brachial pulse wave velocity (PWV) was measured simultaneously between the wrist and upper right arm over a measurement period of 10 min, where the occlusion time was 5 min. The slowing of PWV was determined continuously measuring minimal PWV in comparison to initial PWV value, the percentage of which is then called FMS.

As described by Shechter et al., we defined any FMD value > 11.3% as the normal endothelial function and, accordingly, any FMD value < 11.3% as the impaired endothelial function [15]. We defined the same clinical cut-off for the evaluation of FMS measurement results. Figure 1 shows results of FMD and FMS measurements indicating normal and impaired arterial stiffness (Figure 1).

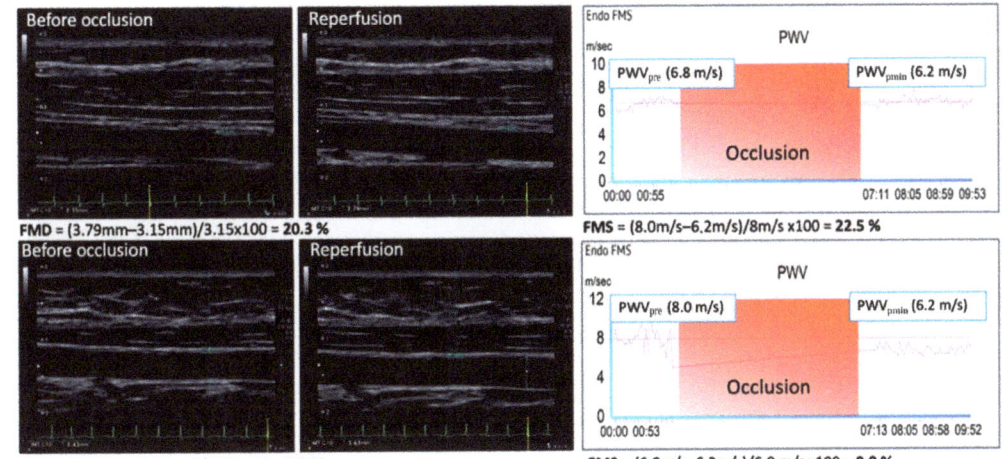

Figure 1. Results of FMD and FMS determination for normal (A) and impaired (B) arterial stiffness. For FMD measurement we used the ultrasound system Canon Aplio 500, which was equipped with a vascular software for 2D-imaging (Preset Carotid), colour and spectral Doppler, an internal electrocardiogram (ECG) monitor and a high-frequency vascular transducer. Diameter of brachial artery was ECG gated measured before and following arterial occlusion for 5 minutes. Flow mediated dilatation was calculated as percentage of change [(Diameter in mm following reperfusion − diameter in mm before occlusion)/diameter in mm before occlusion × 100]. To determine FMS, we used the VICORDER® EndoCheck FMS Model. The brachial PWV was measured simultaneously between wrist and upper right arm. Occlusion was applied for 5 minutes (red phase) and PWV was determined continuously. FMS is calculated form the minimal value measured (PWVmin) in percent of the initial value [(PWV before occlusion − PWVpmin)/PWV before occlusion × 100].

Continuous baseline characteristics are summarized by the median and 25th/75th percentile, and absolute and relative frequencies are provided for categorical data. The diagnostic accuracy was assessed by sensitivity and specificity using the cut-off value of 11.3% for FMD and FMS measurements. Both measurements are described by the median and the 25th/75th percentile. The agreement of the two methods was assessed via Bland–Altman plot.

3. Results

3.1. Cohort Characteristics

Descriptive data of our study population are presented in Table 1.

Table 1. Outline of group characteristics and pregnancy outcome.

Group Characteristics	
BMI [1] (kg/m^2)	25.9 (20.7/31.7)
Age (years)	33.5 (27.2/39.0)
Gestational age at measurement	26 + 5 (22 + 5/31 + 6)
Pre-existent hypertension	3 (15%)
Twin pregnancy	3 (15%)
History of placental disease	1 (5%)
Clinical features at the time of measurement	
None	2 (10%)
Cervical insufficiency	10 (50%)
FGR [2]	4 (20%)
PROM [3]	1 (5%)
Placenta previa	1 (5%)
Pathologic Doppler flow	1 (5%)
Orthostatic circulatory dysregulation	1 (5%)
Placental diseases at admission	4 (20%)
Pregnancy Outcome	
Gestational age at delivery	38 + 0 (34 + 4/39 + 0)
Mode of delivery	
Vaginal delivery	9 (45%)
Elective caesarean section	9 (45%)
Emergency caesarean section	2 (10%)
Placental diseases at delivery	6 (30%)
FGR [2] singleton pregnancy	2 (10%)
sFGR [4] twin pregnancy	2 (10%)
HELLP [5] and sFGR [4] twin pregnancy	1 (5%)
Eclampsia	1 (5%)
Premature birth	9 (45%)

Data are n (%) or median (interquartile range). [1] Body mass index; [2] fetal growth restriction; [3] premature rupture of membranes; [4] selective fetal growth restriction of one child in twin pregnancies; [5] hemolysis elevated liver enzymes and low platelet syndrome.

3.2. Comparison of Measured FMD and FMS Values

Results for the FMD and FMS measurement and the calculated differences are listed for each of the 20 women in Table 2. The FMD values ranged from 5.5% to 15.7%, with a mean of 10.6%. The FMS values ranged from 8 to 17%, with a median of 15%. The difference between FMD and FMS value per test subject varied from 1.2% to 4.4%, with a median of 3.1%.

As shown in Table 3, all cases that identified to have a normal endothelial function by FMD measurement were also characterized to be normal by FMS, revealing a specificity of 100%. In 8 of 11 cases, where the FMD revealed a reduced endothelial function, both methods consistently showed values below 11.3% (sensitivity 72.70%). In 3 of 11 cases, the endothelial function was classified as reduced via FMD, but as normal by the FMS values. In all three cases, the FMD values were above 10% (cases 1, 2 and 19—see Table 2).

Table 2. Outline of measured FMD and FMS values.

	Comparison of Values per Test Subject		
Patient No	FMD (%)	FMS (%)	Difference % (FMS–FMD)
1	10.13	15.00	+4.87
2	10.32	15.00	+4.68
3	3.53	8.00	+4.47
4	15.61	18.00	+2.39
5	4.67	8.00	+3.33
6	21.99	24.00	+2.01
7	8.00	10.00	+2.00
8	12.80	17.00	+4.20
9	17.41	22.00	+4.59
10	2.89	2.00	−0.89
11	2.88	7.00	+4.12
12	9.94	7.00	−2.94
13	15.73	17.00	+1.27
14	2.84	4.00	+1.16
15	16.20	16.00	−0.20
16	18.10	14.00	−4.10
17	13.80	15.00	+1.20
18	9.60	10.00	+0.40
19	10.85	15.00	+4.15
20	13.82	19.00	+5.18

Data for FMD were mean of triplicates performed.

Table 3. Comparison of classification of endothelial function by FMD or FMS using the cut off < 11.3% to determine impaired function.

			FMD		
			>11.3% Indicating Normal Endothelial Function	<11.3% Indicating Reduced Endothelial Function	Total
FMS	>11.3% indicating normal endothelial function	Count	9	3	12
		% of reduced FMD	100.0%	27.3%	60.0%
	<11.3% indicating reduced endothelial function	Count	0	8	8
		% of reduced FMD	0.0%	72.7%	40.0%
Total		Count	9	11	20
		% of reduced FMD	100.0%	100.0%	100.0%

3.3. Agreement between FMD and FMS Method

Figure 1 shows the Bland–Altman plot of agreement between the FMD and FMS method. As shown in the graph, the statistical limits were calculated by using the mean value and standard deviation of the difference between the two methods. The average discrepancy (the bias) between the FMD and FMS method lies at 2.09%. The 95% limits of agreement were 7.39% (bias + 1.96 SD) and −3.21 % (bias − 1.96 SD). A total of 19/20 data points are within ± 2 SD of the mean difference, as recommended by Bland and Altman. (Figure 2).

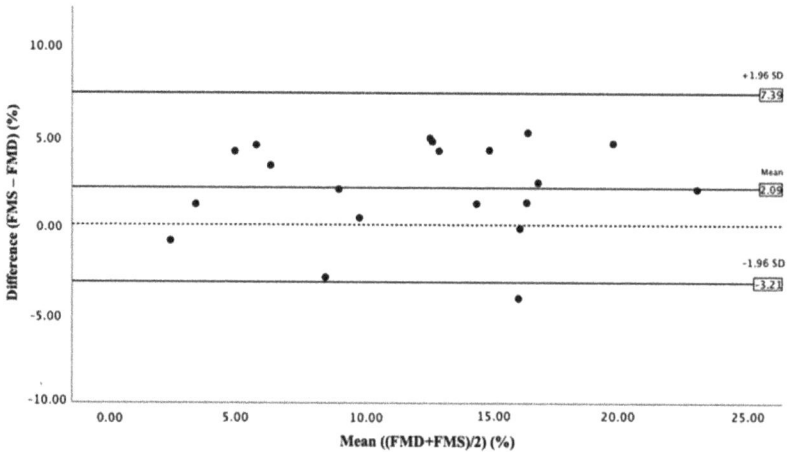

Figure 2. Bland–Altman plot of agreement between FMD and FMS method.

4. Discussion

Hypertensive pregnancy diseases are characterized by a general endothelial dysfunction, and the assessment of the endothelial function will play an increasingly important role in the medical care of these women. Increasing studies demonstrate that the determination of endothelial function by FMD is suitable for the prediction of pregnancy complications in high-risk pregnancies. In a systematic review of vascular structure and function in preeclampsia by Kirollos et al. [5] from 2019, an impaired endothelial function was consistently reported prior to, during and immediately after pregnancy, described by differences in the FMD of 1.7–12.2%. Diverse studies in high-risk women who developed preeclampsia have demonstrated that the endothelial dysfunction precedes the onset of clinical disease [3,4]. Other publications verified that FMD decreases during a preeclamptic pregnancy [6,7].

Additionally to the raising importance of endothelial function determination during pregnancy, the importance of evaluating the vascular function following pregnancies complicated by preeclampsia gains an increasing significance. Clinical observation demonstrates that women with a history of preeclampsia are known for higher cardiovascular morbidity and mortality later in life compared with controls, who had normotensive pregnancies [16]. The American Heart Association—Guidelines recognized preeclampsia as an important risk factor for cardiovascular diseases. This has led to the hypothesis that the endothelial status of these women is characterized by an early onset of aging. In 2018, Breetveld et al. [17] demonstrated that women with a history of preeclampsia remained associated with lower FMD years after pregnancy.

However, in daily clinical practice, measuring FMD is challenging and did not prove to be suitable for routine care. Therefore, a method capable of being implemented in a routine setting and providing reliable and reproducible results on vascular endothelial function is urgently needed and is a fundamental requirement for interventional studies based on an altered endothelial function during pregnancy. The new technique to evaluate the endothelial function using the EndoCheck flow-mediated slowing (FMS) method allows for an automated and operator-independent determination of vascular function. It is based on the same pathophysiological principles as the FMD method. The comparability of both methods was shown before [12] but, so far, the data for pregnant women are missing. Our study provides this data.

We found a high concordance of FMD and FMS values in a cohort of 20 pregnant women. The Bland–Altmann analysis demonstrates that most data points were within ±2 SD of the mean difference, as recommended by Bland and Altman (Figure 2). The mentioned outliner (case 16—see in Table 1) showed the measurements of a healthy pregnant woman without pregnancy complications, where both the FMD and FMS count was above 11.3%.

As there is no generally valid cut-off specified in the literature up to date which distinguishes a normal from a reduced state of endothelial function, we defined the cut-off in our work according to the following study by Shechter et al. [15] from 2014. Herein, the usefulness of FMD to predict long-term cardiovascular events (all-cause mortality, nonfatal myocardial infarction, hospitalization for heart failure or angina pectoris, stroke, coronary artery bypass grafting and percutaneous coronary interventions) in subjects without heart disease was examined. A total of 618 subjects were divided into two groups: FMD $\leq$ 11.3% (n = 309) and FMD > 11.3% (n = 309), where 11.3% was the median FMD in that population. The groups were comparable regarding cardiovascular risk factors, lipoproteins, fasting glucose, C-reactive protein, concomitant medications and Framingham 10-year risk score. In a mean follow-up of 4.6 $\pm$ 1.8 years, 48 of 618 patients (7.7%) developed composite adverse cardiovascular events. All composite adverse cardiovascular endpoints were significantly more common in subjects with FMD below versus above the median FMD (15.2% vs. 1.2%, p = 0.0001). The statistical analysis demonstrated that the median FMD predicted cardiovascular events significantly and independently (p < 0.001) in healthy subjects with no apparent heart disease, in addition to those derived from a traditional risk factor assessment. In accordance, we defined a limit value for the clinical state of the endothelial function of 11.3%, considering that any FMD value > 11.3% indicates a normal endothelial function and, consequently, any FMD value $\leq$ 11.3% for a reduced endothelial function. In order to perform a comparison to the FMS method, we expected the same clinical cut-off for the FMS measurements.

There was a convergence in both methods in 9/9 cases, indicating normal endothelial function (specificity of 100%). In 8/11 cases, a reduced FMD and FMS value was found for both methods (sensitivity of 72.70%). In 3/11 cases (27.30%), the endothelial function was measured as reduced via the FMD method, but as normal via the FMS-method. In those three cases, the FMD values were marginally lower than 11.3%, whereas the FMS values were above the cut-off (cases 1, 2 and 19—see Table 2). Case 1 shows a patient with FGR who suffered from pre-existent hypertension. She took anti-hypertensive medication, which might have affected the measurement. In case 2 and 19, pregnancies are described that were not complicated by the occurrence of any placental diseases.

The major limitation of our study is the small number of pregnant women included. We aimed to include women consecutively in a nonselective approach. As a result of the non-selective approach, individual risk profiles showed large variations (BMI, maternal age, gestational age, parity, etc.). Fortunately, the high consistency of our results comparing the two methods was observed in all pregnant women regardless of their individual risk profile.

5. Conclusions

In conclusion, our data demonstrate the high accordance of FMD and FMS results. We could validate that the FMS measuring by the VICORDER® is suitable for the routine care during pregnancy, yielding reliable clinical results. FMS is an electronic procedure viable for clinical screening and follow-up care in high-risk pregnancies, retrieving results equivalent to those obtained by FMD. We can confirm that large-scale prospective studies with a longitudinal observation of women throughout and after pregnancy to compare clinical outcome can be performed using the investigator independent automated method of the FMS measurement via VICORDER® device.

Author Contributions: C.L., A.M. and T.G. designed the study. C.L. and T.L. carried out the statistical analysis. C.L. drafted the manuscript. T.G. and E.S. supervised and revised the manuscript. All authors have read and agreed to the published version of the manuscript.

Funding: This research received no external funding. We acknowledge support by the German Research Foundation Projekt-Nr. 512648189 and the Open Access Publication Fund of the Thueringer Universitaets- und Landesbibliothek Jena.

Institutional Review Board Statement: The study was conducted according to the guidelines of the Declaration of Helsinki, and the study was approved by the Ethics Committee of the Friedrich–Schiller University, Jena, Germany (2022-2683-Daten).

Informed Consent Statement: Informed consent was obtained from all subjects involved in the study.

Data Availability Statement: All data retrieved are displayed in this manuscript.

Conflicts of Interest: The authors declare no conflict of interest.

References

1. Levine, R.J.; Maynard, S.E.; Qian, C.; Lim, K.H.; England, L.J.; Yu, K.F.; Schisterman, E.F.; Thadhani, R.; Sachs, B.P.; Epstein, F.H.; et al. Circulating angiogenic factors and the risk of preeclampsia. *N. Engl. J. Med.* **2004**, *350*, 672–683. [CrossRef] [PubMed]
2. Valensise, H.; Vasapollo, B.; Gagliardi, G.; Novelli, G.P. Early and late preeclampsia: Two different maternal hemodynamic states in the latent phase of the disease. *Hypertension* **2008**, *52*, 873–880. [CrossRef] [PubMed]
3. Brandão, A.H.; Cabral, M.A.; Leite, H.V.; Cabral, A.C. Endothelial function, uterine perfusion and central flow in pregnancies complicated by Preeclampsia. *Arq. Bras. Cardiol.* **2012**, *99*, 931–935. [CrossRef] [PubMed]
4. Brandão, A.H.; Félix, L.R.; Patrício Edo, C.; Leite, H.V.; Cabral, A.C. Difference of endothelial function during pregnancies as a method to predict preeclampsia. *Arch. Gynecol. Obstet.* **2014**, *290*, 471–477. [CrossRef] [PubMed]
5. Kirollos, S.; Skilton, M.; Patel, S.; Arnott, C. A Systematic Review of Vascular Structure and Function in Pre-eclampsia: Non-invasive Assessment and Mechanistic Links. *Front. Cardiovasc. Med.* **2019**, *6*, 166. [CrossRef] [PubMed]
6. Mori, T.; Watanabe, K.; Iwasaki, A.; Kimura, C.; Matsushita, H.; Shinohara, K.; Wakatsuki, A. Differences in vascular reactivity between pregnant women with chronic hypertension and preeclampsia. *Hypertens. Res.* **2014**, *37*, 145–150. [CrossRef] [PubMed]
7. Oliveira, O.P.; Araujo Júnior, E.; Lima, J.W.; Salustiano, E.M.; Ruano, R.; Martins, W.P.; Costa, F.D.S. Flow-mediated dilation of brachial artery and endothelial dysfunction in pregnant women with preeclampsia: A case control study. *Minerva Ginecol.* **2015**, *67*, 307–313. [PubMed]
8. Meah, V.L.; Backx, K.; Davenport, M.H.; International Working Group on Maternal Hemodynamics. Functional hemodynamic testing in pregnancy: Recommendations of the International Working Group on Maternal Hemodynamics. *Ultrasound Obstet. Gynecol.* **2018**, *51*, 331–340. [CrossRef] [PubMed]
9. Celermajer, D.S.; Sorensen, K.E.; Gooch, V.M.; Spiegelhalter, D.J.; Miller, O.I.; Sullivan, I.D.; Lloyd, J.K.; Deanfield, J.E. Non-invasive detection of endothelial dysfunction in children and adults at risk of atherosclerosis. *Lancet* **1992**, *340*, 1111–1115. [CrossRef] [PubMed]
10. Corretti, M.C.; Anderson, T.J.; Benjamin, E.J.; Celermajer, D.; Charbonneau, F.; Creager, M.A.; Deanfield, J.; Drexler, H.; Gerhard-Herman, M.; Herrington, D.; et al. Guidelines for the ultrasound assessment of endothelial-dependent flow-mediated vasodilation of the brachial artery: A report of the International Brachial Artery Reactivity Task Force. *J. Am. Coll. Cardiol.* **2002**, *39*, 257–265. [CrossRef] [PubMed]
11. Harris, R.A.; Nishiyama, S.K.; Wray, D.W.; Richardson, R.S. Ultrasound assessment of flow-mediated dilation. *Hypertension* **2010**, *55*, 1075–1085. [CrossRef] [PubMed]
12. Ellins, E.A.; New, K.J.; Datta, D.B.; Watkins, S.; Haralambos, K.; Rees, A.; Aled Rees, D.; Halcox, J.P. Validation of a new method for non-invasive assessment of vasomotor function. *Eur. J. Prev. Cardiol.* **2016**, *23*, 577–583. [CrossRef] [PubMed]
13. SMT medical GmbH & Co. KG. VICORDER—EndoCheck FMS—Operator Independent Endothelial Function Testing. Available online: https://www.smt-medical.com/en/products/vicorder-cardio-and-peripheral-vascular-testing/endocheck-model.html (accessed on 30 January 2023).
14. Pereira, T.; Almeida, A.; Conde, J. Flow-Mediated Slowing as a Methodological Alternative to the Conventional Echo-Tracking Flow-Mediated Dilation Technique for the Evaluation of Endothelial Function: A Preliminary Report. *Mayo Clin. Proc. Innov. Qual. Outcomes* **2018**, *2*, 199–203. [CrossRef] [PubMed]
15. Shechter, M.; Shechter, A.; Koren-Morag, N.; Feinberg, M.S.; Hiersch, L. Usefulness of brachial artery flow-mediated dilation to predict long-term cardiovascular events in subjects without heart disease. *Am. J. Cardiol.* **2014**, *113*, 162–167. [CrossRef] [PubMed]
16. Melchiorre, K.; Thilaganathan, B.; Giorgione, V.; Ridder, A.; Memmo, A.; Khalil, A. Hypertensive Disorders of Pregnancy and Future Cardiovascular Health. *Front. Cardiovasc. Med.* **2020**, *7*, 59. [CrossRef] [PubMed]
17. Breetveld, N.M.; Ghossein-Doha, C.; van Neer, J.; Sengers, M.; Geerts, L.; van Kuijk, S.M.J.; van Dijk, A.P.; van der Vlugt, M.J.; Heidema, W.M.; Rocca, H.P.B.-L.; et al. Decreased endothelial function and increased subclinical heart failure in women several years after pre-eclampsia. *Ultrasound Obstet. Gynecol.* **2018**, *52*, 196–204. [CrossRef] [PubMed]

Disclaimer/Publisher's Note: The statements, opinions and data contained in all publications are solely those of the individual author(s) and contributor(s) and not of MDPI and/or the editor(s). MDPI and/or the editor(s) disclaim responsibility for any injury to people or property resulting from any ideas, methods, instructions or products referred to in the content.

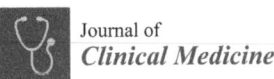

Article

Screening for Preeclampsia and Fetal Growth Restriction in the First Trimester in Women without Chronic Hypertension

Piotr Tousty [1,*], Magda Fraszczyk-Tousty [2], Anna Golara [1], Adrianna Zahorowska [1], Michał Sławiński [3], Sylwia Dzidek [1], Hanna Jasiak-Jóźwik [1], Magda Nawceniak-Balczerska [1], Agnieszka Kordek [2], Ewa Kwiatkowska [4], Aneta Cymbaluk-Płoska [5], Andrzej Torbé [1] and Sebastian Kwiatkowski [1]

1. Department of Gynecology and Obstetrics, Pomeranian Medical University, 70-111 Szczecin, Poland
2. Department of Neonatology and Neonatal Intensive Care, Pomeranian Medical University, 70-111 Szczecin, Poland
3. Department of Laboratory Diagnostics, Public Clinical Hospital No. 2, 70-111 Szczecin, Poland
4. Department of Nephrology, Transplantology and Internal Medicine, Pomeranian Medical University, 70-111 Szczecin, Poland
5. Department of Reconstructive Surgery and Gynecological Oncology, Pomeranian Medical University, 70-111 Szczecin, Poland
* Correspondence: piotr.toscik@gmail.com; Tel.: +48-735-923-533

Abstract: Background: Nowadays, it is possible to identify a group at increased risk of preeclampsia (PE) and fetal growth restriction (FGR) using the principles of the Fetal Medicine Foundation (FMF). It has been established for several years that acetylsalicylic acid (ASA) reduces the incidence of PE and FGR in high-risk populations. This study aimed to evaluate the implementation of ASA use after the first-trimester screening in a Polish population without chronic hypertension, as well as its impact on perinatal complications. Material and methods: A total of 874 patients were enrolled in the study during the first-trimester ultrasound examination. The risk of PE and FGR was assessed according to the FMF guidelines, which include the maternal history, mean arterial pressure (MAP), uterine artery pulsatility index (UtPI), pregnancy-associated plasma protein A (PAPP-A) and placental growth factor (PLGF). Among patients with a risk higher than >1:100, ASA was administered at a dose of 150 mg. Perinatal outcomes were assessed among the different groups. Results: When comparing women in the high-risk group with those in the low-risk group, a statistically significantly higher risk of pregnancy complications was observed in the high-risk group. These complications included pregnancy-induced hypertension (PIH) (OR 3.6 (1.9–7)), any PE (OR 7.8 (3–20)), late-onset PE (OR 8.5 (3.3–22.4)), FGR or small for gestational age (SGA) (OR 4.8 (2.5–9.2)), and gestational diabetes mellitus type 1 (GDM1) (OR 2.4 (1.4–4.2)). The pregnancies in the high-risk group were more likely to end with a cesarean section (OR 1.9 (1.2–3.1)), while the newborns had significantly lower weights (<10 pc (OR 2.9 (1.2–6.9)), <3 pc (OR 10.2 (2.5–41.7))). Conclusions: The first-trimester screening test for PE and FGR is a necessary and effective tool in identifying high-risk pregnancies. ASA prophylaxis among high-risk patients may have the most beneficial effect. Furthermore, this screening tool may significantly reduce the incidence of early-onset PE (eo-PE).

Keywords: preeclampsia; fetal growth restriction; screening; first trimester; aspirin

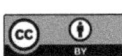

1. Introduction

Preeclampsia (PE) and fetal growth restriction (FGR) are significant causes of maternal and fetal mortality worldwide, leading to iatrogenic preterm labor and prolonged hospitalizations for mothers and newborns [1,2].

Until now, groups at risk of these disorders occurring in the first trimester of pregnancy have been identified based on the maternal history of illnesses and previous pregnancies [3,4]. However, in recent years, the Fetal Medicine Foundation (FMF) has demonstrated that these disorders can be predicted using additional factors. This comprehensive assessment includes biochemical indicators such as the placental growth factor (PLGF) and pregnancy-associated plasma protein A (PAPP-A), biophysical markers such as the mean arterial pressure (MAP) and uterine artery pulsatility index (UtA-PI), and the maternal history. Together, these factors are highly effective predictors of PE, with a detection rate (DR) of 90% for its early-onset variety (eo-PE), 75% for preterm PE, and 42% for term PE with a false positive rate (FPR) of 10%. However, the algorithm's effectiveness in diagnosing FGR is lower, achieving a DR of approximately 50% [5–11].

Currently, there is no available treatment to prolong pregnancy in confirmed PE cases, and the only effective therapeutic option is to terminate the pregnancy. However, the use of acetylsalicylic acid (ASA) in women at an increased risk of developing PE in the first trimester has been shown to reduce the incidence of PE before 37 weeks' gestation (wkGA) by 62% [12]. Furthermore, if women with chronic hypertension and those who received less than 90% of the recommended doses are excluded from the study, the risk reduction would be as high as 95%. Unfortunately, the same study found no significant reduction in the incidence of preterm PE among women with chronic hypertension in the aspirin-taking group (5/49) compared to the placebo (5/61) (OR 1.29, 95% CI 0.33–5.12) [13]. ASA has also been found to be useful in cases of increased risk of small for gestational age (SGA), where it has been shown to reduce the incidence of SGA before 37 wkGA by approx. 40–44%. However, this reduction does not extend to the incidence of SGA after the completion of the 37th wkGA [14]. The current recommendations from the International Federation of Gynecology and Obstetrics (FIGO) suggest the use of ASA in high-risk patients starting before 16 wkGA and continuing until 36 wkGA [15]. The primary objective of this study was to assess the effectiveness of the PE and FGR screening test, according to the FMF, followed by administering ASA to a high-risk group of Polish women without chronic hypertension. It is believed that this group of women may derive the greatest benefit from taking ASA. The secondary goal was to compare the perinatal outcomes between groups based on whether the woman was classified in the ASA-taking group and whether PE or FGR were present. To the best of our knowledge, there have been no previous evaluations of ASA use in women at high risk of developing PE and FGR in the Polish population.

2. Patients and Methods

This prospective study, conducted from 2019 to 2022, included 908 Caucasian women with healthy singleton pregnancies who were examined in the Pomeranian Medical University's Second Autonomous Public Clinical Hospital, in the Department of Obstetrics and Gynecology. Patients with chronic hypertension were excluded, resulting in a final enrollment of 874 patients. A first-trimester screening test was performed in each patient to assess aneuploidy, fetal defects, and the risk of developing PE and FGR. The study was conducted following the FMF principles. The Polish healthcare system features a publicly funded prenatal screening program for women aged 35+, who accounted for a significant percentage of the study population. Basic anthropometric measurements were taken, medical histories were obtained, the arterial pressure was measured twice in each arm, and a transabdominal probe was used to determine the UtA-PI. Subsequently, blood samples were collected from each patient for PAPP-A and PlGF concentration measurements, using the Cobas e 801 (Roche Diagnostics, Warsaw, Poland) analyzer. Each patient was then assessed for the risk of eo-PE and FGR based on the FMF algorithms (FMF—2012 software, version 2.8.1). The algorithm for the eo-PE risk assessment consists of a comprehensive assessment of maternal characteristics together with UtPI, MAP, UtPI, and PLGF, with or without PAPP-A, and it is currently based on a paper from 2018 [5]. The authors defined eo-PE according to the International Society for the Study of Hypertension in Pregnancy (ISSHP) criteria [16]. The algorithm for assessing FGR also consists of evaluating the same parameters used to evaluate eo-PE, but it is based on a 2010 paper, where other parameters currently not used in predictions were evaluated (for example, placental protein 13 (PP13) and A Disintegrin and Metalloprotease (ADAM12)). For FGR, the authors used the definition of a birth weight below the fifth percentile [11]. Patients at a high risk (>1:100) of developing eo-PE or FGR were advised to take doses of 150 mg of ASA until 36 wkGA. Perinatal outcomes, such as pregnancy-induced hypertension (PIH), gestational diabetes mellitus (GDM), FGR (in accordance with the Delphi criteria—see Table 1) [17], an SGA diagnosis (estimated fetal weight (EFW) or a fetal abdominal circumference (AC) between the 3rd and 10th percentiles (pc) without any features of FGR), and the presence of PE, were assessed.

Table 1. Definition of FGR in accordance with the Delphi criteria.

Early FGR: GA < 32 weeks, in the absence of congenital anomalies	Late FGR: GA ≥ 32 weeks, in the absence of congenital anomalies
AC/EFW < 3rd centile or UA-AEDF Or 1. AC/EFW < 10th centile combined with 2. UtA-PI > 95th centile and/or 3. UA-PI > 95th centile	AC/EFW < 3rd centile Or at least two out of three of the following: 1. AC/EFW < 10th centile 2. AC/EFW crossing centiles > 2 quartiles on growth centiles * 3. CPR < 5th centile or UA-PI > 95th centile

Note: * Growth centiles are non-customized centiles; AC: fetal abdominal circumference; AEDF: absent end-diastolic flow; CPR: cerebroplacental ratio; EFW: estimated fetal weight; GA, gestational age; PI: pulsatility index; UA: umbilical artery; UtA: uterine artery.

For PE, the criterion used was as defined by the ISSHP. PE was diagnosed if the following criteria were met after 20 wkGA: systolic blood pressure ≥ 140 mm Hg or diastolic blood pressure ≥ 90 mm Hg, along with proteinuria, defined as daily protein loss > 300 mg (or protein:creatinine ratio > 30 mg/mmol). If no proteinuria was found, then at least one of the following criteria had to be satisfied:

1. Hematological disorders (thrombocytopenia, DIC, hemolysis).
2. Serum creatinine content > 1.1 mg/dL or a 2-fold increase in its baseline level where no other kidney disease is observed.
3. Increased serum liver enzymes ≥ 2 times the upper limit of the standard or severe right upper quadrant or epigastric pain.
4. Neurological signs or visual impairment.
5. Pulmonary edema.
6. Intrauterine growth restriction [16].

For each newborn, the following information was assessed: birth week, sex, delivery method, 5-min Apgar score, and basic anthropometric measurements such as the neonatal birth weight. Fenton growth charts (www.ucalgary.ca/fenton accessed on 17 July 2023) were used to determine the birth weight percentiles. The flowchart of the study is shown in Figure 1.

The study was conducted in compliance with the Declaration of Helsinki and received approval from the Institutional Review Board of the Pomeranian Medical University in Szczecin (KB-0012/122/12 of 29 October 2012). Table 2 presents the essential characteristics of the study group, including anthropometric measurements, medical histories of comorbidities, obstetric history, family history, and addictions.

Table 2. Characteristics of the study group.

Feature	n (%)
Maternal age and weight	
Age > 35 yo	311 (35.6%)
Age > 40 yo	48 (5.5%)

Table 2. Cont.

Feature	n (%)
BMI	
Underweight (<18.5)	31 (3.5%)
Normal weight (18.5–24.9)	550 (62.9%)
Overweight (≥25)	199 (22.8%)
Obesity (≥30)	93 (10.6%)
Comorbidities and addictions	
SLE	6 (0.7%)
APS	9 (1%)
Diabetes mellitus type 1	4 (0.5%)
Smoking	39 (4.5%)
Obstetrical history	
Parous previous PE	11 (1.3%)
Previous FGR or SGA fetuses	16 (1.8%)
Family history of PE	5 (0.6%)
Nulliparous	390 (44.6%)
IVF	12 (1.4%)

Note: APS: antiphospholipid syndrome; **BMI: body mass index**; FGR: fetal growth restriction; IVF: In vitro fertilization; SGA: small for gestational age; **SLE: systemic lupus erythematosus**; PE: preeclampsia; yo: years old.

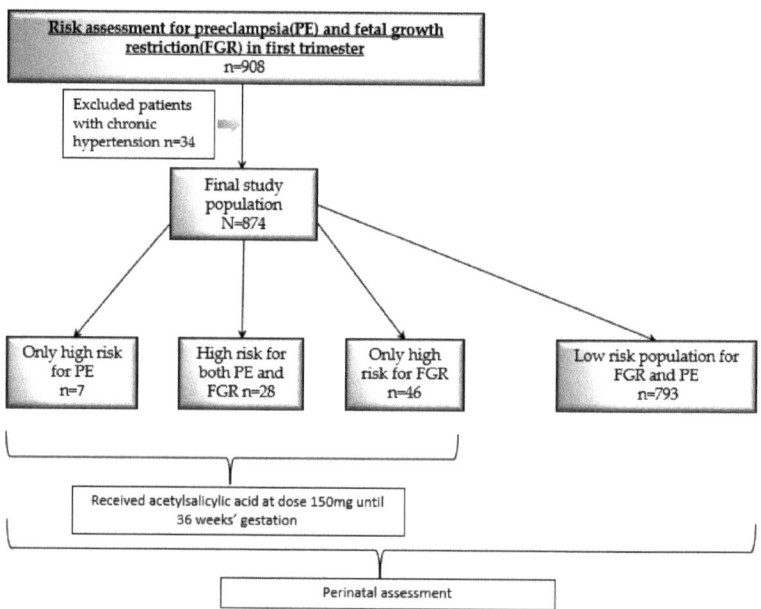

Figure 1. Study flow chart.

3. Statistical Analysis

Data from the study were subjected to statistical analysis. Quantitative data were analyzed using non-parametric Mann–Whitney U tests, while qualitative data were analyzed using either the chi-squared test or Fisher's exact test. Multivariate logistic regression was performed to calculate the area under the curve (AUC) and odds ratio (OR) for selected parameters. The analysis was conducted using the Statistica software (version 13, StatSoft, Kraków, Poland).

4. Results

Table 3 provides an overview of the differences between patients categorized as being at either high or low risk of PE (left-hand side) or FGR (right-hand side) during the first trimester. A high risk of PE was found in 35 of 874 patients (4%). This group included 4 of 19 patients who developed any form of PE (21%) and 6 of 51 patients who were diagnosed with FGR or SGA (11.7%). Patients at high risk for PE demonstrated a statistically significant association with nulliparity (OR 2.4 (1.2–5)). In terms of perinatal outcomes, patients at high risk for PE exhibited a higher likelihood of developing PIH (OR 3.8 (1.6–9.1)), all PE (OR 7.1 (2.2–22.6)), lo-PE (OR 7.6 (2.4–24.4)), and FGR or SGA (OR 3.7 (1.4–9.2)). Additionally, these pregnancies were more frequently concluded with a cesarean section (OR 2.1 (0.98–4.4)), although this result approached statistical significance. However, the high-risk PE group did not show statistically significant differences in terms of maternal age, maternal weight, the development of GDM, pre-pregnancy diabetes, stillbirths, smoking, eo-PE, preterm births, the birth status of the newborn assessed by the Apgar scale, the sex of the newborn, or birth weight ($p > 0.05$).

Table 3. Selected midgestational parameters and perinatal outcomes among pregnant patients at high risk of FGR or PE during the first trimester, excluding those with chronic hypertension.

	High Risk for PE n (%)	Low Risk for PE n (%)	p	OR (95%CI)	High Risk for FGR n (%)	Low Risk for FGR n (%)	p	OR (95%CI)
	n = 35	n = 839	-		n = 74	n = 800		
			Maternal characteristics, comorbidities and obstetric history					
Age > 35	12 (34.3%)	299 (35.7%)	0.87	-	31 (41.9%)	280 (35%)	0.24	-
Age > 40	1 (2.9%)	47 (5.6%)	0.48	-	3 (4.1%)	45 (5.6%)	0.76	-
Underweight (BMI < 18.5)	1 (2.9%)	30 (3.6%)	0.81	-	3 (4.1%)	28 (3.5%)	0.93	-
Normal weight (BMI 18.5–24.9)	21 (60%)	529 (63.1%)	0.71	-	51 (68.9%)	499 (62.5%)	0.27	-
Overweight (BMI ≥ 25)	6 (17.1%)	193 (23%)	0.42	-	10 (13.5%)	189 (23.7%)	0.08	-
Obesity (BMI ≥ 30)	7 (20%)	86 (10.3%)	0.07	-	10 (13.5%)	83 (10.4%)	0.41	-
Nulliparous	23 (65.7%)	367 (43.7%)	0.01	2.4 (1.2–5)	45 (60.8%)	345 (43.1%)	0.003	2 (1.3–3.3)
Smoking	0	39 (5.5%)	0.31	-	11 (16.2%)	28 (4.2%)	<0.001	4.4 (2.1–9.3)
PGDM	1 (2.9%)	3 (0.4%)	0.39	-	1 (1.4%)	3 (0.4%)	0.77	-
			Maternal and perinatal outcome					
GDM1	9 (25.7%)	106 (12.6%)	0.03	-	19 (25.7%)	96 (12%)	<0.001	3.1 (1.8–5.2)
GDM2	2 (5.7%)	93 (11.1%)	0.47	-	7 (9.5%)	88 (11%)	0.68	-
PIH	7 (20%)	52 (6.2%)	0.001	3.8 (1.6–9.1)	15 (20.3%)	44 (5.5%)	<0.001	4.4 (2.3–8.3)
All PE	4 (11.4%)	15 (1.8%)	<0.001	7.1 (2.2–22.6)	8 (10.8%)	11 (1.4%)	<0.001	8.7 (3.4–22.4)
eo-PE	0	1 (0.12%)	-	-	0	1 (0.13%)	-	-
lo-PE	4 (11.4%)	14 (1.7%)	<0.001	7.6 (2.4–24.4)	8 (10.8%)	10 (1.3%)	<0.001	9.6 (3.7–25.1)
Cesarean delivery	25 (71.4%)	458 (54.8%)	0.05	2.1 (0.98–4.4)	50 (67.6%)	433 (54.3%)	0.03	1.8 (1.1–2.9)
Preterm birth	2 (5.7%)	62 (7.4%)	0.71	-	6 (8.1%)	58 (7.3%)	0.79	-
			Newborn outcome					
FGR or SGA	6 (17.1%)	45 (5.4%)	0.003	3.7 (1.4–9.2)	15 (20.3%)	36 (4.5%)	<0.001	5.4 (2.8–10.4)
Stillbirth	0	3 (0.4%)	0.26	-	1 (1.4%)	2 (0.25%)	0.61	-
Newborn sex (male)	20 (57.1%)	454 (54.1%)	0.72	-	42 (56.8%)	432 (54%)	0.65	-
Apgar score < 7 at 5 min	1 (2.9%)	15 (1.9%)	0.82	-	2 (2.7%)	15 (1.9%)	0.96	-
Birth weight < 10 pc	3 (8.6%)	29 (3.5%)	0.26	-	7 (9.5%)	25 (3.1%)	0.005	3.2 (1.3–7.7)
Birth weight < 3 pc	1 (2.9%)	7 (0.8%)	0.75	-	4 (5.4%)	4 (0.5%)	<0.001	11.3 (2.8–46.3)

Note: all PE: all preeclampsia types; BMI: body mass index; CI: confidence interval; eo-PE: early-onset preeclampsia; FGR: fetal growth restriction; GDM1: gestational diabetes mellitus type 1; GDM2: gestational diabetes mellitus type 2; lo-PE: late-onset preeclampsia; OR: odds ratio; pc: percentile; PGDM: pregestational diabetes mellitus; PIH: pregnancy-induced hypertension; SGA: small for gestational age.

In contrast, a high risk of FGR was found in 74 of 874 patients (8.4%). This group included 8 of 19 patients who developed any form of PE (42.1%) and 15 of 51 patients who were diagnosed with FGR or SGA (29.4%). Patients at high risk of FGR during the first trimester were statistically significantly more likely to be nulliparous (OR 2 (1.3–3.3)) and smokers (OR 4.4 (2.1–9.3)). Concerning perinatal outcomes, patients at high risk for FGR demonstrated a higher likelihood of developing GDM1 (OR 3.1 (1.8–5.2)), PIH (OR 4.4 (2.3–8.3)), all PE (OR 8.7 (3.4–22.4)), lo-PE (OR 9.6 (3.7–25.1)), and FGR or SGA (OR 5.4 (2.8–10.4)). Additionally, these pregnancies were more likely to result in a cesarean delivery (OR 1.8 (1.1–2.9)), and the neonatal birth weight was more likely to be <10th percentile (OR 3.2 (1.3–7.7)) and <3rd percentile (OR 11.3 (2.8–46.3)). No statistical significance was found for maternal age, maternal weight, pre-pregnancy diabetes, GDM2, stillbirth, eo-PE, preterm birth, newborn sex, newborn status as assessed by the Apgar scale, or newborn sex among patients at high risk for FGR.

Table 4 presents the differences observed between patients diagnosed with or without PE (left-hand side) and diagnosed with or without FGR or SGA (right-hand side). In the whole group, 19 cases of PE (2.1%) were diagnosed. Patients diagnosed with PE demonstrated a higher likelihood of having FGR or SGA (OR 8.3 (3–22.9)), with their pregnancies being more frequently concluded via cesarean section (OR 3.1 (1.01–9.3)). Furthermore, their newborns were more likely to have a birth weight < 3rd percentile (OR 16.6 (3.1–88.3)). Among patients diagnosed with PE, statistically significantly higher values were observed for MoM UtPI (OR 8.5 (2.4–30.5)) and MoM MAP (OR 32.4 (14.4–55.3)) in the first trimester, while MoM PLGF was significantly lower (OR 0.2 (0.03–0.9)). However, no statistical significance was found for maternal age, maternal weight, nulliparity, pre-pregnancy diabetes, GDM, stillbirth, preterm birth, newborn status as assessed by the Apgar scale, newborn sex, birth weight < 10 pc, or MoM PAPP-A among patients diagnosed with PE.

Table 4. Selected midgestational parameters and perinatal outcomes among pregnant patients diagnosed with PE and those diagnosed with FGR or SGA, excluding those with chronic hypertension.

	PE Diagnosis n (%)	without PE Diagnosis n (%)	p	OR (95%CI)	FGR or SGA Diagnosis n (%)	without FGR or SGA Diagnosis n (%)	p	OR (95%CI)
	n= 19	n= 855			n= 51	n= 823		
Maternal characteristics, comorbidities and obstetric history								
Age > 35	7 (36.8%)	304 (35.6%)	0.91	-	17 (33.3%)	304 (37%)	0.75	-
Age > 40	2 (10.5%)	46 (5.4%)	0.33	-	1 (2%)	47 (5.7%)	0.25	-
Underweight (BMI < 18.5)	1 (5.3%)	30 (3.5%)	0.82	-	5 (9.8%)	26 (3.2%)	0.04	3.3 (1.2–9.1)
Normal weight (BMI 18.5–24.9)	13 (68.4%)	537 (62.9%)	0.61	-	35 (68.6%)	515 (62.6%)	0.4	-
Overweight (BMI ≥ 25)	2 (10.5%)	197 (23.1%)	0.31	-	9 (17.7%)	190 (23.1%)	0.32	-
Obesity (BMI ≥ 30)	3 (15.8%)	90 (10.5%)	0.72	-	2 (3.9%)	92 (11.2%)	0.14	-
Nulliparous	12 (63.2%)	378 (44.2%)	0.1	-	35 (68.6%)	355 (43.1%)	<0.001	2.9 (1.6–5.3)
Smoking	0	39 (5.4%)	0.66	-	4 (8%)	35 (5.1%)	0.58	-
PGDM	0	4 (0.5%)	0.16	-	0	4	-	-
Maternal and perinatal outcome								
GDM1	2 (10.5%)	113 (13.2%)	0.73	-	9 (17.7%)	106 (12.9%)	0.43	-
GDM2	0	95 (11.1%)	0.24	-	3 (5.9%)	92 (11.2%)	0.28	-
PIH	-	-	-	-	7 (13.7%)	50 (6.1%)	0.06	-
All PE	-	-	-	-	6 (11.8%)	13 (1.6%)	<0.001	8.3 (3–22.9)
eo-PE	-	-	-	-	0	1 (0.1%)	-	-
lo-PE	-	-	-	-	6 (11.8%)	12 (1.5%)	<0.001	9 (3.2–25.1)
Cesarean delivery	15 (79%)	469 (55%)	0.04	3.1 (1.01–9.3)	30 (58.8%)	453 (55.2%)	0.62	-
Preterm birth	3 (15.8%)	61 (7.1%)	0.15	-	8 (15.7%)	56 (6.8%)	0.04	2.5 (1.1–5.7)

Table 4. Cont.

	PE Diagnosis n (%)	without PE Diagnosis n (%)	p	OR (95%CI)	FGR or SGA Diagnosis n (%)	without FGR or SGA Diagnosis n (%)	p	OR (95%CI)
				Newborn outcome				
FGR or SGA	6 (31.6%)	45 (5.3%)	<0.001	8.3 (3–22.9)	-	-	-	-
Stillbirth	0	3 (0.4%)	0.8	-	2 (3.9%)	1 (0.1%)	-	-
Newborn sex (male)	6 (31.6%)	468 (54.7%)	0.05	2.6 (0.98–7)	23 (45.1%)	451 (54.8%)	0.18	-
Apgar score <7 at 5 min	0	17 (2%)	0.82	-	2 (3.9%)	15 (1.8%)	0.6	-
Birth weight < 10 pc	2 (10.5%)	30 (3.5%)	0.11	-	21 (41.2%)	11 (1.3%)	<0.001	51.4 (22.8–116)
Birth weight < 3 pc	2 (10.5%)	6 (0.7%)	<0.001	16.6 (3.1–88.3)	4 (7.8%)	4 (0.5%)	<0.001	17.4 (4.2–71.7)
			First trimester biochemical or biophysical measurement					
	Median (min-max)	Median (min-max)	p	OR (95%CI)	Median (min-max)	Median (min-max)	p	OR (95%CI)
MoM UtPI	1.26 (0.6–1.8)	0.98 (0.4–2.3)	<0.001	8.5 (2.4–30.5)	1.06 (0.7–1.7)	0.98 (0.4–2.3)	0.03	2.6 (1.1–6.4)
UtPI	2.1 (0.9–2.86)	1.5 (0.6–3.8)	0.002	3.5 (1.6–7.8)	1.8 (1.1–2.6)	1.5 (0.6–3.8)	0.01	2 (1.2–3.5)
MoM PAPP-A	0.87 (0.2–3.1)	0.96 (0.2–4.8)	0.32	-	0.79 (0.2–2.8)	0.96 (0.2–4.8)	0.12	-
PAPP-A (IU/l)	2.8 (0.5–12.4)	3.4 (0.5–21.4)	0.53	-	3.3 (0.5–14)	3.4 (0.5–21.4)	0.49	-
MoM PLGF	0.78 (0.2–1.63)	0.9 (0.1–3.2)	0.04	0.2 (0.03–0.9)	0.82 (0.2–1.9)	0.9 (0.1–3.2)	0.005	0.24 (0.1–0.7)
PLGF (ng/mL)	39.4 (12.6–98)	50.4 (11–357)	0.04	0.97 (0.94–0.99)	46 (11–100)	50.5 (60–357)	0.01	0.98 (0.96–0.99)
MoM MAP	1.12 (0.9–1.4)	1.03 (0.7–1.4)	<0.001	32.4 (14–55.3)	1.03 (0.8–1.3)	1.03 (0.7–1.4)	0.88	-
MAP (mm Hg)	95 (78.3–113)	87 (60–123)	<0.001	1.09 (1.04–1.14)	85 (72–112)	88 (60–123)	0.27	-

Note: all PE: all preeclampsia types; BMI: body mass index; CI: confidence interval; eo-PE: early –onset preeclampsia; FGR: fetal growth restriction; GDM1: gestational diabetes mellitus type 1; GDM2: gestational diabetes mellitus type 2; lo-PE: late –onset preeclampsia; MoM: multiple of the median; OR: odds ratio; pc: percentile; PAPP-A: Pregnancy Associated Plasma Protein-A; PGDM: pregestational diabetes mellitus; PIH: pregnancy induced hypertension; PLGF: placental growth factor; SGA: small for gestational age; UtPI: uterine artery pulsatility index.

There were 51 cases of FGR or SGA (5.8%) in the entire study group. Significantly more patients diagnosed with FGR or SGA were underweight (OR 3.3 (1.2–9.1)) and nulliparous (OR 2.9 (1.6–5.3)). In this group, the incidence of all PE (OR 8.3 (3–22.9)), lo PE (OR 9 (3.2–25.1)), and preterm birth (OR 2.5 (1.1–5.7)) was significantly higher. Regarding newborns, neonatal birth weight was more often <10th percentile (OR 51.4 (22.8–116.5)) and <3rd percentile (OR 17.4 (4.2–71.7)). Patients diagnosed with FGR or SGA exhibited statistically significantly higher MoM UtPI values (OR 2.6 (1.1–6.4)) and lower MoM PLGF values (OR 0.24 (0.1–0.7)) in the first trimester. However, among the patients diagnosed with FGR or SGA, no statistical significance was found for age, normal maternal weight, overweight, obesity, pre-pregnancy diabetes, GDM, smoking, stillbirth, PIH, eo-PE, incidence of cesarian delivery, newborn sex, newborn status as assessed by the Apgar scale, MoM PAPP-A, and MoM MAP values in the first trimester.

Table 5 summarizes the differences between patients at high or low risk of PE or/and FGR in the first trimester. A high risk of FGR and/or PE was found in 81 of 874 patients (9%). This group included 8 of 19 patients who developed any form of PE (42.1%) and 15 of 51 patients who were diagnosed with FGR or SGA (29.4%). Patients in the high-risk group were significantly more likely to be nulliparous (OR 1.9 (1.2–3)) and smokers (OR 3.9 (1.9–8.2)). In terms of perinatal outcomes, the high-risk group had a higher incidence of gestational diabetes mellitus type 1 (GDM1) (OR 2.4 (1.4–4.2)), pregnancy-induced hypertension (PIH) (OR 3.6, (1.9–7)), all types of PE (OR 7.8 (3–20)), late-onset PE (lo-PE) (OR 8.5 (3.3–22.4)), and FGR or SGA (OR 4.8 (2.5–9.2)). Furthermore, pregnancies in the high-risk group were more likely to result in a cesarean delivery (OR 1.9 (1.2–3.1)). Neonates born to high-risk patients had a higher likelihood of being <10 percentile (OR 2.9 (1.2–6.9)) for birth weight and <3 percentile (OR 10.2 (2.5–41.7)). No statistical significance was found for maternal age, maternal weight, pre-pregnancy diabetes, GDM2, eo-PE, preterm births, stillbirth, <7 Apgar score, or newborn sex. For correlations between first-trimester biochemical and biophysical parameters and the birth weight and birth week in all of the discussed groups, please refer to Table S1 in the Supplementary Materials.

Table 5. Selected midgestational parameters and perinatal outcomes among pregnancies at high risk of FGR and/or PE in the first trimester, excluding those with chronic hypertension.

	High Risk for PE or/and FGR n (%)	Low Risk for PE and FGR n (%)	p	OR (95%CI)
	n = 81	n = 793	-	
Maternal characteristics, comorbidities, and obstetrical history				
Age > 35	35 (43.2%)	276 (34.8)	0.13	-
Age > 40	3 (3.7%)	45 (5.7%)	0.45	-
Underweight (BMI < 18.5)	3 (3.7%)	28 (3.5%)	0.93	-
Normal weight (BMI 18.5–24.9)	53 (65.4%)	497 (62.8%)	0.63	-
Overweight (BMI ≥ 25)	13 (16.1%)	186 (23.5%)	0.12	-
Obesity (BMI ≥ 30)	12 (14.8)	81 (10.2%)	0.2	-
Nulliparous	48 (59.3%)	342 (43.1%)	<0.01	1.9 (1.2–3)
Smoking	11 (14.7%)	28 (4.2%)	<0.001	3.9 (1.9–8.2)
PGDM	1 (1.2%)	3 (0.4%)	0.82	-
Maternal and perinatal outcomes				
GDM1	20 (24.7%)	95 (12%)	<0.01	2.4 (1.4–4.2)
GDM2	7 (8.6%)	88 (11.1%)	0.49	-
PIH	14 (17.3%)	43 (5.43%)	0.001	3.6 (1.9–7)
All PE	8 (9.9%)	11 (1.4%)	<0.001	7.8 (3–20)
eo-PE	0	1 (0.13%)	0.15	-
lo-PE	8 (9.8%)	10 (1.3%)	<0.001	8.5 (3.3–22.4)
Cesarean delivery	56 (69.1%)	427 (54%)	0.009	1.9 (1.2–3.1)
Preterm birth	6 (7.4%)	58 (7.3%)	0.97	-
Newborn outcome				
FGR or SGA	15 (18.5%)	36 (4.5%)	<0.001	4.8 (2.5–9.2)
Stillbirth	1 (1.2%)	2 (0.25%)	0.15	-
Newborn sex (male)	45 (55.5%)	429 (54.1%)	0.8	-
Apgar score < 7 at 5 min	2 (2.5%)	15 (1.9%)	0.71	-
Birth weight < 10 pc	7 (8.6%)	25 (3.1%)	0.01	2.9 (1.2–6.9)
Birth weight < 3 pc	4 (4.9%)	4 (0.5%)	<0.001	10.2 (2.5–41.7)

Note: all PE: all preeclampsia types; BMI: body mass index; CI: confidence interval; eo-PE: early-onset preeclampsia; FGR: fetal growth restriction; GDM1: gestational diabetes mellitus type 1; GDM2: gestational diabetes mellitus type 2; lo-PE: late-onset preeclampsia; OR: odds ratio; pc: percentile; PGDM: pregestational diabetes mellitus; PIH: pregnancy-induced hypertension; SGA: small for gestational age.

Table 6 presents the DR for screening for all forms of PE, as well as FGR or SGA, in a Polish population without chronic hypertension, followed by the implementation of ASA in the high-risk group. For all forms of PE, the DR was 48% and 61% at an FPR of 5% and 10%, respectively, with an area under the curve (AUC) of 0.85 (0.81–0.89 95%CI). Regarding FGR and SGA, the DR was 20% and 24% at an FPR of 5% and 10%, respectively, with an

AUC of 0.70 (0.67–0.73 95%CI). Figure 2 shows receiver operating characteristic (ROC) curves for the relevant parameters.

Table 6. Performance of the Fetal Medicine Foundation's algorithm for the different groups.

	AUC	CI (95%)	Sensitivity for the FPR	
Variables			5%	10%
Any PE	0.85	(0.81–0.89)	48	61
FGR or SGA	0.71	(0.67–0.75)	20	24

Note: AUC: area under the curve; CI: confidence interval; FGR: fetal growth restriction; FPR: false positive ratio; PE: preeclampsia; SGA: small for gestational age.

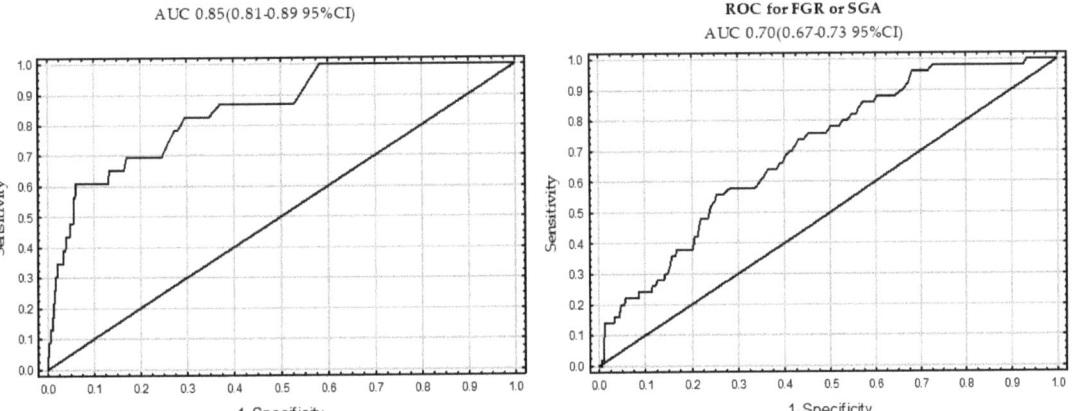

Figure 2. Receiver operating characteristic (ROC) curves for the any form of preeclampsia and fetal growth restriction or small for gestational age.

5. Discussion

Our study is the first in Poland to evaluate the efficacy of implementing ASA in pregnancies without chronic hypertension at high risk of PE and FGR, according to the screening principles published after the ASPRE study. The ASPRE study showed the advantages of ASA use in the general population, resulting in a 62% reduction in the incidence of preterm PE and up to an 82% reduction in early-onset (eo-PE) cases, although the latter result bordered on statistical significance [12]. A secondary analysis of the ASPRE study indicated that, if women with chronic hypertension were excluded from the study, consistent ASA use (>90% of the doses) could potentially achieve a 95% reduction in PE incidence [13,18].

In our study, none of the women classified as high-risk for eo-PE developed this form of PE. This finding may be attributed to the delayed diagnosis of PE in the later weeks of pregnancy due to the effects of ASA. eo-PE is known to be associated with the abnormal remodeling of spiral arteries, inflammation, and subsequent vascular endothelial damage [19–21]. It is speculated that implementing ASA before 16 wkGA in high-risk pregnancies for placental pathologies such as PE or FGR promotes normal spiral artery remodeling and stabilizes the vascular endothelium. As a result, it prevents the development of early-onset forms of PE or FGR or postpones their diagnosis in favor of late-onset forms. This shift in diagnosis leads to significantly improved perinatal outcomes by reducing fetal and maternal morbidity and mortality [22,23].

However, these beneficial effects of ASA are not observed in pregnancies with chronic hypertension. This discrepancy may be due to pre-existing vascular endothelial dysfunction and an ongoing inflammation, which make the development of PE likely even with less severe impairment of spiral vascular remodeling, exacerbating the already existing vascular damage [24].

Our study results demonstrated that the DR for all the forms of PE in our population was 61% at an FPR of 10%, even considering the use of acetylsalicylic acid (ASA), which could potentially affect the DR. To date, the algorithm proposed by the FMF, which incorporates a multivariate analysis including maternal characteristics and history and biochemical and biophysical measurements, is considered the best method for PE detection [5]. It is important to note that the DRs assumed by the FMF algorithm may vary depending on the population in which it is implemented. Previous studies have reported DRs ranging from 41% to 57% at an FPR of 10% when the FMF first-trimester screening test is performed for all forms of PE. However, the DR differs when diagnosing preterm PE or eo-PE, with the same algorithm achieving much higher DR values of up to 90% at an FPR of 10% [25–28]. Despite this high DR, there is still debate around the world regarding the method for PE screening in the first trimester, as well as the recommended dose of ASA. Scientific societies do not present a unified statement, but, after the ASPRE publication, many countries have changed their recommendations to the approach proposed by the FMF [29]. Our study shows that we still do not have a perfect method for predicting the occurrence of all forms of PE, especially those with a late onset, and many occur in low-risk patients.

When authors compare the FMF algorithm with those proposed by the American College of Obstetricians and Gynecologists (ACOG) and the National Institute for Health and Care Excellence (NICE), the FMF algorithm appears to be the most effective at a relatively low FPR. Following the NICE recommendations, we can detect 41% of preterm PE cases and 34% of term PE cases at an FPR of 10%. On the other hand, according to the new ACOG recommendations, the DR is much higher, reaching up to 90%. However, in the latter case, the FPR can be as high as 60% or more, which may lead to the low acceptance of ASA use among this group of patients and potentially reduce compliance with the recommended treatment [30–32]. In our study, we did not present DRs for these forms of PE as there were no eo-PE cases in the group taking ASA. Nonetheless, our results demonstrated that the first-trimester screening test for PE allowed for the identification of the high-risk pregnancy group. A positive test result for PE was associated with a more than seven-fold increase in the risk of developing PE in this group, and up to one in five patients would develop pregnancy complications such as PIH or FGR or be diagnosed with fetal SGA.

Consequently, our study suggests that we are making progress in detecting and preventing PE, particularly in its early-onset form. However, the prediction of FGR or SGA is a slightly different challenge. The algorithm proposed by the FMF demonstrates a lower DR of 21–44% for term SGA and 46–55% for detecting preterm SGA [14,33]. In our study, we did not achieve satisfactory results in terms of detecting SGA or FGR, with a DR of only 24% at an assumed FPR of 10%. Given these findings, the question arises as to whether we can prevent the occurrence of these disorders despite the low percentage of identified higher-risk pregnancies.

ASA comes to our aid; however, the reduction in the incidence of SGA or FGR is not as significant as it is in the case of PE. Studies suggest that, in cases of increased risk identified in the first trimester, there may be a decrease of approximately 40–44% in the preterm form of these disorders. This decrease is mainly attributed to the reduced incidence of preterm PE and eo-PE. However, no such correlations are observed in cases without PE diagnosis or with a lower incidence of term SGA [10,14,22,23,33,34]. In our study, we demonstrated that pregnant women at an increased risk of FGR were significantly more likely to develop pregnancy complications such as PIH, all PE forms, and FGR, or to be diagnosed with SGA. Furthermore, their pregnancies were more likely to conclude with a cesarean section, and newborns were more likely to have a weight of <10 pc and <3 pc.

What should we recommend to a patient at high risk of developing PE or FGR in the first trimester? It is crucial that we actively collaborate with these patients to ensure the consistent and regular intake of ASA. While ASA might not always be effective, it is currently our only option in preventing the occurrence of these disorders. Consistent intake of ASA is the key to success [13,18]. Second, the close monitoring of these high-risk pregnancies is necessary. As our study has demonstrated, the incidence of other pregnancy complications is much higher in this group. Appropriate and prompt diagnosis may help to improve perinatal outcomes by reducing fetal morbidity and mortality [28].

In Poland, the main current focus of the first-trimester screening test is the detection of structural abnormalities and chromosomal abnormalities through ultrasounds and blood sampling for PAPP-A and Beta human chorionic gonadotropin (BHCG). However, not all women are eligible for reimbursement of the test costs, and not all sonographers are certified to identify risks related to PE and FGR. As our study showed, expanding the first-trimester screening test to include additional measurements not only facilitated the implementation of ASA prophylaxis in pregnancies at higher risk of these disorders but also enabled the identification of the high-risk pregnancy group, thus enabling appropriate management.

6. Strength and Limitations

This paper's strength lies in the inclusion of a large number of women over the age of 35, who are already at higher risk of pregnancy complications due to their age. Another strength is the exploration of screening tests in Poland following the ASPRE trail and the identification of the high-risk group, which has not been validated in the country so far.

As for weaknesses, it should be noted that the study group lacked cases of eo-PE, preventing the determination of DR and AUC for this complication. This may be attributed to the significant reduction in the risk of eo-PE in high-risk populations without chronic hypertension who have received ASA. The use of ASA in our study can be considered controversial, as it has impacted the obtained results. A comparison between high-risk groups with and without ASA administration would be desirable. However, conducting such a study presents ethical challenges. In the present work, we were more interested in showing how screening in the first trimester can help isolate pregnancies that are at the highest risk of perinatal complications. It is also important to mention the potential for errors in the diagnosis of FGR or SGA, especially in the 3–10 pc range. Furthermore, the differentiation between elective and emergency cesarean sections was not addressed, and the monitoring of ASA adherence by the patients was not included, which could have enhanced the value of this study.

7. Conclusions

Our results show the importance and effectiveness of the first-trimester screening test for PE and FGR, particularly in high-risk pregnancies where ASA prophylaxis may have the most beneficial effect. Moreover, the implementation of ASA prophylaxis in pregnancies without chronic hypertension may be especially important in reducing the incidence of eo-PE, as suggested by the absence of such a complication in our high-risk population.

Screening for PE and FGR additionally shows that, even in the absence of an ASA effect, we isolated high-risk pregnancies, meaning that the patients may then receive better perinatal care. However, it should be noted that studies involving a greater number of patients would be necessary to confirm this finding in the Polish population.

Supplementary Materials: The following supporting information can be downloaded at: https://www.mdpi.com/article/10.3390/jcm12175582/s1, Table S1. Correlations between first-trimester biophysical and biochemical markers and selected perinatal parameters among groups at high risk of PE or FGR or those who developed PE or FGR.

Author Contributions: Conceptualization, S.K. and P.T.; methodology, M.F.-T., P.T., M.S. and E.K.; investigation, M.F.-T., M.N.-B., A.G., A.Z. and S.D.; data curation, P.T., A.G., A.Z., M.S., S.D. and H.J.-J.; writing—original draft preparation, P.T. and M.F.-T.; writing—review and editing, P.T., M.F.-T., S.K., A.K. and A.T.; supervision, S.K., A.T., E.K. and A.C.-P. All authors have read and agreed to the published version of the manuscript.

Funding: This research received no external funding.

Institutional Review Board Statement: The study was conducted in accordance with the Declaration of Helsinki, and approved by the Institutional Review Board of the Pomeranian Medical University in Szczecin (KB-0012/122/12 of 29 October 2012).

Informed Consent Statement: Informed consent was obtained from all subjects involved in the study.

Data Availability Statement: The data presented in this study are available upon request from the corresponding author. The data are not publicly available, as not all patients agreed to publicly disclose their data.

Conflicts of Interest: The authors declare no conflict of interest.

References

1. Kuklina, E.V.; Ayala, C.; Callaghan, W.M. Hypertensive disorders and severe obstetric morbidity in the United States. *Obstet. Gynecol.* **2009**, *113*, 1299–1306. [CrossRef]
2. Duley, L.; Meher, S.; Hunter, K.E.; Seidler, A.L.; Askie, L.M. Antiplatelet agents for preventing pre-eclampsia and its complications. *Cochrane Database Syst. Rev.* **2019**, *2019*, CD004659. [CrossRef] [PubMed]
3. Hypertension in Pregnancy: Diagnosis and Management NICE Guideline. 2019. Available online: www.nice.org.uk/guidance/ng133 (accessed on 17 July 2023).
4. Low-Dose Aspirin Use for the Prevention of Preeclampsia and Related Morbidity and Mortality. ACOG. Available online: https://www.acog.org/clinical/clinical-guidance/practice-advisory/articles/2021/12/low-dose-aspirin-use-for-the-prevention-of-preeclampsia-and-related-morbidity-and-mortality (accessed on 17 July 2023).
5. Tan, M.Y.; Syngelaki, A.; Poon, L.C.; Rolnik, D.L.; O'Gorman, N.; Delgado, J.L.; Akolekar, R.; Konstantinidou, L.; Tsavdaridou, M.; Galeva, S.; et al. Screening for pre-eclampsia by maternal factors and biomarkers at 11–13 weeks' gestation. *Ultrasound Obstet. Gynecol.* **2018**, *52*, 186–195. [CrossRef] [PubMed]
6. O'Gorman, N.; Wright, D.; Syngelaki, A.; Akolekar, R.; Wright, A.; Poon, L.C.; Nicolaides, K.H. Competing risks model in screening for preeclampsia by maternal factors and biomarkers at 11–13 weeks gestation. *Am. J. Obstet. Gynecol.* **2016**, *214*, 103.e1–103.e12. [CrossRef] [PubMed]
7. O'Gorman, N.N.; Wright, D.; Poon, L.C.; Rolnik, D.L.; Syngelaki, A.; Wright, A.; Akolekar, R.; Cicero, S.; Janga, D.; Jani, J.; et al. Accuracy of competing-risks model in screening for preeclampsia by maternal factors and biomarkers at 11–13 weeks' gestation. *Ultrasound Obstet. Gynecol.* **2017**, *49*, 751–755. [CrossRef]
8. Akolekar, R.; Syngelaki, A.; Poon, L.; Wright, D.; Nicolaides, K.H. Competing Risks Model in Early Screening for Preeclampsia by Biophysical and Biochemical Markers. *Fetal Diagn. Ther.* **2013**, *33*, 8–15. [CrossRef] [PubMed]
9. Poon, L.C.Y.; Akolekar, R.; Lachmann, R.; Beta, J.; Nicolaides, K.H. Hypertensive disorders in pregnancy: Screening by biophysical and biochemical markers at 11–13 weeks. *Ultrasound Obstet. Gynecol.* **2010**, *35*, 662–670. [CrossRef]
10. Poon, L.C.; Syngelaki, A.; Akolekar, R.; Lai, J.; Nicolaides, K.H. Combined Screening for Preeclampsia and Small for Gestational Age at 11–13 Weeks. *Fetal Diagn. Ther.* **2012**, *33*, 16–27. [CrossRef]
11. Karagiannis, G.; Akolekar, R.; Sarquis, R.; Wright, D.; Nicolaides, K.H. Prediction of Small-for-Gestation Neonates from Biophysical and Biochemical Markers at 11–13 Weeks. *Fetal Diagn. Ther.* **2010**, *29*, 148–154. [CrossRef]
12. Rolnik, D.L.; Wright, D.; Poon, L.C.; O'Gorman, N.; Syngelaki, A.; de Paco Matallana, C.; Akolekar, R.; Cicero, S.; Janga, D.; Singh, M.; et al. Aspirin versus Placebo in Pregnancies at High Risk for Preterm Preeclampsia. *N. Engl. J. Med.* **2017**, *377*, 613–622. [CrossRef]
13. Poon, L.C.; Wright, D.; Rolnik, D.L.; Syngelaki, A.; Delgado, J.L.; Tsokaki, T.; Leipold, G.; Akolekar, R.; Shearing, S.; De Stefani, L.; et al. Aspirin for Evidence-Based Preeclampsia Prevention trial: Effect of aspirin in prevention of preterm preeclampsia in subgroups of women according to their characteristics and medical and obstetrical history. *Am. J. Obstet. Gynecol.* **2017**, *217*, 585.e1–585.e5. [CrossRef]
14. Tan, M.Y.; Poon, L.C.; Rolnik, D.L.; Syngelaki, A.; de Paco Matallana, C.; Akolekar, R.; Cicero, S.; Janga, D.; Singh, M.; Molina, F.S.; et al. Prediction and prevention of small-for-gestational-age neonates: Evidence from SPREE and ASPRE. *Ultrasound Obstet. Gynecol.* **2018**, *52*, 52–59. [CrossRef]
15. Poon, L.C.; Shennan, A.; Hyett, J.A.; Kapur, A.; Hadar, E.; Divakar, H.; McAuliffe, F.; da Silva Costa, F.; von Dadelszen, P.; McIntyre, H.D.; et al. The International Federation of Gynecology and Obstetrics (FIGO) initiative on pre-eclampsia: A pragmatic guide for first-trimester screening and prevention. *Int. J. Gynaecol. Obstet. Off. Organ Int. Fed. Gynaecol. Obstet.* **2019**, *145* (Suppl. S1), 1–33. [CrossRef] [PubMed]
16. Brown, M.A.; Magee, L.A.; Kenny, L.C.; Karumanchi, S.A.; McCarthy, F.P.; Saito, S.; Hall, D.R.; Warren, C.E.; Adoyi, G.; Ishaku, S.; et al. Hypertensive Disorders of Pregnancy: ISSHP Classification, Diagnosis, and Management Recommendations for International Practice. *Hypertension* **2018**, *72*, 24–43. [CrossRef] [PubMed]
17. Gordijn, S.J.; Beune, I.M.; Thilaganathan, B.; Papageorghiou, A.; Baschat, A.A.; Baker, P.N.; Silver, R.M.; Wynia, K.; Ganzevoort, W. Consensus definition of fetal growth restriction: A Delphi procedure. *Ultrasound Obstet. Gynecol.* **2016**, *48*, 333–339. [CrossRef]

18. Wright, D.; Poon, L.C.; Rolnik, D.L.; Syngelaki, A.; Delgado, J.L.; Vojtassakova, D.; de Alvarado, M.; Kapeti, E.; Rehal, A.; Pazos, A.; et al. Aspirin for Evidence-Based Preeclampsia Prevention trial: Influence of compliance on beneficial effect of aspirin in prevention of preterm preeclampsia. *Am. J. Obstet. Gynecol.* **2017**, *217*, 685.e1–685.e5. [CrossRef] [PubMed]
19. Phipps, E.A.; Thadhani, R.; Benzing, T.; Karumanchi, S.A. Pre-eclampsia: Pathogenesis, novel diagnostics and therapies. *Nat. Rev. Nephrol.* **2019**, *15*, 275–289. [CrossRef]
20. Brosens, I.; Puttemans, P.; Benagiano, G. Placental bed research: I. The placental bed: From spiral arteries remodeling to the great obstetrical syndromes. *Am. J. Obstet. Gynecol.* **2019**, *221*, 437–456. [CrossRef]
21. Aouache, R.; Biquard, L.; Vaiman, D.; Miralles, F. Oxidative Stress in Preeclampsia and Placental Diseases. *Int. J. Mol. Sci.* **2018**, *19*, 1496. [CrossRef]
22. Roberge, S.; Villa, P.; Nicolaides, K.; Giguère, Y.; Vainio, M.; Bakthi, A.; Ebrashy, A.; Bujold, E. Early administration of low-dose aspirin for the pre-vention of preterm and term preeclampsia: A systematic review and meta-analysis. *Fetal. Diagn. Ther.* **2012**, *31*, 141–146. [CrossRef] [PubMed]
23. Roberge, S.; Nicolaides, K.; Demers, S.; Hyett, J.; Chaillet, N.; Bujold, E. The role of aspirin dose on the prevention of preeclampsia and fetal growth restriction: Systematic review and meta-analysis. *Am. J. Obstet. Gynecol.* **2017**, *216*, 110–120.e6. [CrossRef]
24. Battarbee, A.N.; Sinkey, R.G.; Harper, L.M.; Oparil, S.; Tita, A.T.N. Chronic hypertension in pregnancy. *Am. J. Obstet. Gynecol.* **2020**, *222*, 532–541. [CrossRef] [PubMed]
25. Zwertbroek, E.F.; Groen, H.; Fontanella, F.; Maggio, L.; Marchi, L.; Bilardo, C.M. Performance of the FMF First-Trimester Preeclampsia-Screening Algorithm in a High-Risk Population in The Netherlands. *Fetal Diagn. Ther.* **2021**, *48*, 103–111. [CrossRef]
26. Boutin, A.; Guerby, P.; Gasse, C.; Tapp, S.; Bujold, E. Pregnancy outcomes in nulliparous women with positive first-trimester preterm preeclampsia screening test: The Great Obstetrical Syndromes cohort study. *Am. J. Obstet. Gynecol.* **2020**, *224*, 204.e1–204.e7. [CrossRef]
27. Lobo, G.A.R.; Nowak, P.M.; Panigassi, A.P.; Lima, A.I.F.; Araujo Júnior, E.; Nardozza, L.M.M.; Pares, D.B.S. Validation of Fetal Medicine Foun-dation algorithm for prediction of pre-eclampsia in the first trimester in an unselected Brazilian population. *J. Matern.-Fetal Neonatal Med.* **2019**, *32*, 286–292. [CrossRef]
28. Cordisco, A.; Periti, E.; Antoniolli, N.; Lozza, V.; Conticini, S.; Vannucci, G.; Masini, G.; Pasquini, L. Clinical implementation of pre-eclampsia screening in the first trimester of pregnancy. *Pregnancy Hypertens.* **2021**, *25*, 34–38. [CrossRef] [PubMed]
29. Tousty, P.; Fraszczyk-Tousty, M.; Dzidek, S.; Jasiak-Jóźwik, H.; Michalczyk, K.; Kwiatkowska, E.; Cymbaluk-Płoska, A.; Torbé, A.; Kwiatkowski, S. Low-Dose Aspirin after ASPRE—More Questions Than Answers? Current International Approach after PE Screening in the First Trimester. *Biomedicines* **2023**, *11*, 1495. [CrossRef] [PubMed]
30. O'Gorman, N.; Wright, D.; Poon, L.C.; Rolnik, D.L.; Syngelaki, A.; De Alvarado, M.; Carbone, I.F.; Dutemeyer, V.; Fiolna, M.; Frick, A.; et al. Multicenter screening for pre-eclampsia by maternal factors and biomarkers at 11–13 weeks' gestation: Comparison with NICE guidelines and ACOG recommendations. *Ultrasound Obstet. Gynecol.* **2017**, *49*, 756–760. [CrossRef]
31. Tan, M.Y.; Wright, D.; Syngelaki, A.; Akolekar, R.; Cicero, S.; Janga, D.; Singh, M.; Greco, E.; Wright, A.; Maclagan, K.; et al. Comparison of diagnostic accuracy of early screening for pre-eclampsia by NICE guidelines and a method combining maternal factors and biomarkers: Results of SPREE. *Ultrasound Obstet. Gynecol.* **2018**, *51*, 743–750. [CrossRef]
32. Green, M.; Shennan, A. Aspirin should be targeted to those who need it. *BJOG Int. J. Obstet. Gynaecology.* **2021**, *128*, 157. [CrossRef]
33. Mosimann, B.; Pfiffner, C.; Amylidi-Mohr, S.; Risch, L.; Surbek, D.; Raio, L. First trimester combined screening for preeclampsia and small for gestational age—A single centre experience and validation of the FMF screening algorithm. *Swiss. Med. Wkly.* **2017**, *147*, w14498. [CrossRef] [PubMed]
34. Bujold, E.; Roberge, S.; Lacasse, Y.; Bureau, M.; Audibert, F.; Marcoux, S.; Forest, J.-C.; Giguère, Y. Prevention of preeclampsia and intrauterine growth restriction with aspirin started in early pregnancy: A meta-analysis. *Obstet. Gynecol.* **2010**, *116*, 402–414. [CrossRef] [PubMed]

Disclaimer/Publisher's Note: The statements, opinions and data contained in all publications are solely those of the individual author(s) and contributor(s) and not of MDPI and/or the editor(s). MDPI and/or the editor(s) disclaim responsibility for any injury to people or property resulting from any ideas, methods, instructions or products referred to in the content.

MDPI
St. Alban-Anlage 66
4052 Basel
Switzerland
www.mdpi.com

Journal of Clinical Medicine Editorial Office
E-mail: jcm@mdpi.com
www.mdpi.com/journal/jcm

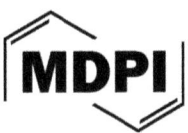

Disclaimer/Publisher's Note: The statements, opinions and data contained in all publications are solely those of the individual author(s) and contributor(s) and not of MDPI and/or the editor(s). MDPI and/or the editor(s) disclaim responsibility for any injury to people or property resulting from any ideas, methods, instructions or products referred to in the content.

www.ingramcontent.com/pod-product-compliance
Lightning Source LLC
LaVergne TN
LVHW070605100526
838202LV00012B/572